Anesthesia for Dental and Oral Maxillofacial Surgery

Anesthesia for Dental and Oral Maxillofacial Surgery

Spencer D. Wade

Caroline M. Sawicki

Megann K. Smiley

Michael A. Cuddy

Steven Vukas

Paul J. Schwartz

WILEY Blackwell

Library of Congress Cataloging-in-Publication Data

Names: Wade, Spencer D., editor.
Title: Anesthesia for dental and oral maxillofacial surgery / [edited by]
  Spencer D. Wade, Caroline M. Sawicki, Megann K. Smiley, Michael A.
  Cuddy, Steven Vukas, Paul J. Schwartz.
Description: Hoboken, New Jersey : Wiley-Blackwell, [2024] | Includes
  bibliographical references and index.
Identifiers: LCCN 2024005300 (print) | LCCN 2024005301 (ebook) | ISBN
  9781394164899 (paperback) | ISBN 9781394164905 (ePDF) | ISBN
  9781394164912 (ePUB) | ISBN 9781394164929 (oBook)
Subjects: MESH: Anesthesia, Dental–methods | Oral Surgical Procedures |
  Tooth Diseases–surgery | Jaw–surgery | Face–surgery |
  Anesthetics–therapeutic use
Classification: LCC RK510 (print) | LCC RK510 (ebook) | NLM WO 460 | DDC
  617.9/676–dc23/eng/20240301
LC record available at https://lccn.loc.gov/2024005300
LC ebook record available at https://lccn.loc.gov/2024005301

Cover Design: Wiley
Cover Image: © Spencer D Wade, fotograzia/Getty Images

Set in 9.5/12.5pt STIXTwoText by Straive, Pondicherry, India

SKY10071320_040224

To my beautiful daughter, Ava Kristina Wade, thank you for providing the inspiration behind this book and the motivation to finish.

Spencer D. Wade
Editor-in-Chief

Contents

Editorial Board

Editor-in-Chief

SPENCER D. WADE, DDS, MS
Dentist Anesthesiologist
Diplomate, American Dental Board of Anesthesiology
Clinical Assistant Professor
New York University College of Dentistry, New York, New York, USA
Oral Health Center for People with Disabilities

Co-Authors

CAROLINE M. SAWICKI, DDS, PhD
Pediatric Dentist
Board Eligible, American Board of Pediatric Dentistry
Clinical Assistant Professor
University of North Carolina Adams School of Dentistry, Chapel Hill, North Carolina, USA
Division of Pediatric and Public Health

MEGANN K. SMILEY, DMD, MS
Dentist Anesthesiologist
Diplomate, American Dental Board of Anesthesiology
Columbus, Ohio
Nationwide Children's Hospital, Columbus, Ohio, USA
Department of Anesthesiology and Pain Medicine
The Ohio State University College of Dentistry
Division of Pediatric Dentistry, Columbus, Ohio, USA

MICHAEL A. CUDDY, DMD
Dentist Anesthesiologist
Diplomate, American Dental Board of Anesthesiology
Associate Professor
University of Pittsburgh School of Dental Medicine, Pittsburgh, Pennsylvania, USA
Department of Dental Anesthesiology

STEVEN VUKAS, DMD, MD
Oral and Maxillofacial Surgeon
Diplomate, American Board of Oral and Maxillofacial Surgery
Assistant Professor
University of Pittsburgh School of Dental Medicine, Pittsburgh, Pennsylvania, USA
Department of Oral and Maxillofacial Surgery
Department of Dental Anesthesiology

PAUL J. SCHWARTZ, DMD
Oral and Maxillofacial Surgeon
Dentist Anesthesiologist
Diplomate, American Board of Oral and Maxillofacial Surgery
Diplomate, American Dental Board of Anesthesiology
Diplomate, National Board of Dental Anesthesiology
Assistant Professor
University of Pittsburgh School of Dental Medicine, Pittsburgh, Pennsylvania, USA
Department of Oral and Maxillofacial Surgery
Department of Dental Anesthesiology

Content Editors

STEVEN GANZBERG, DMD, MS
Dentist Anesthesiologist
Diplomate, American Dental Board of Anesthesiology
Professor and Chair, Retired
The Ohio State University, Columbus, Ohio, USA
Division of Oral and Maxillofacial Surgery and Dental Anesthesiology
University of California, Los Angeles, California, USA
Division of Dental Anesthesiology

Acknowledgments and Contributors

DANIEL L. ORR II, DDS, MS Anesthesiology, PhD, JD, MD
Dentist Anesthesiologist
Oral and Maxillofacial Surgeon
Lawyer
Diplomate, American Dental Board of Anesthesiology
Diplomate, American Board of Oral and Maxillofacial Surgery
Diplomate, American Board of Legal Medicine
Professor Emeritus
University of Nevada Las Vegas School of Dental Medicine
Las Vegas, Nevada, USA

TIMOTHY M. ORR, DMD, JD
Dentist Anesthesiologist
Lawyer
Diplomate, American Dental Board of Anesthesiology
Diplomate, American Board of Legal Medicine
Austin, Texas, USA

KYLE J. KRAMER, DDS, MS
Dentist Anesthesiologist
Diplomate, American Dental Board of Anesthesiology
Clinical Associate Professor
Indiana University School of Dentistry
Indianapolis, Indiana, USA
Department of Oral Surgery and Hospital Dentistry

Preface

Message From the Authors

Anesthesia for Dental and Oral Maxillofacial Surgery was developed to provide essential information in basic medical knowledge and anesthesia care. This valuable resource will act as a convenient perioperative reference and serve as an excellent study guide in preparation for written and oral board examinations in Dental Anesthesiology and Oral and Maxillofacial Surgery.

This text is not only designed for the resident or new graduate studying for their oral or written boards, but is also useful to those out in practice who want to refresh themselves on anesthetic concepts. It is set up in bullet point format to give you, the reader, high-yield information at a glance and space to highlight, draw, and write in your own explanations to help connect the dots. This will personalize the book to your own learning style to enhance your learning experience.

This book is not going to be a substitute for residency experience and dedicated studying throughout your training. Many of the topics included here are covered in greater depth in other anesthesia textbooks. However, this text should give you solid foundational knowledge as well as guide your studying where knowledge deficits arise.

For questions regarding the content or if there are future topics you think would be beneficial, please email the Editor-in-Chief:

spencerwadedds@gmail.com

Disclaimer: This book is not a substitute for crafting an anesthetic plan on a specific patient/procedural basis.

Oral/Written Boards

It is a great honor and significant career accomplishment to earn a board certification in your chosen specialty. Board certification is certainly worth the time and sacrifice to achieve.

Time management is the most important aspect of preparation when it comes to an oral or written board certification examination. Having an efficient strategy for finding vital topics pertinent to the exam is critical to doing well. One way to demonstrate mastery of core skills and knowledge is to show that you understand how to use resources efficiently and appropriately.

In-Service Training Examination (ITE)

These are secure examinations developed by specific specialty boards for residents in training. The content areas cover the breadth of the specialty with basic science and clinical questions. The exam tests your foundational knowledge in the entire training curriculum. These exams predominately function in gauging your knowledge among your peers, as well as track your progression in the curriculum.

The Written Board Examination

Passing this exam is a prerequisite for being able to sit for the Oral Examination.

Written Examinations are psychometrically valid computer-based exams administered to test your knowledge in core principles of the specialty. Questions range from direct, factual information to specific clinical techniques, and span from basic to complex in breadth.

The Oral Examination

Once you have successfully completed the Written Examination, you are eligible to begin your application for the Oral Examination. This exam is designed to test your clinical judgment and ability to apply and verbalize the cognitive knowledge that was successfully demonstrated on the Written Examination.

The format of the Oral Examination allows you to demonstrate your ability to assess and manage patients presenting for treatment, as well as your ability to effectively communicate these relevant issues with both patients and colleagues.

The Oral Examination seeks to evaluate your ability to analyze and act appropriately and expediently in all situations. The exam encompasses several aspects of anesthesiology practice, including perioperative management and proper responses to urgent and emergency situations.

You will be given case scenarios and asked to interpret and discuss findings, make a clinical judgment, and defend your position. You may request additional information that is relevant to aid in your assessment and management.

The focus of each discussion can change as new issues develop in a given case. You will be evaluated throughout the preoperative, operative, and postoperative periods.

Oral Board Examination Tips

The Oral Examination, in Dental Anesthesiology and Oral and Maxillofacial Surgery can be intimidating and require intense preparation. Adequate preparation is measured in many months of study post-residency. For most candidates, this will be the first oral exam they have ever encountered. Residents who participate in frequent verbal discussions with their attendings regarding clinical scenarios will find themselves better prepared to succeed in this type of exam, and such discussions are strongly encouraged throughout your training. Many residents and candidates also find it useful to take turns asking each other potential board questions to practice talking through the management of patients.

On the whole, it is wise to take the exam soon after completion of residency. You will be more likely to remember detailed information about complicated patients and surgical management. Once you enter private practice, your scope naturally narrows, and some of these minute details can get lost and forgotten.

General Tips

- Your oral exam begins the moment you meet your examiners. Greet your examiners with a smile, look interested, pay attention to every detail of your examiner's instruction. You will be nervous and your examiners will do their best to put you at ease. They will do everything they can to help you relax and perform well.
- Make sure to look and act professional. Business casual is appropriate for the oral exam.
- Realize that your visual appearance and your body language are vital forms of communication during the exam. Your body language should be deliberate; it should exude confidence and communicate that you are happy to be there.
- Make every attempt to answer questions as rapidly and completely as you can. The clearer and more concise you are, the more likely you are to finish the cases and positively impact your grade.

- If you do not know the answer to a specific question, admit this but try to quickly offer information appropriate to the topic which demonstrates your knowledge of the subject and how you would address the situation.
- Always be prepared to articulate your rationale and be prepared to defend your course of action.
- It is important to verbalize your thought process for every stage of case management. Do not assume that the examiners know why you are ordering particular labs and tests, or how you reached a particular conclusion. When in doubt, talk it out.

The Board exam, especially the oral exam, has evolved considerably over time. They are no longer adversarial with intimidating examiners probing the candidates' cognitive and psychological limits. Specialty boards in both Dental Anesthesiology and Oral and Maxillofacial Surgery are directed by our brightest, most accomplished practitioners who truly care about presenting the exam that will fairly evaluate you to join the ranks of the specialty. To be board certified is an extraordinary accomplishment and identifies you as someone who meets the standards of training, education, and professionalism necessary to earn the title of Diplomate.

Dentist Contributions to Anesthesiology

- For millennia, the fear of the pain of surgery was not worth the procedure
- Death was often the preferred option to surgery
- Early efforts included strangulation, freezing, alcohol, opiates, and hallucinogens; none were predictably safe or effective
- Since the 1960s, a series of published articles documented dental outpatient GA safety. Initial mortality estimates of 1/400 000 are now at 1/720 000, supporting an astounding record of safety

The History of Anesthesiology

- 1799: Sir Humphry Davy published that N_2O may be an advantage in surgery
- 1842: Crawford W. Long, MD, observed, *but did not make known*, the effects of N_2O
- 1842: William E. Clark administered ether for a dental extraction, *but did not make known*
- 1844: Horace Wells, DDS, *observed and made known* ("discovered") the predictably safe and effective analgesic effects of N_2O. Wells is the Discoverer of Anesthesia
- 1846: William T.G. Morton, DDS, used ether to assist with tooth extraction and, later that year, neck tumor removal
- 1847: First sexual assault by Parisian dentist convicted on two counts of assault on two anesthetized girls
- 1848: First published anesthesia death involving chloroform for ingrown toenail surgery

- 1865: William T.G. Morton, DDS, provides over 3000 ether anesthetics during the Civil War
- 1868: Alfred Coleman, DDS, invented the first CO_2 absorber
- 1883: G.V. Black, DDS, promoted the use of bromide of ethyl as an anesthetic
- 1902: Charles Teeter, DDS, introduced the first machine capable of delivering N_2O/O_2, ether, and chloroform. Later, Teeter was elected President of both the ASA and IARS
- 1912: Jay Heidbrink, DDS, first used color-coded anesthesia gas tanks and invented the pin index safety system
- 1910: Edgar Rudolph Randolph "Painless" Parker, DDS, advocated for the routine use of local anesthesia in dentistry. The ADA did not recommend local anesthesia until the 1930s
- 1940: Adrian Orr Hubbell, DDS, introduced sodium thiopental as an effective agent for outpatient surgery
- 1944: Leonard Monheim, DDS, published "A,B,C" preanesthesia risk categories
- 1963: The ASA published the Physical Status Classification
- 1963: Hoffmann-La Roche introduced Diazepam. The oral formulation became the most prescribed drug in the world
- 1970s: Medicine begins to adopt half of the 1844 dental paradigm for outpatient anesthesia, i.e. allowing a patient to leave from and return to home after GA and surgery the same day
- 2010s: Medicine begins to adopt the other half of dentistry's 1844 model, i.e. GA in facilities outside the OR

Glossary of Abbreviations

AA	Anesthesiologist assistant	BSSO	Bilateral sagittal split osteotomy
AAOMS	American Association of Oral and Maxillofacial Surgeons	BUN	Blood urea nitrogen
		BW	Birth weight
AAP	American Academy of Pediatrics	°C	Celsius
ABG	Arterial blood gas	CABG	Coronary artery bypass grafting
ABO/Rh	Blood group classification	CAD	Coronary artery disease
ABOMS	American Board of Oral and Maxillofacial Surgery	CaO_2	Arterial oxygen content
		CBF	Cerebral blood flow
ACC	American College of Cardiology	CBC	Complete blood count
ACE	Angiotensin-converting enzyme	CC	Correlation coefficient
ACEi	Angiotensin-converting enzyme inhibitors	CCB	Calcium channel blocker
ACLS	Advanced cardiac life support	CD	Cluster of differentiation (CD4 cells)
ACTH	Adrenocorticotropic hormone	CDC	Centers for Disease Control and Prevention
ADA	American Dental Association	CHD	Congenital heart disease
ADBA	American Dental Board of Anesthesiology	CHF	Congestive heart failure
ADH	Antidiuretic hormone or vasopressin	CI	Confidence interval
ADHD	Attention-deficit/hyperactivity disorder	CKD	Chronic kidney disease
ADSA	American Dental Society of Anesthesiology	CL	Cleft lip
AED	Automated external defibrillator	CLP	Cleft palate
AHA	American Heart Association	cm	Centimeter
AHI	Apnea–hypopnea index	CMP	Comprehensive metabolic panel
AIDS	Acquired immunodeficiency syndrome	$CMRO_2$	Cerebral metabolic oxygen consumption rate
AMA	American Medical Association	CMS	Centers for Medicare and Medicaid Services
AMS	Altered mental status	CN	Cranial nerve
AOP	Apnea of prematurity	CO	Cardiac output
APL	Adjustable pressure limiting	CO_2	Carbon dioxide
ARB	Angiotensin receptor blockers	COMT	Catechol-O-methyltransferase
ASA	American Society of Anesthesiologists	COPD	Chronic obstructive pulmonary disease
ASC	Ambulatory surgery center	COX	Cyclooxygenase
ASD	Atrial septal defect **or** autism spectrum disorder	CNS	Central nervous system
ASDA	American Society of Dentist Anesthesiologists	CPAP	Continuous positive airway pressure
AV	Atrioventricular	CPP	Cerebral perfusion pressure
AVNRT	Atrioventricular nodal reentrant tachycardia	CPR	Cardiopulmonary resuscitation
AVRT	Atrioventricular reentrant tachycardia	CRH	Corticotropin-releasing hormone
BAR	Blunt autonomic response	CNRA	Certified Registered Nurse Anesthetist
BBB	Blood–brain barrier	CSF	Cerebral spinal fluid
BiPAP	Bilevel positive airway pressure	CT	Computed tomography
BMI	Body mass index	CV	Cardiovascular
BMP	Basic metabolic panel	CVA	Cerebrovascular accident
BMS	Bare metal stent	CVR	Cerebrovascular resistance
BNP	B-type natriuretic peptide	DA	Dentist anesthesiologist
BP	Blood pressure	DAPT	Dual antiplatelet therapy
BPD	Bronchopulmonary dysplasia	DASI	Duke Activity Status Index

DBP	Diastolic blood pressure	ICD	Implantable cardioverter defibrillator
DDAVP	Desmopressin	ICP	Intracranial pressure
DDS	Doctorate of Dental Surgery	IDDM	Insulin-dependent diabetes mellitus
DEA	Drug Enforcement Agency	IE	Infective endocarditis
DES	Drug eluting stent	IM	Intramuscular
DHEA	Dehydroepiandrosterone	IN	Intranasal
dL	Deciliter	INR	International normalized ratio
DMARD	Disease-modifying antirheumatic drugs	IV	Intravenous
DMD	Doctor of Medicine in Dentistry	IVH	Intraventricular hemorrhage
DNA	Deoxyribonucleic acid	J	Joule
DO	Doctor of Osteopathic Medicine	kg	Kilogram
DO_2	Oxygen delivery	l	Liter
DOS	Day of surgery	LBW	Lean body weight
DPG	2,3 diphosphoglyceric acid	LFT	Liver function tests
DPP-4	Dipeptidyl peptidase-4 inhibitors	LMA	Laryngeal mask airway
DVT	Deep vein thrombosis	LMWH	Low molecular weight heparin
ECG	Electrocardiography	LR	Lactated ringer's
Echo	Echocardiogram	LV	Left ventricle
ED	Emergency department	LVAD	Left ventricular assist device
EDV	End diastolic volume	LVEF	Left ventricular ejection fraction
EEG	Electroencephalogram	LVF	Left ventricular function
EGD	Esophagogastroduodenoscopy	LVH	Left ventricular hypertrophy
ESRD	End-stage renal disease	m	Meter
ESV	End systolic volume	m.	Muscle
$ETCO_2$	End tidal carbon dioxide	MAC	Minimum alveolar concentration **or** monitored anesthesia care
ETT	Endotracheal tube		
FA	Alveolar concentration of anesthetic gas	MACE	Major adverse cardiac events
FDA	Food and Drug Administration	MAOIs	Monoamine oxidase inhibitors
FEV_1	Forced expiratory volume over one second	MAP	Mean arterial pressure
FGF	Fresh gas flow	MD	Doctor of Medicine
FI	Inspired concentration of inhaled anesthetic	MDI	Metered dose inhaler
FIO_2	Fraction of inspired oxygen	MET	Metabolic equivalent
FOI	Fiberoptic intubation	mEq	Milliequivalent
FRC	Functional residual capacity	MH	Malignant hyperthermia
FVC	Forced vital capacity	MI	Myocardial infarction
g	Gram	MIO	Mean incisal opening
G6PD	Glucose-6-phosphate dehydrogenase	ml	Milliliter
G_A	Gestational age	mm	Millimeter
GA	General anesthesia	mm.	Muscles
GABA	γ-Aminobutyric acid	MMA	Maxillary and mandibular advancement
GER	Gastroesophageal reflux	MMF	Maxillomandibular fixation
GERD	Gastroesophageal reflux disease	mmHg	Millimeters of mercury
GFR	Glomerular filtration rate	MRI	Magnetic resonance imaging
GI	Gastrointestinal	MRSA	Methicillin-resistant staphylococcus aureus
GLP-1	Glucagon-like peptide 1 receptor agonists	MTHFR	Methylenetetrahydrofolate reductase
h	hour(s)	ms	Millisecond
HAART	Highly active antiretroviral therapy	mV	Millivolt
HbA1c	Hemoglobin A1c	MV	Minute ventilation
HBF	Hepatic blood flow	n.	Nerve
HCL	Hydrochloric acid	N_2O	Nitrous oxide
HIV	Human immunodeficiency virus	N/A	Not applicable
HMG-CoA	3-hydroxy-3-methylglutaryl coenzyme A	NAS	Neonatal abstinence syndrome
HR	Heart rate	NEC	Necrotizing enterocolitis
HTN	Hypertension	NETT	Nasal endotracheal tube
IANB	Inferior alveolar nerve block	NG	Nasal-gastric

NGA	Natural guarded airway	RAD	Reactive airway disease
NICU	Neonatal intensive care unit	RAE	Right angle endotracheal
NIDDM	Non-insulin dependent diabetes mellitus	RBCs	Red blood cells
NIV	Noninvasive ventilation	RBF	Renal blood flow
NMB	Neuromuscular blockade	RDS	Respiratory distress syndrome
NMDA	N-methyl-D-aspartate	RQ	Respiratory quotient (Typically ~0.8)
NMJ	Neuromuscular junction	Rh	Rh immunoglobulin
NNT	Numbers needed to treat	ROM	Range of motion
NOE	Nasal-orbital-ethmoid	ROP	Retinopathy of prematurity
NPA	Nasal pharyngeal airway	ROSC	Return of spontaneous circulation
NPH	Neutral Protamine Hagedorn	RR	Respiratory rate
NPO	Latin "Nil per os" or nothing by mouth	RSI	Rapid sequence induction
NSAID	Nonsteroidal anti-inflammatory drugs	RSV	Respiratory syncytial virus
NYHA	New York Heart Association	RV	Right ventricle
OB	Obstetrics	RVH	Right ventricular hypertrophy
ODD	Oppositional defiant disorder	RVOT	Right ventricular outflow tract
OETT	Oral endotracheal tube	RVR	Rapid ventricular response
OG	Oral-gastric	SA	Sinoatrial
OM	Otitis media	SBP	Systolic blood pressure
OMS	Oral and maxillofacial surgeon	SDB	Sleep disordered breathing
OPA	Oral pharyngeal airway	SGA	Supraglottic airway
OR	Operating room	SGL2	Sodium glucose cotransporter-2 inhibitors
OSA	Obstructive sleep apnea	SHS	Secondhand smoke
$PaCO_2$	Arterial partial pressure of carbon dioxide	SIDS	Sudden infant death syndrome
PACU	Post-anesthesia care unit	SL	Sublingual
PaO_2	Arterial partial pressure of oxygen	SpO_2	Percent of oxygen-saturated hemoglobin
P_AO_2	Alveolar partial pressure of oxygen	SNRIs	Serotonin norepinephrine reuptake inhibitors
PAP	Pulmonary arterial pressure	SSRIs	Selective serotonin reuptake inhibitors
P_{atm}	Barometric pressure (760 mmHg)	SV	Stroke volume
PCI	Percutaneous coronary intervention	SVR	Systemic vascular resistance
PDEi	Phosphodiesterase inhibitors	SVT	Supraventricular tachycardia
PE	Pulmonary embolism	T&A	Tonsillectomy and/or adenoidectomy
PEA	Pulseless electrical activity	T_3	Triiodothyronine
PEEP	Positive end-expiratory pressure	T_4	Thyroxine
PEG	Percutaneous endoscopic gastrostomy	TAAA	Thoracoabdominal aortic aneurysm
PFO	Patent foramen ovale	TCAs	Tricyclics
PFT	Pulmonary function test	TIA	Transient ischemic attack
pH	Potential of hydrogen (Measuring degree of acidity)	TIVA	Total intravenous anesthesia
PH_2O	Partial pressure of water (47 mmHg)	TMJ	Temporomandibular joint
PO	Latin "Per os" or by mouth	TSH	Thyroid-stimulating hormone
PONV	Postoperative nausea vomiting	TV	Tidal volume
PPE	Personal protective equipment	TZDs	Thiazolidinediones
PPM	Permanent pacemaker	UPPP	Uvulopalatopharyngoplasty
pRBCs	Packed red blood cells	UTI	Urinary tract infection
PRN	Latin "Pro re nata" or as needed	URI	Upper respiratory infection
PPIs	Proton pump inhibitors	URTI	Upper respiratory tract infection
PPV	Positive pressure ventilation	VF	Ventricular fibrillation
PSI	Pounds per square inch	V/Q	Ventilation/perfusion
PT	Prothrombin time	VSD	Ventricular septal defect
PTT	Partial thromboplastin time	VT	Ventricular tachycardia
PVC	Polyvinyl chloride	VTE	Venous thromboembolism
PVCs	Premature ventricular contractions	vWF	von Willebrand factor
PVR	Pulmonary vascular resistance	WBCs	White blood cells
pVT	Pulseless ventricular tachycardia	WPW	Wolff–Parkinson–White
q	Latin abbreviation of "quaque" or every	ZMC	Zygomaticomaxillary complex

Section 1
Statistics I Physics I Equipment

1.1 Statistics

- Sampling
  - Samples are subsets of the population
  - Ideal samples are truly representative of the population
- Probability
  - The possibility of an outcome from any random event
  - Numerical value between 0 and 1
- Mean
  - The average value of a data set
- Median
  - The middle value of a set of data which has been arranged in order of magnitude
- Mode
  - The most frequent value in a data set
- Standard Deviation
  - Quantifies the variability of values from the mean
- Standard Error
  - Measures the accuracy of the sample mean to the population mean
- Correlation Coefficient
  - The strength of linear relationship between two variables
- Confidence Interval
  - A range of values defined that there is a specific probability that the true value of a parameter lies within it
- Number Needed to Treat
  - The estimated number of patients that need to be treated to impact one patient
- P-value
  - The primary goal of any statistical test/analysis is to determine if a result is statistically significant which is done by a p-value
  - A p-value less than 0.05 is generally considered statistically significant

Normal Distribution (Figure 1.1)

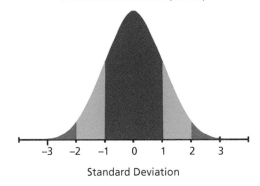

1 Standard Deviation (68.2%)

2 Standard Deviations (95%)

3 Standard Deviations (99.7%)

Standard Deviation

Figure 1.1

Variables

- Independent Variable
  - The variable being manipulated in a study
  - Typically on the X-axis
- Dependent Variable
  - The variable whose measurements depend on the independent variable
  - Typically on the Y-axis
- Continuous Variable
  - Numerical value that can include decimals
  - Examples
    o Income
    o Distance

Anesthesia for Dental and Oral Maxillofacial Surgery, First Edition. Spencer D. Wade, Caroline M. Sawicki, Megann K. Smiley, Michael A. Cuddy, Steven Vukas, and Paul J. Schwartz.
© 2024 John Wiley & Sons, Inc. Published 2024 by John Wiley & Sons, Inc.

- Categorical Variable
  - Distinct categories of data
  - Examples
    - ○ Demographics
    - ○ Days of the week
  - Can include a number range

Basic Statistical Tests

- Student's T-test
  - Used when two categorical variables are tested against a continuous variable
    - ○ Drug 1 vs. drug 2's (Categorical) effect on tumor size (Continuous)
- Chi-Square (χ^2) Test
  - Used when ≥2 categories are tested against ≥2 categorical outcomes
    - ○ Drug 1 vs. drug 2's (Categorical) in eliminating depression (Categorical)
- Analysis of Variance
  - Used when >2 categorical variables are tested against a continuous variable
    - ○ Drug 1 vs. drug 2 vs. drug 3's (Categorical) effect on tumor size (Continuous)

Research Methodologies (Figure 1.2)

- Systematic Review
  - Synthesizing summaries and conclusions from the results of independent studies
- Randomized Controlled Clinical Trial
  - Randomly assigns participants to two or more groups where at least one group receives treatment
    - ○ E.g. The treatment group(s) receive a drug and the control group receives a placebo

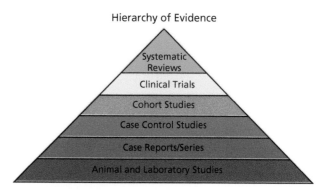

Figure 1.2

- Cohort Study
  - Subjects are grouped based on a risk factor to evaluate disease presence
  - Retrospective cohort
    - ○ Risk factor exposure and disease prevalence are recorded
  - Prospective cohort
    - ○ Following patients forward to see if disease will develop after exposure to a risk factor
- Case Control Study
  - Subjects with a disease are investigated to find cause or risk factors and compared to subjects who do not have the disease
- Case Series
  - Subjects with a disease are investigated to find cause or risk factors
  - There is no control group

1.2 Anesthetic Monitoring Standards

From The Committee of Origin: Standards and Practice Parameters on the Standards for Basic Anesthetic Monitoring by the American Society of Anesthesiologists

Standard I (Figure 1.3)

"Qualified anesthesia personnel shall be present in the room throughout the conduct of all general anesthetics, regional anesthetics and monitored anesthesia care."

Figure 1.3

Standard II (Figure 1.4)

"During all anesthetics, the patient's oxygenation, ventilation, circulation, and temperature shall be continually evaluated."

Figure 1.4

1.3 Pulse Oximetry

Function

- Uses photoplethysmography and pulsatile blood flow to derive oxygen saturation of hemoglobin (Figure 1.5)
  - Deoxyhemoglobin 660 nm
  - Oxyhemoglobin 940 nm

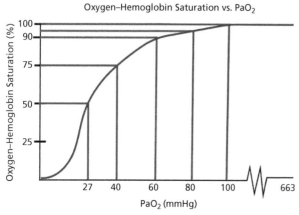

Oxygen–Hemoglobin Saturation vs. PaO$_2$

O$_2$ Saturation	PaO$_2$ (mmHg)	O$_2$ Saturation	PaO$_2$ (mmHg)
100%	100+	90%	60
97%	90	75%	40
95%	80	50%	27

Figure 1.5

Clinical Considerations

- *Factors affecting oxygen–hemoglobin affinity covered on page 47*
  - Falsely Low Reading
    - Nail polish
      - Debatable [1, 2]
    - Shivering
    - Poor circulation
    - Hypotension
    - Vasoconstrictors
    - Methemoglobinemia
      - *Methemoglobinemia covered on page 285*
    - Sulfhemoglobinemia from sulfonamides [3]
- Falsely High Reading
  - Carbon monoxide poisoning
    - SpO$_2$ will read 95+% regardless of true PaO$_2$
    - Venous blood will appear cherry pink
    - Carbon monoxide binds with 200× greater affinity to hemoglobin than oxygen forming carboxyhemoglobin
    - Carboxyhemoglobin has a similar absorption wavelength to oxyhemoglobin
    - Common clinical/exam scenario for this occurring is the first case on a Monday after the anesthesia machine has been left on over the weekend, desiccating the absorbent, which in turn will react with volatile agents to produce carbon monoxide

1.4 Electrocardiography

Function

- Measures electrical cardiac activity (Figure 1.6)
- *Dysrhythmia management covered in Section VI*

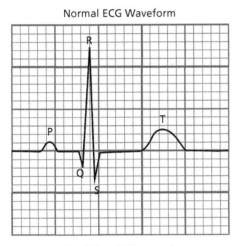

Normal ECG Waveform

Small Box: 0.04 seconds
Big Box: 0.2 seconds

Figure 1.6

Clinical Considerations

- Dysrhythmia Detection
  - Lead II is considered best for routine monitoring
- Ischemia Detection [4]
  - Lead II and V_5, 80% sensitivity
  - Lead II, V_4, and V_5, 90% sensitivity
- P-Wave
  - Atrial depolarization
    - Typically upright and originates from the SA node
    - Normal
      - Upright
    - Inverted or absent P-wave
      - Likely due to rhythm propagation occurring inferior to the SA node or junctional rhythm
- P–R Interval
  - Conduction delay at the AV node
  - Normal
    - ~120–200 ms
  - Prolonged
    - First-degree heart block
- QRS Complex
  - Ventricular depolarization
  - Normal/narrow
    - ~80–100 ms
  - Delayed
    - 100–120 ms
    - Incomplete right or left bundle branch block
    - Nonspecific intraventricular conduction delay
  - Wide
    - >120 ms
    - Bundle branch block
    - Severe vagal stimulation
    - Second- or third-degree heart block
      - Can sometimes still be narrow depending on location of ectopic pacemaker
    - Premature ventricular contractions
    - Ventricular dysrhythmias
- T-Wave
  - Ventricular repolarization
  - Peaked T-wave
    - Sign of hyperkalemia
  - Inverted T-wave
    - Sign of ischemia

- QT Interval
  - Time from ventricular depolarization to repolarization
  - Normal
    - ~350–440 ms
  - Prolonged
    - Drug-induced
    - Prolonged QT syndrome

- R–R Interval
  - Time between QRS complexes
  - Dependent on heart rate
  - Normal
    - 0.6–1.0 seconds
      - 60 beats/min: RR is 1.0 seconds
      - 100 beats/min: RR is 0.6 seconds

1.5 Blood Pressure Monitors

Noninvasive Blood Pressure Cuff

- Function
  - Measures blood pressure by an inflatable cuff
  - Automated cuffs most commonly use oscillometry (Figure 1.7)
- Clinical Considerations
  - The extremity should be measured at the level of the heart
  - Bladder length should cover 80% of the upper arm circumference [5]
  - Bladder width should be >40% of upper arm circumference [5]
  - A cuff that is too small will give an artificially high reading
  - A cuff that is too big will give an artificially low reading
  - Morbidly obese patients may require a wrist cuff for accurate measurements

- Cuff unable to read
  - Patient movement
  - Leak/disconnect in the cuff
  - Significant hypotension
  - Surgeon leaning on cuff
  - Kink in tubing
- During head and neck procedures, consider placing cuff on a lower extremity or wrist to avoid surgeon interference and easier access

Arterial Line

- Function
  - Measures beat-to-beat arterial blood pressure by a transducer (Figure 1.8)
  - Access for ABG/blood samples
    - *Lab testing covered in Section III*

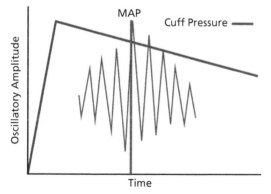

Determining Blood Pressure on Automated BP Cuffs

MAP is determined by the maximum oscillatory amplitude
An algorithm then extrapolates SBP and DBP from MAP

Figure 1.7

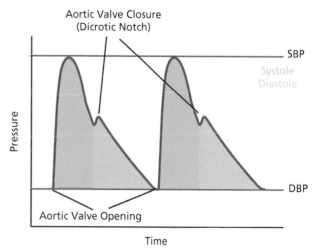

Normal Arterial Wave Form

Figure 1.8

- Clinical Considerations
  - Zero the transducer at the level of the heart
    - If the transducer is elevated, it will give an artificially low reading
    - If transducer is lowered, it will give an artificially elevated reading
  - Unstable hemodynamics
  - Long cases
    - Reduce burden of repeated noninvasive cuff inflation
  - Repeated blood sampling

1.6 Temperature Monitoring

Function

- Measures body temperature
- Recommended:
  - Malignant hyperthermia (MH) triggering agents are administered
  - General anesthetics longer than 30 minutes
  - Temperature changes are anticipated [5]

Clinical Considerations

- The goal is to measure as closely to core body temperature as possible
- Pulmonary Artery
  - Gold standard for temperature measurement
  - Highly invasive and impractical for most head and neck cases
- Esophageal
  - Accurate
  - Difficult to utilize during most head and neck cases
- Nasopharyngeal
  - Accurate if inserted at least 10 cm past naris
  - Irrigation fluid around placement can lead to inaccuracy
- Axillary
  - Fair accuracy if carefully placed with arms tucked
  - Not prone to surgical manipulation during head and neck procedures
- Skin
  - Poor accuracy due to weak blood flow to skin
  - Flexibility with placement
- ↑ Temp
  - Malignant hyperthermia
  - Iatrogenic heating
  - Infection/sepsis
- ↓ Temp
  - Hypothermia
    - Cold operating room
    - Patient exposure
    - Radiation loss
    - General anesthetics
      - Vasodilation
      - Direct inhibition of the hypothalamus
  - Irrigation fluid on probe
  - Dislodgement of probe

1.7 Ventilation Monitoring

Pretracheal/Precordial Stethoscope

- Function
  - Continuous direct monitor of ventilation and cardiac rhythm
- Clinical Considerations
  - Mask induction
  - Natural airway, and also useful for intubated cases
  - Alternative/adjunct when nasal cannula $ETCO_2$ is unreliable
    - Mouth breathing
    - Nasal congestion/obstruction
    - Deviated septum
    - Choanal atresia

Capnography

- Function
  - Indirectly measures $PaCO_2$
- Clinical Considerations
  - Confirm endotracheal intubation
  - Evaluate ventilation status
  - Detect circuit disconnects
  - Monitors CPR efficacy
  - ↑ $ETCO_2$
    - Hypoventilation
      - ↑ Narcotics/sedatives
      - Volatile agents
      - Paralytic agents
    - Malignant hyperthermia
    - Sepsis
    - Hyperthyroidism
    - Desiccated CO_2 absorbent
  - ↓ $ETCO_2$
    - Hyperventilation
    - Pulmonary embolism
    - Severe hypovolemia
    - Low cardiac output
  - Absent or near 0 $ETCO_2$
    - Not ventilating
    - Esophageal intubation
    - Equipment malfunction
    - Cardiac arrest
    - Monitor disconnect
    - Kinked sampling line
    - Water condensation in sampling line/trap
    - Significant circuit leak

1.8 Capnograms (Figures 1.9 & 1.10)

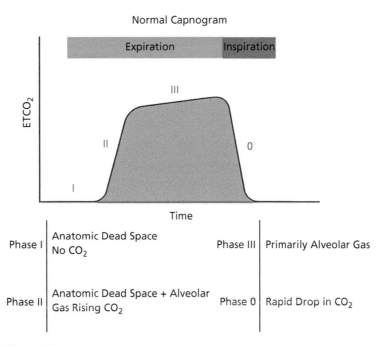

Figure 1.9

Common Capnograms

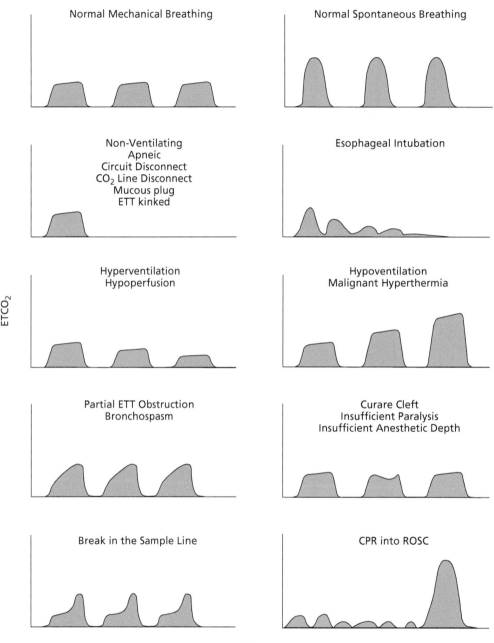

Figure 1.10

1.9   Fluid and Gas Physics

- Fluids never perfectly follow laminar or turbulent flow but always a combination (Figure 1.11)

Reynolds Number

Identifies if the fluid follows more turbulent or laminar principles

$$RE = \frac{\rho u L}{\mu}$$

RE - Reynolds Number
ρ - Fluid Density
u - Flow Speed
L - Length of Tubing
μ - Fluid Viscosity

RE < 1000 will have more laminar flow properties
RE > 1000 will have more turbulent flow properties

Figure 1.11

Laminar Flow

- Fluids of laminar flow follow Poiseuille's law (Figure 1.12)
- ↑ Flow Rate
  - ↑ Pressure difference
    - ○ ↑ IV bag height
    - ○ Compression bag
  - ↑ Orifice diameter
    - ○ Larger ETT size
    - ○ Large IV catheter size
      - Most significant as it is to the fourth power
    - ○ ↓ Tubing length
    - ○ ↓ Fluid viscosity

Poiseuille's Law

Fluid flow through a tube is directly proportional to the pressure of the liquid and to the fourth power of the radius of the tube and inversely proportional to its viscosity and the length of the tube

$$Q = \frac{\Delta P \pi r^4}{8 \eta l}$$

Q - Flow Rate
ΔP - Pressure Difference
η - Fluid Viscosity
l - Length
r - Radius

Figure 1.12

1.10 Medical Gas

Characteristics (Figure 1.13)

E-Cylinder Volume and Pressure

Volume in gas phase is directly proportional to pressure

Oxygen	E cylinder holds 660 l at 2000 PSI*
Medical Air	E cylinder holds 660 l at 2000 PSI*
Nitrous Oxide	E cylinder holds 1590 l** at 750 PSI*

*After tank regulators decrease the pressure to 45 PSI
**Holds more volume as N_2O is partially stored as a liquid under these conditions

Figure 1.13

Nitrous Oxide

- Critical temperature is 36.5 °C
  - Temperature at which gas cannot be liquefied by pressure alone

- N_2O E cylinder will read 750 PSI until less than 400 l remains
  - Must weigh tank to know exact amount of N_2O if reading is 750 PSI
  - Proportional decrease in tank pressure below 750 PSI
    - A reading of 375 PSI will have 200 l N_2O remaining

Gas Supply Colors (Figure 1.14)

- International color for oxygen is white

Color Coded Gas
System in the USA

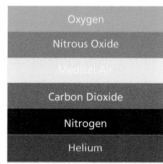

Oxygen
Nitrous Oxide
Medical Air
Carbon Dioxide
Nitrogen
Helium

Figure 1.14

1.11 Mapleson Circuit

Characteristics (Figure 1.15)

- Fresh Gas Flow
  - Influx of anesthetic gases, oxygen, and air to the circuit
- Reservoir Bag
  - Inflates and holds excess anesthetic gases, oxygen, and air
- Adjustable Pressure-Limiting Valve
  - Adjusts the pressure within the circuit

- Advantages
  - Can supply a mixture of anesthetic gases
  - Allows for positive pressure ventilation
  - Can attach advanced airways
- Disadvantages
  - Requires high fresh gas flow (FGF) to avoid rebreathing CO_2
  - Environmental pollution

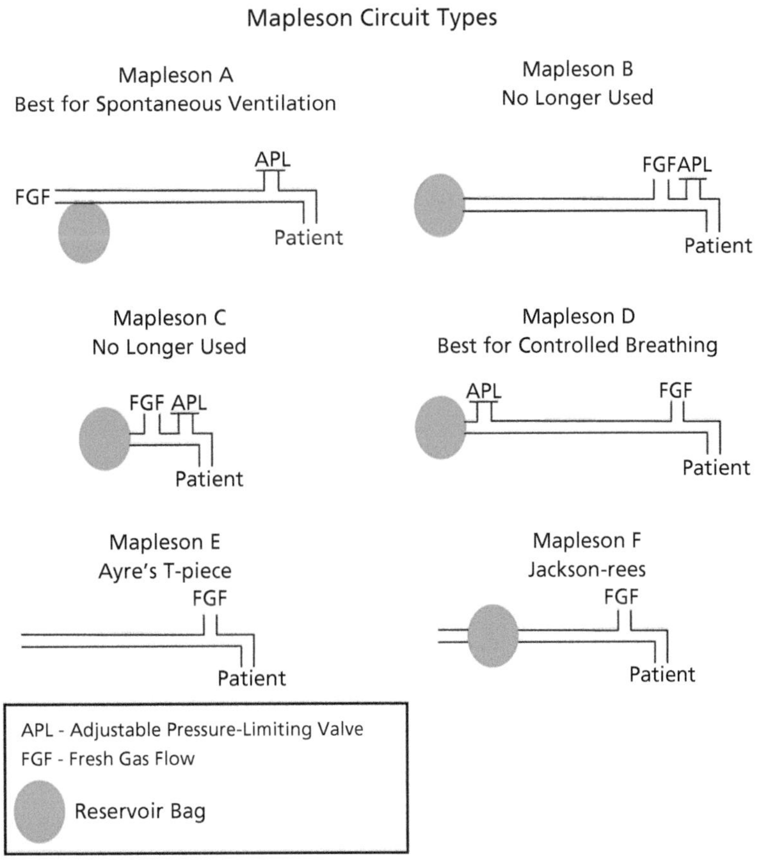

Mapleson Circuit Types

Figure 1.15

1.12   Circle System

- System that modern anesthesia machines use
- Minimizes the environmental waste and CO_2 rebreathing of Mapleson Circuits

Humidifiers

- Types
  - Passive humidifier
    - Traps exhaled humidity and heat
    - Releases it upon inspiration
  - Active humidifier
    - Adds humidity directly to circuit
    - More effective than passive
- Advantages
  - Maintains ciliary function
    - ↓ Atelectasis
    - ↓ Shunting
    - ↓ Sputum retention
- Disadvantages
  - ↑ Humidity can cause valves to malfunction
  - Active humidifier
    - ↑ Nosocomial infections [6]
    - ↑ Complexity

Carbon Dioxide Absorbent

- Absorbs CO_2
- $Ca(OH)_2$ is the main component
- Sevoflurane reacts with NaOH and KOH to form compound A [7]
  - *Likely little relevance under typically clinical conditions*
- Desflurane reacts with desiccated NaOH and KOH to form carbon monoxide [8]
  - Newer absorbents have $Ca(OH)_2$ with small safe amounts of NaOH/KOH, which prevents significant formation of compound A nor carbon monoxide [9]
- Advantages
  - ↓ Pollution/waste
  - ↓ Anesthetic gas use
  - ↓ Flows can be used
- Disadvantages
  - ↑ System's resistance
  - Can potentially release compound A or carbon monoxide to the patient

1.13 Anesthesia Machine Safety Features

Color system	Gas tanks and lines have unique colors which represent the medical gas they store or transport
	See page 16 for color coding
Pin index safety system	Prevents the wrong E cylinder attachment to the anesthesia machine (Figure 1.16)
Diameter index safety system	*Prevents the wrong yolk attachment to the wall supply*
Pressure differential	*Preferential use of gas wall supply (55 PSI) over an E cylinder (45 PSI)*
E tank regulators	*Reduces E cylinder pressure to 45 PSI to reduce the risk of barotrauma*
Pressure gauge	*Allows the anesthesia provider to know the pressure and, subsequently, the volume of gas remaining in tanks*
Low oxygen alarm	*Machine alarms if oxygen concentration falls significantly*
Fail safe valve	*Triggers when oxygen pressure is low*
	Completely occludes nitrous from entering the system
Second-stage regulators	*Reduces anesthetic gas pressures to ~15 PSI*
Adjustable pressure-limiting valve	*Adjusts the pressure within the circuit*
	Most modern machines have an upper limit of 70 cm H_2O to avoid barotrauma
Oxygen flush valve	*Allows immediate burst of oxygen*
	Bypasses second-stage regulator, flowmeters, and vaporizers to common gas outlet at 55 PSI
	Can cause barotrauma if used excessively
Oxygen guard	*Designed to ensure a minimum concentration of oxygen is delivered with nitrous oxide*
Oxygen knob	*Usually larger, fluted, green, and protrudes further than other gas knobs*

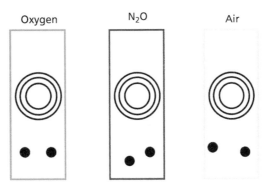

Pin Index
Safety System

Oxygen   N$_2$O   Air

Figure 1.16

Flowmeters	*Older machines use glass tapered tubes (Thorpe tubes) with bobbins (Figure 1.17)*
Flowmeter arrangement	*Oxygen is always the most downstream flowmeter* *Prevents hypoxic gas mixture*
Gas sampling	*Allows analysis of gases during inhalation and exhalation*
Battery	*Allows the anesthesia machine to run for an extra 30–60 minutes during a power outage*

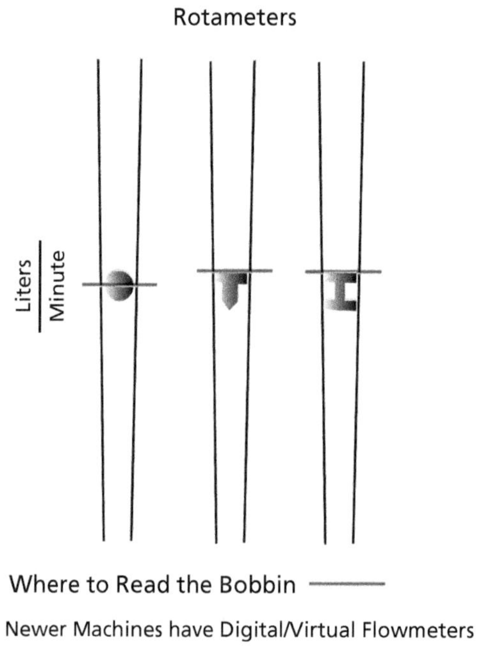
Rotameters
Liters
Minute
Where to Read the Bobbin
Newer Machines have Digital/Virtual Flowmeters

Figure 1.17

1.14 Vaporizer

- Allows for precise titration of volatile agents
- Modern vaporizers are specifically designed for one agent
- Modern vaporizers are variable bypass vaporizers that compensate for both temperature and total gas flow

Vapor Pressure (Figures 1.18 & 1.19)

Vapor Pressure

The Pressure Exerted by the Gas Phase in a Closed Container

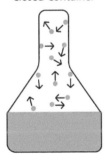

Vapor Pressure is Only Dependent on the Substance's Physical Properties and Temperature

Figure 1.18

Vapor Pressure at 20 °C

	Vapor Pressure (mmHg)
Halothane	~240
Isoflurane	~240
Sevoflurane	~160
Enflurane	~180
Desflurane	~660

Figure 1.19

- Board Facts
  - A halothane vaporizer could potentially utilize isoflurane as their vapor pressures are close
  - Sevoflurane in a halothane vaporizer would cause a gross underdose as sevoflurane's vapor pressure is much lower; thus, less exists in the gas phase and thus less would get to the patient. Furthermore, the MAC requirement of halothane is much lower than a MAC of sevoflurane so the anesthesia provider would likely set a lower output concentration of anesthetic

Safety Features

- Filling Adaptor
  - Volatile agent bottles need an adaptor or "key" to a specific vaporizer
  - Prevents inadvertent mixture of anesthetic liquid in the wrong vaporizer
- Temperature-Compensating Valve
  - ↑ Temperature → ↑ Vapor pressure
  - Valve will ↓ inlet gas flow as more volatile agent will be in gas phase
- High Altitude Compensation
  - Delivers a higher percent at a lower pressure so partial pressure will remain the same
    - Exception is desflurane which is explained later
- Board Facts
  - At half P_{atm} (380 mmHg), sevoflurane is set to 2%, but it is really 4% due to decreased barometric pressure as more sevoflurane will be in the gas phase. However, 4% of 380 mmHg is equivalent to 2% of 760 mmHg (~15 mmHg)

Desflurane Vaporizer

- Characteristics
  - Unlike other vaporizers, delivers a constant percentage of desflurane regardless of barometric pressure

- The vaporizer warms desflurane to a vapor pressure of ~1500 mmHg. Allows more predictable delivery as desflurane boils close to room temperature
- Board Facts
  - At half P_{atm} (380 mmHg), desflurane is set to 6%, but it is really 6% at a lower atmospheric pressure so the patient is receiving half the intended dose
- Need to manually adjust vaporizer to compensate for elevation changes

1.15 Ventilator

- Allows for automated, mechanical respiratory assistance to the patient

Common Ventilator Modes

- Volume Controlled Ventilation
  - The patient is ventilated at a set volume regardless of inspiratory effort
- Pressure Control Ventilation
  - The patient is ventilated at a set pressure regardless of inspiratory effort
- Synchronized Intermittent-Mandatory Ventilation (Figure 1.20)
  - The ventilator will deliver a set number of breaths per minute
  - Also allows for spontaneous breathing by the patient
  - Ideally synchronized to spontaneous efforts
- Volume Support Ventilation
  - The spontaneously ventilating patient is supported by additional volume from the ventilator
- Pressure Support Ventilation
  - The spontaneously ventilating patient is supported by additional pressure from the ventilator

Components and Safety Features

- Ventilator Pressure Relief Valve
  - Ventilators have their own adjustable pressure-limiting (APL) valve or "spill valve" to prevent excessive pressure from causing barotrauma
- Low-Pressure Alarm
  - Detects drop in peak inspiratory pressure
    o Circuit disconnection
    o Significant leak
    o Inadvertent extubation
- High-Pressure Alarm
  - Detects rise in peak inspiratory pressure
    o Inadequate anesthetic level
    o Mucous plug/obstruction
    o Bronchospasm
    o Mainstem intubation
- Low-Volume Alarm/Apnea Alarm
  - Detects drop in tidal volume and/or minute ventilation
- Ascending Bellows
  - Safest in detecting circuit disconnects compared to descending bellows as bellows will be noticeably collapsed
- Drive Gas
  - In case there is a leak within the ventilator, the patient would receive 100% oxygen
- Board Facts
  - Avoid using the oxygen flush valve during inspiration as it may cause barotrauma

Synchronized Intermittent-Mandatory Ventilation

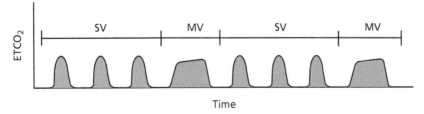

MV - Mandatory Ventilation
SV - Spontaneous Ventilation

Figure 1.20

1.16   Infusion Pump

- Allows for precise and continuous intravenous infusion of medications

Components and Safety Features

- Syringe Verification
  - Verifies the correct size and type of syringe placed
- Syringe Attached Verification
  - Verifies that the syringe is appropriately attached
- Low Medication Alarm
  - Detects low medication volume remaining in syringe

- Occlusion Alarm
  - Detects when there is occlusion in line preventing medication infusion
    - Clamp on infusion line
    - IV line kinked
    - Infiltration
- Battery
  - Allows the infusion pump to not require an external power source

References

1 Rodden, A.M., Spicer, L., Diaz, V.A., and Steyer, T.E. (2007). Does fingernail polish affect pulse oximeter readings? *Intensive Crit. Care Nurs.* 23 (1): 51–55. https://doi.org/10.1016/j.iccn.2006.08.006.

2 Hakverdioğlu Yönt, G., Akin Korhan, E., and Dizer, B. (2014). The effect of nail polish on pulse oximetry readings. *Intensive Crit. Care Nurs.* 30 (2): 111–115. https://doi.org/10.1016/j.iccn.2013.08.003.

3 Aravindhan, N. and Chisholm, D.G. (2000). Sulfhemoglobinemia presenting as pulse oximetry desaturation. *Anesthesiology* 93 (3): 883–884. https://doi.org/10.1097/00000542-200009000-00040.

4 London, M.J., Hollenberg, M., Wong, M.G. et al. (1988). Intraoperative myocardial ischemia: localization by continuous 12-lead electrocardiography. *Anesthesiology* 69 (2): 232–241.

5 Pickering, T.G., Hall, J.E., Appel, L.J. et al. (2005). Recommendations for blood pressure measurement in humans: an AHA scientific statement from the Council on High Blood Pressure Research Professional and Public Education Subcommittee. *J. Clin. Hypertens. (Greenwich)* 7 (2): 102–109. https://doi.org/10.1111/j.1524-6175.2005.04377.x.

6 Sessler, D.I. (2021). Perioperative temperature monitoring. *Anesthesiology* 134 (1): 111–118. https://doi.org/10.1097/ALN.0000000000003481.

7 Kranabetter, R., Leier, M., Kammermeier, D. et al. (2004). The effects of active and passive humidification on ventilation-associated nosocomial pneumonia. *Anaesthesist* 53 (1): 29–35. https://doi.org/10.1007/s00101-003-0607-7.

8 Higuchi, H., Adachi, Y., Arimura, S. et al. (2000). Compound A concentrations during low-flow sevoflurane anesthesia correlate directly with the concentration of monovalent bases in carbon dioxide absorbents. *Anesth. Analg.* 91 (2): 434–439. https://doi.org/10.1097/00000539-200008000-00039.

9 Keijzer, C., Perez, R.S., and de Lange, J.J. (2005). Carbon monoxide production from desflurane and six types of carbon dioxide absorbents in a patient model. *Acta Anaesthesiol. Scand.* 49 (6): 815–818. https://doi.org/10.1111/j.1399-6576.2005.00690.x.

Section 2
Anatomy I Physiology

2.1 Body Fluids

Fluid Compartments

- H_2O is ~60% of total body weight (Figure 2.1)

Total Body Water Distribution

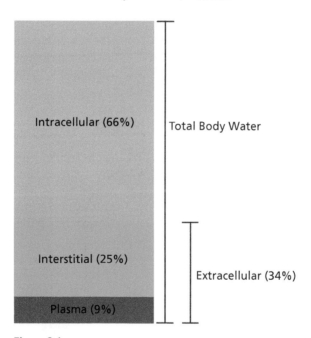

Figure 2.1

Anesthesia for Dental and Oral Maxillofacial Surgery, First Edition. Spencer D. Wade, Caroline M. Sawicki, Megann K. Smiley, Michael A. Cuddy, Steven Vukas, and Paul J. Schwartz.

2.2 Intravenous Fluids

Fluid Composition

	pH	Na⁺	K⁺	Cl⁻
Plasma	*7.4*	*135 – 145*	*3.5 – 5*	*98 – 108*
0.9% Saline	*5.5*	*154*	*0*	*154*
Lactated ringers	*6.5*	*130*	*4*	*109*
5% Dextrose	*4.0*	*0*	*0*	*0*
Plasma-Lyte® *Normosol®*	*7.4*	*140*	*5*	*98*

Crystalloids

- 0.9% Saline
  - Generally used to dilute pRBCs over past concern for Ca²⁺ chelation in other crystalloids, but this has been debunked [1]
    - Advantages
      - Useful if hyponatremic
    - Disadvantages
      - Electrolyte composition not very similar to plasma
- Lactated Ringers
  - Advantages
    - Closer composition to plasma than 0.9% saline
  - Disadvantages
    - Not useful when concerned about hyperkalemia

- 5% Dextrose
  - Advantages
    - ↓PONV
  - Disadvantages
    - Poor to use a sole agent as it is hypotonic due to the lack of electrolytes
- Plasma-Lyte®/Normosol®
  - Advantages
    - Very similar composition to plasma
  - Disadvantages
    - Expensive

Colloids

- Larger molecules, rapid expansion of intravascular space
- Types
  - 5% albumin
  - Hydroxyethyl starch
  - Hetastarch
- Advantages [2, 3]
  - Possible advantage during volume resuscitation
    - Debatable/debunked
- Disadvantages [4, 5]
  - More expensive than crystalloids
  - ↑ Risk of allergic reaction
  - AKI, particularly with hetastarch
  - May increase bleeding time

2.3 Head and Neck Blood Supply (Figures 2.2 & 2.3)

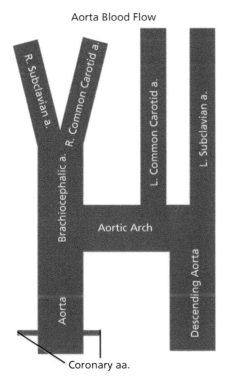

Aorta Blood Flow

R. Subclavian a.

R. Common Carotid a.

L. Common Carotid a.

L. Subclavian a.

Brachiocephalic a.

Aortic Arch

Descending Aorta

Aorta

Coronary aa.

Figure 2.2

External Carotid Artery Branches

Superficial Temporal a.

Maxillary a.

Posterior Auricular a.

Occipital a.

Facial a.

External Carotid a.

Lingual a.

Ascending Pharyngeal a.

Superior Thyroid a

Figure 2.3

2.4   Sensory Nerves (Figure 2.4)

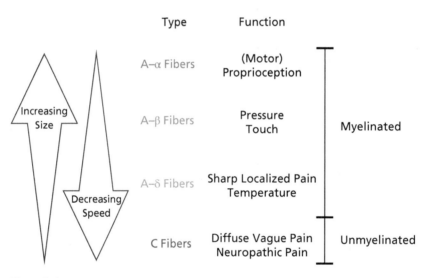

Figure 2.4

2.5   Cranial Nerves

CN I	*Olfactory*
CN II	*Optic*
CN III	*Oculomotor*
CN IV	*Trochlear*
CN V	*Trigeminal*
CN VI	*Abducens*
CN VII	*Facial*
CN VIII	*Vestibulocochlear*
CN IX	*Glossopharyngeal*
CN X	*Vagus*
CN XI	*Spinal Accessory*
CN XII	*Hypoglossal*

CN I (Olfactory)

- Traverses the cribriform plate of the ethmoid bone
- Special Sensory
  - Smell

CN II (Optic)

- Traverses the optic foramen of the sphenoid bone
- Special Sensory
  - Vision

CN III (Oculomotor)

- Originates in the midbrain
- Traverses the superior orbital fissure of the sphenoid bone
- Motor
  - Eye movement
    - Superior rectus m.
    - Inferior rectus m.
    - Medial rectus m.
    - Inferior oblique m.
  - Pupillary constriction
    - Circular m.
  - Pupillary accommodation
    - Ciliary m.
  - Raises eyelid
    - Levator palpebrae superioris m.

CN IV (Trochlear)

- Originates in the midbrain
- Traverses the superior orbital fissure of the sphenoid bone
- Motor
  - Eye movement down and abducted
    - Superior oblique m.

CN V (Trigeminal)

- Originates in the midbrain, pons, and medulla
- Forms the trigeminal ganglion
- Diverges into Three Branches: (Figure 2.5)
  - Ophthalmic branch (V_1)
  - Maxillary branch (V_2)
  - Mandibular branch (V_3)

Trigeminal Nerve
Sensory Distribution

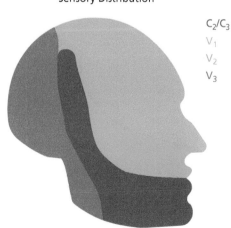

C_2/C_3
V_1
V_2
V_3

Figure 2.5

Ophthalmic Branch (V$_1$)

- Traverses the superior orbital fissure of the sphenoid
- Sensory
  - Eye
  - Scalp
  - Forehead

Maxillary Branch (V$_2$)

- Traverses the foramen rotundum of the sphenoid
- Enters pterygopalatine fossa
- Branches off to form posterior superior alveolar nerve, middle superior alveolar nerve, and anterior superior alveolar nerve before continuing through infraorbital foramen
- Sensory
  - Teeth
  - Palate
  - Gingiva
- Continues through infraorbital foramen as infraorbital nerve
- Sensory
  - Nose
  - Cheeks
  - Upper lip

Mandibular Branch (V$_3$)

- Traverses the foramen ovale of the sphenoid
- Enters the infratemporal fossa
- Motor
  - Muscles of mastication:
    - Medial pterygoid m.
    - Lateral pterygoid m.
    - Masseter m.
    - Temporalis m.
- Further branches into buccal n, auriculotemporal n., lingual n., and mylohyoid n. before entering the mandibular foramina (Figure 2.6)

CN VI (Abducens)

- Abducens nerve
- Originates in the pons
- Traverses the superior orbital fissure of the sphenoid
- Motor
  - Eye abduction
    - Lateral rectus m.

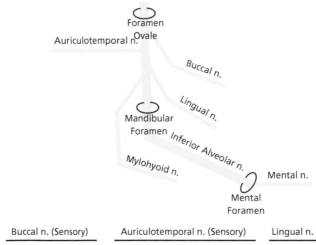

Buccal n. (Sensory)	Auriculotemporal n. (Sensory)	Lingual n. (Sensory)
Buccal Mucosa Mandibular Molars	Side of Face Ear Scalp	Anterior 2/3 of Tongue Floor of Mouth Lingual Gingiva Dentition

Mylohyoid n. (Motor)	Inferior Alveloar n. (Sensory)	Mental n. (Sensory)
Mylohyoid m. Anterior Belly of Digastric m.	Jaw Dentition Gingiva	Lower Lip Chin

Figure 2.6

CN VII (Facial)

- Originates in the pons
- Traverses the facial canal and stylomastoid foramen of the temporal bone
- Terminates at gland or muscle innervated
- Sensory and visceral provided by the chorda tympani n. (CN V)
- Special Sensory
  - Anterior 2/3 of tongue taste
- Motor
  - Facial mm.
    - Except muscles of mastication
  - Posterior belly of digastric m.
- Visceral
  - Submandibular gland
  - Sublingual gland

CN VIII (Vestibulocochlear)

- Originates in the midbrain, pons, and medulla
- Traverses the internal acoustic meatus of the temporal bone
- Terminates at inner ear
- Special Sensory
  - Balance
  - Hearing

CN IX (Glossopharyngeal)

- Originates in the medulla
- Traverses the jugular foramen between the occipital and temporal bones
- Special Sensory
  - Posterior 1/3 tongue taste
- Sensory
  - Pharynx
- Motor
  - Stylopharyngeus m.
- Visceral
  - Parotid gland
  - Carotid sinus

CN X (Vagus)

- Originates from the medulla
- Traverses the jugular foramen between the occipital and temporal bones
- Follows internal jugular vein and internal carotid artery down the neck (Figure 2.7)
- Pharyngeal nerve branches in the neck
- Pharyngeal Nerve
  - Motor
    - Pharyngeal mm.
      - Except stylopharyngeus muscle (CN IX)
    - Palatoglossus m.

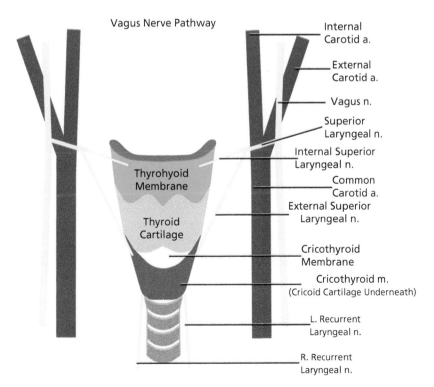

Figure 2.7

- Superior laryngeal nerve branches in the neck just inferior to the pharyngeal nerve which further branches into internal superior laryngeal nerve and external superior laryngeal nerve
- Internal Superior Laryngeal Nerve
  - Sensory
    - Above vocal cords
- External Superior Laryngeal Nerve
  - Motor
    - Cricothyroid m.
- Vagus nerve keeps traversing down the common carotid where the right vagus nerve wraps around the subclavian artery giving off the right recurrent laryngeal nerve and the left vagus nerve wraps around the aortic arch giving off the left recurrent laryngeal nerve
- Recurrent Laryngeal Nerve
  - Sensory
    - Below vocal cords
  - Motor
    - Intrinsic muscles of larynx except cricothyroid m.
    - Posterior cricoarytenoid m.
      - Abduct vocal cords
    - Lateral cricoarytenoid m.
      - Adduct vocal cords
    - Cricothyroid m.
      - Tenses vocal cords
    - Thyroarytenoid m.
      - Relaxes cords
- The portions of the nerve that do not become the recurrent laryngeal n. continue inferiorly to innervate abdominal and thoracic viscera

CN XI (Spinal Accessory)

- Originates from the medulla
- Traverses the jugular foramen between the occipital and temporal bones
- Motor
  - Sternocleidomastoid m.
  - Trapezius m.

CN XII (Hypoglossal)

- Originates from the medulla
- Traverses the hypoglossal canal of the occipital bone
- Motor
  - Tongue mm.
    - Except palatoglossus m. (CN X)

2.6 Neuromuscular Junction

Anatomy

- Synapse between presynaptic motor neuron and post-synaptic muscle by the NMJ
- Motor Unit
  - The muscle fibers innervated by one motor axon
  - Precise muscles have a 1 : 5 motor unit ratio
    - Fingers
    - Eyes
  - Larger muscles have a 1 : 2000 motor unit ratio
    - Back
    - Legs

Muscle Contraction

- Neuromuscular Action Potential
  - Acetylcholine is released into the synaptic space to bind postsynaptic type 1 nicotinic receptors (Figure 2.8)
  - Na^+ influxes through ligand-gated channels, raising the resting potential from −70 to −55 mV, initiating rapid depolarization of the postsynaptic membrane (Figure 2.9)
  - At −55 mV, voltage-gated Na^+ channels open to further depolarize the cell to +30 mV, creating an action potential
- Muscle Contraction
  - The action potential runs across the cell membrane and down the T-tubule to the sarcoplasmic reticulum
  - Sarcoplasmic reticulum voltage-gated channels open and release Ca^{2+} into the cytosol
  - The released Ca^{2+} then binds to troponin to allow actin and myosin to form a "bridge" and thus muscle contraction
- Signal Termination
  - In addition to diffusion of acetylcholine out of the synapse, acetylcholinesterase hydrolyzes acetylcholine in the synaptic cleft, allowing the postsynaptic membrane to slowly repolarize back to baseline with the aid of Na^+/K^+ ATPase

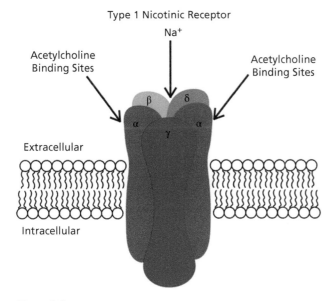

Figure 2.8

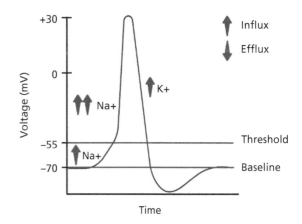

Figure 2.9

2.7 Parasympathetic Nervous System

Anatomy

- Part of the autonomic nervous system
- Cell bodies are in nuclei of the brainstem (CN III, IV, VII, and IX) and S_2–S_4 lateral horns
- Ganglion closer to target organ for more directed effects when compared to sympathetic nervous system

Physiology (Figures 2.10 & 2.11)

- Preganglionic and postganglionic fibers release acetylcholine

Receptors

- Muscarinic Receptor
  - G-protein coupled receptors
  - 5 Types
    - Only M_2 and M_3 discussed here

M_2	↓ *Heart rate*
	↓ *Atrioventricular node conduction*
M_3	*Bronchoconstriction*
	Miosis
	Peripheral vasodilation
	↑ *Secretions*
	Urination

Parasympathetic Nervous System

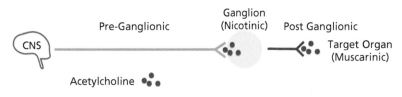

Figure 2.10

Acetylcholine Synthesis and Termination

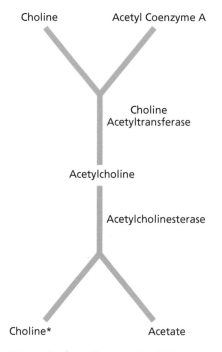

*Reuptake from the synaptic cleft

Figure 2.11

2.8   Sympathetic Nervous System

Anatomy

- Part of the autonomic nervous system
- Cell bodies are in T_1–L_2 intermediolateral columns
- Synapse with paravertebral ganglia early for widespread activation
- Ganglion Types
  - Paravertebral
    - 22 pairs
    - Superior cervical
    - Inferior cervical
    - Stellate ganglia
  - Prevertebral
    - Celiac
    - Superior mesenteric
    - Inferior mesenteric
  - Terminal Ganglia
    - Adrenal medulla

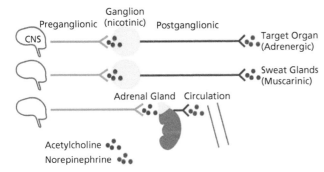

Figure 2.12

Physiology (Figures 2.12 & 2.13)

- Preganglionic fibers release acetylcholine and postganglionic fibers release norepinephrine
  - Exceptions
    - Postganglionic fibers of sweat glands release acetylcholine
      - Preganglionic fibers release acetylcholine at adrenal medulla which releases catecholamines directly into circulation

Norepinephrine/Epinephrine Synthesis and Termination

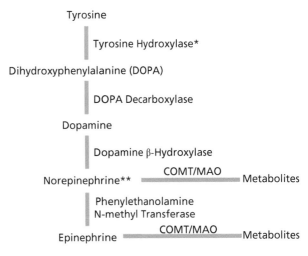

*Rate limiting step
**Signal termination primarily by reuptake, not metabolism
COMT - Catechol-O-methyltransferase
MAO - Monoamine oxidase

Figure 2.13

Receptors

- Adrenergic Receptors
  - All are G-coupled protein receptors

α_1	Mydriasis
	Hypertension
	Glycogenesis
	Gluconeogenesis
α_2	Vasoconstriction (Direct-acting)
	Vasodilation (Central-acting)
	Sedation
β_1	↑ Cardiac contractility
	↑ Heart rate
	Renin release
	Lipolysis
β_2	Vasodilation (Skeletal muscles)
	Bronchodilation
	Insulin release
	Lipolysis
	Gluconeogenesis
β_3	Lipolysis

2.9 Brain

Anatomy

- Cerebrum
  - Frontal lobe
    - Motor movements
    - Logic and reasoning
  - Temporal lobe
    - Speech
    - Listening
  - Parietal lobe
    - Sensory processing
  - Occipital lobe
    - Vision
- Cerebellum
  - Balance
  - Coordination
- Thalamus
  - Connection between the cerebrum and input from the rest of the body
  - Input and processing center for sensory and motor impulses
- Hypothalamus
  - Homeostasis
  - Hormone synthesis and secretion
- Brainstem
  - Midbrain
    - Eye movement
    - Sensory processing
  - Medulla oblongata
    - Blood pressure and heart rate control
    - Area postrema
    - Respiratory center
  - Pons
    - Respiratory center
- Amygdala
  - Role in fear and anxiety
- Hippocampus
  - Memory formation
- Pituitary
  - Hormone synthesis and secretion
- Pineal Gland
  - Regulates circadian rhythm
- Meninges (Outer to Inner)
  - Dura mater
    - Falx cerebri
      - Separates cerebral hemispheres
    - Tentorium cerebelli
      - Separates supratentorial (cerebrum) and infratentorial (cerebellum and brainstem) spaces
  - Arachnoid mater
  - Pia mater
- Microscopic
  - Neurons
  - Glia
    - Astrocytes
    - Oligodendrocytes
      - Produce myelin
    - Microglia
      - Immune cells of the CNS
  - Blood–brain barrier
    - Protective barrier between the vascular system and the brain
    - Allows the passage of nutrients, oxygen, and removal of waste

Function

- Homeostasis
- Sensation
- Movement
- Consciousness

Cerebral Blood Flow (CBF)

- ~10–15% of cardiac output
  - Normal CBF is 50 ml blood/100 g/min
- Circle of Willis provides intracranial collateral blood flow (Figure 2.14)

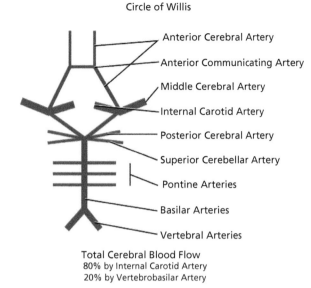

Circle of Willis

- Anterior Cerebral Artery
- Anterior Communicating Artery
- Middle Cerebral Artery
- Internal Carotid Artery
- Posterior Cerebral Artery
- Superior Cerebellar Artery
- Pontine Arteries
- Basilar Arteries
- Vertebral Arteries

Total Cerebral Blood Flow
80% by Internal Carotid Artery
20% by Vertebrobasilar Artery

Figure 2.14

Cerebral Blood Flow Regulation (Figure 2.15)

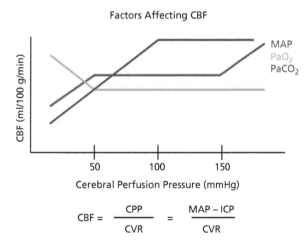

Factors Affecting CBF

MAP
PaO$_2$
PaCO$_2$

$$CBF = \frac{CPP}{CVR} = \frac{MAP - ICP}{CVR}$$

Figure 2.15

- Cerebral Perfusion Pressure (CPP)
  - Directly related to cerebral blood flow
  - Depends on intracranial and mean arterial pressures
- Intracranial pressure (ICP)
  - Usually low and stable: ICP = MAP − CPP
- Mean Arterial Pressure
  - <50 mmHg MAP → ↓ CPP → ↓ CBF
  - 50–150 mmHg → Little to no change
  - >150 mmHg MAP → ↑ CPP → ↑ CBF
  - Autoregulation of CPP range will be higher in chronic hypertension
- Cerebrovascular Resistance (CVR)
  - Indirectly correlated to cerebral blood flow
    - PaCO$_2$
      - ↑ PaCO$_2$ → ↓ CVR → ↑ CBF
      - ↓ PaCO$_2$ → ↑ CVR → ↓ CBF
    - PaO$_2$
      - <60 mmHg O$_2$ → ↓ CVR → ↑ CBF
      - >60 mmHg O$_2$ → Little to no change in CVR and CBF
  - Anesthetic agents
    - All IV agents ↓ CVR → ↑ CBF except ketamine
    - All inhalational agents ↓ CVR → ↑ CBF except N$_2$O

Innervation

- N/A

Cerebrospinal Fluid

- Circulates within ventricles and the subarachnoid space of the brain and spine
- Function
  - Protection
  - Removes metabolic waste
  - Delivers nutrients
- Synthesis
  - By the choroid plexus in the lining of ventricles
- Absorption
  - Arachnoid villi

Anterior Pituitary Hormones

Follicle–stimulating hormone	*Spermatogenesis (Males)* *Follicular growth (Females)*
Luteinizing hormone	*↑ Testosterone (Males)* *↑ Estrogen and progesterone (Females)* *Ovulation (Females)*
Adrenocorticotropic hormone	*↑ Cortisol* *↑ Aldosterone* *↑ Androgens*
Thyroid-stimulating hormone	*↑ Thyroid hormone*
Prolactin	*↑ Milk production*
Growth hormone	*Stimulates tissue growth and development*

Posterior Pituitary Hormones

- The hormones are synthesized in the hypothalamus, but released by the posterior pituitary

Vasopressin	*↑ H$_2$O reabsorption in the distal tubules and collecting ducts of the kidney* *Vasoconstriction*
Oxytocin	*Uterine contraction* *Lactation*

2.10   Spinal Cord

Anatomy

- Spinal Cord
  - Adults: Extends to L_1–L_2
  - Peds: Extends to L_3
- Spinal Nerves
  - 31 pairs
    - 8 Cervical
    - 12 Thoracic
    - 5 Lumbar
    - 5 Sacral
    - 1 Coccygeal
- Meninges
  - Surround, protect, and support the spinal cord
  - Outer to inner
    - Dura mater
    - Arachnoid mater
    - Pia mater
- Epidural Space
  - Between the dura mater and the vertebrae
- Vertebrae (33)
  - 7 Cervical
  - 12 Thoracic
  - 5 Lumbar
  - 1 Sacrum (5 fused vertebrae)
  - 1 Coccyx (4 fused vertebrae)
- Microscopic
  - Similar to cerebral
  - Neurons
  - Astrocytes
    - Form the blood spinal cord barrier
  - Oligodendrocytes
    - Produce myelin
  - Microglia
    - Immune cells of the CNS
- Spinal Cord Cross-Section (Figure 2.16)
  - Ventral horn
    - Houses cell bodies of motor neurons
  - Dorsal horn
    - Transmits sensory information rostrally
  - Dorsal root ganglion
    - Houses cell bodies of peripheral sensory nerves

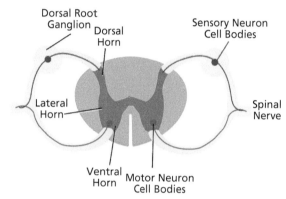

Figure 2.16

  - Lateral horn
    - T_1–L_2 (Intermediolateral columns)
      - Cell bodies of sympathetic nervous system
    - S_2–S_4
      - Cell bodies of parasympathetic nervous system
  - Spinal nerves
    - Combination of motor and sensory information

Function

- Transmits motor, sensory, and autonomic innervation between the peripheral and central nervous system

Blood Flow

- Anterior spinal arteries
- Posterior spinal arteries
- Radicular arteries

Innervation

- N/A

Endocrine/Exocrine

- N/A

2.11 Cardiac

Anatomy

- Two atria
- Two ventricles
- Atrioventricular Valves
  - Allows blood flow from the atria to the ventricles during diastole
  - Mitral valve
    - Conduit from the left atrium to the left ventricle
  - Tricuspid valve
    - Conduit from the right atrium to the right ventricle
  - Chordae tendineae
    - Fibrous strands that connect the papillary muscle to atrioventricular valves
    - ↓ Prolapse/regurgitation into the atria during systole
  - Papillary muscles
    - Attached to the chordae tendineae
- Semilunar Valves
  - Allows blood to flow from the ventricles to the great vessels during systole
  - Aortic valve
    - Conduit from the left ventricle atrium to the aorta
  - Pulmonic valve
    - Conduit from the right ventricle to the pulmonary artery
- Great Vessels
  - Pulmonary veins
    - Return oxygenated blood to the left atrium
  - Superior and Inferior vena cavae
    - Return deoxygenated blood to the right atrium
  - Pulmonary artery
    - Transports deoxygenated blood to the lungs
  - Aorta
    - Transports oxygenated blood to the body
- Pericardium
  - Protective fibrous outer bilayer membrane
- Microscopic
  - Myocytes
  - Fibroblasts
  - Smooth muscle cells
  - Endothelial cells

Function

- Delivers oxygen, hormones, and nutrients to tissues
- Transports away caron dioxide and metabolic waste
- Regulates blood pressure

Cardiac Blood Flow (Figure 2.17)

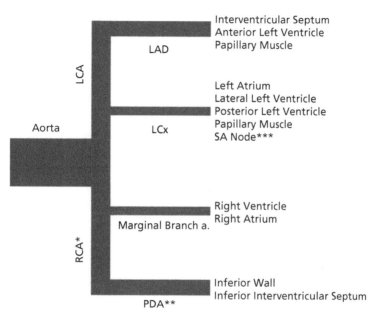

Coronary Blood Flow

LCA → LAD	Interventricular Septum Anterior Left Ventricle Papillary Muscle
LCA → LCx	Left Atrium Lateral Left Ventricle Posterior Left Ventricle Papillary Muscle SA Node***
RCA* → Marginal Branch a.	Right Ventricle Right Atrium
RCA* → PDA**	Inferior Wall Inferior Interventricular Septum

LCA - Left Coronary Artery
RCA - Right Coronary Artery
LCx - Left Circumflex Artery
LAD - Left Anterior Descending Artery
PDA - Posterior Descending Artery

*RCA supplies the AV Node in most the population and the SA node in 60% of the population
** PDA arises from the RCA in 80% of the population and the LCA in 20% of the population
***LCx supplies SA node in 40% of the population

Figure 2.17

Innervation

- Non-innervated heart rate is 110–120 beats/min
- Parasympathetic
  - M_2 receptors from vagus nerve
    - ↓ Heart rate
    - ↓ Contractility
- Sympathetic
  - Direct β_1 stimulation by cardiac accelerator fibers (T_1–T_4) or circulating catecholamines
    - ↑ Heart rate
    - ↑ Contractility

Cardiac Output (Figure 2.18)

Cardiac Output = Heart Rate × Stroke Volume

$$Cardiac\ Index = \frac{Cardiac\ Output}{Body\ Surface\ Area}$$

Normal Values
Adult Cardiac Output: ~5 l/min
Adult Cardiac Index: ~2.5 – 4.0 l/min/m²

Figure 2.18

- Heart Rate (HR)
  - ↑ M_2 → ↓ HR → ↓ CO
  - ↓ M_2 → ↑ HR → ↑ CO
  - ↑ β_1 → ↑ HR → ↑ CO
  - ↓ β_1 → ↓ HR → ↓ CO
  - Baroreceptors
    - Regulate heart rate in relationship to blood pressure
    - ↑ Blood pressure → ↓ Heart rate
    - ↓ Blood pressure → ↑ Heart rate
    - Aortic arch baroreceptor innervated by CN X
    - Carotid sinus baroreceptor innervated by CN IX
- Stroke Volume (SV)
  - Amount of blood ejected from the left ventricle into aorta per systolic contraction (Figure 2.19)
- Normal values
  - Adult: 70–110 ml
  - Pediatric: 2 ml/kg
- Factors affecting SV
  - Preload
    - ↑ Preload → ↑ EDV → ↑ SV
    - ↓ Preload → ↓ EDV → ↓ SV
  - Afterload
    - ↑ Afterload → ↑ ESV → ↓ SV
    - ↓ Afterload → ↓ ESV → ↑ SV

Stroke Volume = End Diastolic Volume (EDV) – End Systolic Volume (ESV)

Figure 2.19

- Inotropy
  - ↑ Inotropy → ↓ ESV → ↑ SV
  - ↓ Inotropy → ↑ ESV → ↓ SV

Flow-Volume Loop (Figure 2.20)

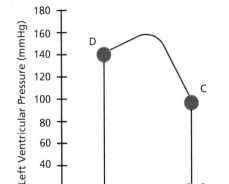

Cardiac Flow Volume Loop

A: Mitral Valve Opens   A–B: Diastolic Filling
B: Mitral Valve Closes   B–C: Isovolumetric Contraction
C: Aortic Valve Opens   C–D: Left Ventricle Ejection
D: Aortic Valve Closes   D–A: Isovolumetric Relaxation

Figure 2.20

Conduction

- Sinoatrial Node
  - Primary cardiac pacemaker
- Internodal Pathways
  - Propagates signal to AV node
    - Anterior internodal pathway
    - Middle internodal pathway
    - Posterior internodal pathway

- Atrioventricular Node
  - Brief conduction delay to allow complete ventricular filling
  - Secondary cardiac pacemaker
  - Intrinsic rate of 40–60 beats/minute
- Bundle of His
  - Branches
    - Left bundle branch
      - Anterior superior fascicles
      - Posterior inferior fascicles
    - Right bundle branch
      - Only one fascicle
  - Intrinsic rate of 25–40 beats/minute
- Purkinje Fibers
  - Intrinsic rate of 25–40 beats/minute

Cardiac Action Potentials (Figures 2.21 & 2.22)

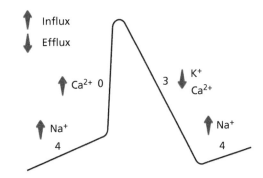

Cardiac Pacemaker Action Potetial

Phase 4	Slow, spontaneous influx of sodium through "funny" channels until threshold
Phase 0	Once threshold is reached, voltage-gated calcium channels open to depolarize
Phase 3	Potassium and calcium efflux out of the cell to repolarize the cell

Figure 2.21

Cardiac Myocyte Action Potential

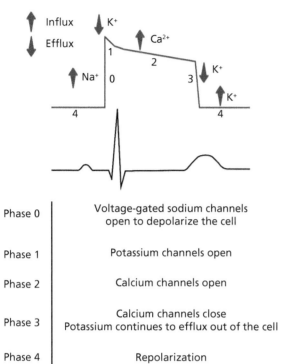

Phase 0	Voltage-gated sodium channels open to depolarize the cell
Phase 1	Potassium channels open
Phase 2	Calcium channels open
Phase 3	Calcium channels close Potassium continues to efflux out of the cell
Phase 4	Repolarization

Figure 2.22

Endocrine/Exocrine

B-Type natriuretic peptide	*Released by atrial myocytes in response to atrial distension*
	↑ Diuresis
	↑ Vasodilation
	↑ Vascular permeability

2.12   Pulmonary

Anatomy

- Nose
- Mouth
- Pharynx
- Larynx
  - Cartilages of the airway
    - Unpaired cartilages
      - Epiglottis
      - Thyroid
      - Cricoid
    - Paired
      - Arytenoid
      - Corniculate
      - Cuneiform
- Trachea
  - Tracheal rings
  - Carina
- Carina
  - Bifurcation of trachea into main stem bronchi
- Lungs
  - Right lung
    - Right bronchus is more vertical, shorter, and wider than the left bronchus and more likely to be inadvertently intubated
    - Three Lobes (superior, middle, inferior)
  - Left lung
    - Two Lobes (superior, inferior)
- Microscopic
  - Alveoli
  - Squamous epithelium
  - Goblet cells
    - Secrete mucous to protect surface and trap bacteria/foreign matter
  - Type 1 pneumocytes
    - Epithelial cells
    - Most abundant cell type
    - Primarily involved in gas exchange
  - Type 2 pneumocytes
    - Produce surfactant
    - Divide to produce type 1 pneumocytes

Function

- Deliver oxygen
- Remove waste gases
- Acid–base balance
- Phonation
- Warms and humidifies air
- Filtration against pathogens

Pulmonary Blood Flow

- Larynx
  - Superior laryngeal artery
  - Inferior laryngeal artery
- Bronchi
  - Bronchial arteries
    - Direct blood supply to the lungs
    - Branches off the aorta
  - Bronchial veins
    - Drains the lungs
    - Drains into azygos and hemiazygos veins
- Lungs
  - Pulmonary arteries
    - Transports deoxygenated blood from right ventricle to lungs
  - Pulmonary veins
    - Four total
    - Transports oxygenated blood from the lungs to the left atrium

Innervation

- Larynx
  - Sensory
    - o Internal superior laryngeal n.
    - o Recurrent laryngeal n.
  - Motor
    - o Recurrent laryngeal n.
    - o External superior laryngeal n.
- Lungs
  - Parasympathetic
    - o Vagus n.
      - Bronchoconstriction
      - ↑ Secretions
  - Sympathetic
    - o ~T_1–T_4
      - Bronchodilation
      - ↓ Secretions
- Diaphragm
  - Motor
    - o Phrenic nerves (C_3–C_5)

Ventilation

- Conducting Zone
  - Mouth/nose → Trachea → Bronchi → Bronchioles → Terminal bronchioles
  - Warms, filters, and humidifies the air
  - Anatomic dead space
    - o Volume of ventilated air with no gas exchange due to lack of pulmonary perfusion
    - o Average anatomic dead space ~2 ml/kg
- Respiratory Zone
  - Respiratory bronchioles → Alveolar ducts → Alveoli
  - Alveoli present with pulmonary perfusion for gas exchange
- Inspiratory Muscles
  - Diaphragm
    - o Accounts for most of the intrathoracic volume change
  - External intercostal mm.
  - Forced inspiration mm.
    - o Sternocleidomastoid mm.
    - o Scalene mm.
    - o Pectoralis mm.
- Expiratory Muscles
  - Generally passive
  - Forceful expiration
    - o Abdominal rectus mm.
    - o External oblique mm.
    - o Internal oblique mm.
    - o Internal intercostal mm.

Shunts and Dead Space (Figure 2.23)

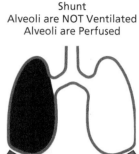

Figure 2.23

Oxygen–Hemoglobin Dissociation Curve (Figure 2.24)

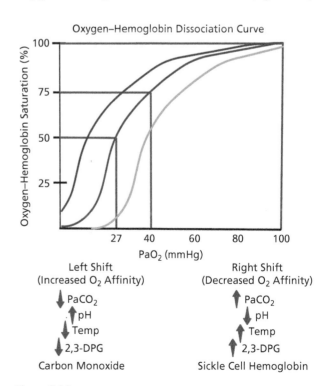

Figure 2.24

Blood Oxygen Calculations (Figure 2.25)

> ### Blood Oxygen Calculations
>
> $$CaO_2 = (0.003 \times PaO_2) + (1.34 \times \text{Hemoglobin} \times SaO_2)$$
>
> $$DO_2 = CaO_2 \times CO$$
>
> $$OE = \frac{CaO_2 - CvO_2}{CaO_2}$$
>
> $$P_AO_2 = FiO_2(Patm - PH_2O) - \frac{PaCO_2}{RQ}$$
>
> $$\text{Calculated A-a Gradient} = P_AO_2 - PaO_2$$
> $$\text{Predicted A-a Gradient} = (Age + 10)/4$$
>
> CaO_2: Total Arterial Content of Blood
> CvO_2: Central Venous Oxygen Saturation
> SaO_2: Hemoglobin–Oxygen Saturation
> P_AO_2: Alveolar Partial Pressure of Oxygen
> PaO_2: Arterial Partial Pressure of Oxygen
>
> PH_2O: 47 mmHg
> Patm: 760 mmHg
> DO_2: Oxygen Delivery
> OE: Oxygen Extraction
> RQ: Respiratory Quotient

Figure 2.25

Acid–Base Balance (Figure 2.26)

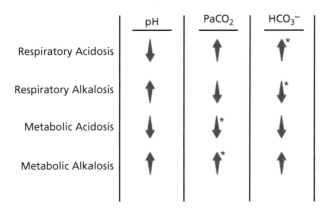

	pH	PaCO₂	HCO₃⁻
Respiratory Acidosis	↓	↑	↑*
Respiratory Alkalosis	↑	↓	↓*
Metabolic Acidosis	↓	↓*	↓
Metabolic Alkalosis	↑	↑*	↑

*Compensatory change

Figure 2.26

- The lungs can raise or lower plasma pH by adjusting exhalation of CO_2
- The kidneys can raise or lower plasma pH by adjusting reabsorption of HCO_3^- and excretion of H^+
- $PaCO_2$ and HCO_3^- will generally trend in the same direction to maintain a physiologic pH

Endocrine/Exocrine

Surfactant	*↓ Surface tension within alveoli*
Angiotensin-converting enzyme	*Converts angiotensin I to angiotensin II*

2.13 Renal

Anatomy

- Bean-shaped organ located retroperitoneal below the ribs at T_{12}–T_{13}
- 1% of the population has a horseshoe kidney
- Cortex
  - Outer-most parenchymal layer
- Medulla
  - Inner-most parenchymal layer
- Calyces, Renal Pelvis, Ureters
  - Urine transport away from the parenchyma
- Microscopic
- Nephron
  - Functional unit of the kidney (Figure 2.29)

Function

- Electrolyte and acid–base balance
- Urine formation
- Blood pressure regulation
- Secretion of erythropoietin
- Activation of vitamin D

Renal Blood Flow

- Renal arteries
- Renal veins

Innervation

- Parasympathetic
  - CN X
- Sympathetic
  - ~T_{10}–L_1

Renal Volume Management (Figures 2.27 & 2.28)

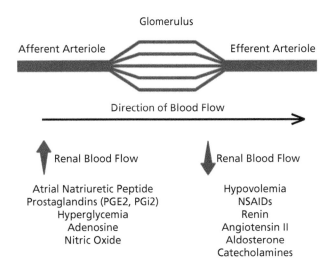

Figure 2.27

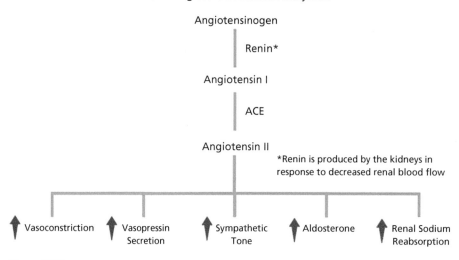

Renin Angiotensin Aldosterone System

Angiotensinogen

Renin*

Angiotensin I

ACE

Angiotensin II

*Renin is produced by the kidneys in response to decreased renal blood flow

Vasoconstriction | Vasopressin Secretion | Sympathetic Tone | Aldosterone | Renal Sodium Reabsorption

Figure 2.28

Urine Concentration (Figure 2.29)

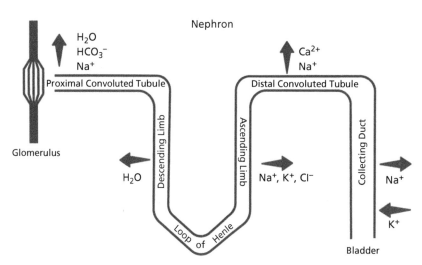

Urine Concentration and Dilution

Nephron

H_2O
HCO_3^-
Na^+

Ca^{2+}
Na^+

Proximal Convoluted Tubule

Distal Convoluted Tubule

Glomerulus

Descending Limb

Ascending Limb

Collecting Duct

H_2O

Na^+, K^+, Cl^-

Na^+

K^+

Loop of Henle

Bladder

Figure 2.29

- Proximal Convoluted Tubule
  - Primary site of Na^+, HCO_3^-, and H_2O reabsorption
- Descending Limb
  - H_2O diffuses out passively by aquaporins
  - Allows the urine to concentrate
- Ascending Limb
  - Actively transport of Na^+, K^+, Cl^- out of the lumen
  - Impermeable to H_2O
- Distal Convoluted Tubule
  - Primary site of Ca^{2+} reabsorption
  - Na^+ reabsorption
  - Macula densa is located here
- Collecting Duct
  - Na^+/K^+ cotransporter
  - Aquaporins concentrate urine

Acid–Base Balance

- See Figure 2.26

Endocrine/Exocrine

Renin	*Governed by the juxtaglomerular apparatus*
	Released in response to reduced renal blood flow
	Converts Angiotensinogen to Angiotensin I to increase blood pressure
Erythropoietin	*Stimulates red blood cell formation*
Vitamin D	*Involved in vitamin D activation*

2.14   Hepatic and Biliary

Anatomy

- Liver
  - Lobes
    - Left
    - Right
    - Caudate
    - Quadrate
  - Ligaments
    - Falciform
    - Round
- Bile ducts
  - Transports bile from liver to gallbladder
- Gallbladder
  - Reservoir for bile
- Microscopic
  - Hepatocytes
  - Kupffer cells
    - Macrophages of the liver
  - Lobule
  - Acinus
    - Functional unit of the liver

Function

- Bile formation and secretion
- Glucose homeostasis
- Fat metabolism
- Protein synthesis
- Synthesis of most clotting factors
- Urea cycle
- Iron and vitamin storage
- Detoxification and metabolism of drugs
  - *Metabolism of drugs covered on page 123*

Hepatic Blood Flow (Figure 2.30)

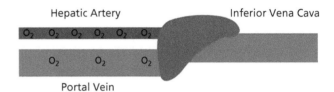

Hepatic Blood Flow

Hepatic Artery   Inferior Vena Cava

Portal Vein

HBF ~25% of Cardiac Output

Portal Vein	Hepatic Artery
~75% of HBF	~25% of HBF
Deoxygenated	Oxygenated

The portal vein and hepatic artery each contribute
~50% of oxygen/nutrients to the liver

Figure 2.30

Innervation [6]

- Parasympathetic
  - CN X
- Sympathetic
  - ~T_7–T_{12}

Endocrine/Exocrine

Protein synthesis	*All plasma proteins synthesized in the liver EXCEPT:*
	Gamma globulins
	Some Factor VIII
	von Willebrand factor
Bile	*Secreted by the liver and stored in the gall bladder*
	Emulsifies lipids and fat-soluble vitamins and lipids

2.15 Gastrointestinal

Anatomy

- Mouth
- Pharynx
- Esophagus
- Stomach
- Small Intestine
  - Duodenum
  - Jejunum
  - Ileum
- Large Intestine
  - Ascending colon
  - Transverse colon
  - Descending colon
  - Sigmoid colon
  - Rectum
- Microscopic
  - Epithelial cells
  - Secretory cells
  - Absorptive cells
  - Smooth muscle
  - Skeletal muscle

Function

- Eating
- Drinking
- Speaking
- Swallowing
- Food storage
- Digestion
- Nutrient uptake
- Water absorption

Blood Flow

- *Head and neck blood flow covered in Figure 2.3*
- Inferior thyroid artery
- Thoracic aortic branches
- Azygos veins
- Hemiazygos veins
- Gastric arteries
- Gastric veins
- Mesenteric arteries
- Mesenteric veins

Innervation

- *Head and neck innervation covered on pages 31–34*
- Parasympathetic
  - CN X
  - S_2–S_4
- Sympathetic
  - ~T_5–L_2

Endocrine

Table 2.1

Cholecystokinin	↑ *Release from gall bladder*
	↓ *Gastric emptying*
	↑ *Pancreatic enzyme release*
Glucagon-like Peptide-1 (GLP)	↑ *Insulin secretion*
Gastrin	↑ *Secretion of HCl*
Motilin	↑ *Gastric, small intestine motility*
Secretin	↑ *Release of HCO_3^- into duodenum*
Somatostatin	↓ *Gastric emptying*
Vasoactive Intestinal Peptide (VIP)	↓ *Gastric sections*
	↑ *Smooth muscle relaxation*
	↑ *Water, electrolyte, bicarbonate secretion*

Exocrine

Table 2.2

Amylase Sucrase Maltase Lactase	*Carbohydrate breakdown*
Pepsinogen gastric acid Trypsin peptidases Bile	*Protein breakdown*
	Emulsify lipids and fat-soluble vitamins
	A, D, E, K
Intrinsic factor	*B_{12} absorption in ileum*
Bicarbonate	*Buffer against acidic foods and gastric acid*

2.16   Pancreas

Anatomy

- Retroperitoneal gland
- Head
- Neck
- Body
- Tail
- Microscopic
  - Exocrine glands
  - δ islet cells
  - β cells
  - α cells

Function

- Blood sugar regulation
- Aids digestion

Blood Supply

- Splenic artery
- Splenic vein

Innervation

- Parasympathetic
  - CN X
  - S_2–S_4
- Sympathetic
  - ~T_5–T_{12}

Endocrine/Exocrine (Figure 2.31)

- The pancreas is primarily an exocrine organ

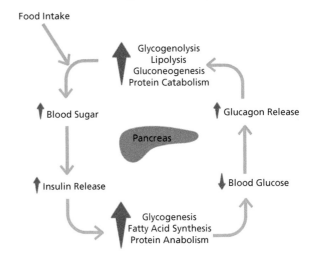

Insulin Glucagon Feedback Loop

Figure 2.31

Insulin	Secreted in response to high blood glucose by β islet cells
	↑ Glycogenesis
	↑ Fatty acid synthesis
	↓ Gluconeogenesis
	↑ Protein anabolism
Glucagon	Secreted in response to low blood glucose by α islet cells
	↑ Glycogenolysis
	↑ Lipolysis
	↑ Gluconeogenesis
	↑ Protein catabolism
	↓ Glycogenesis
Somatostatin	Secreted in response to food ingestion by δ islet cells
	↓ Glucagon
	↓ Insulin
	↓ Growth hormone
	↓ TSH
	↓ Many GI hormones and secretions covered in Table 2.1
Digestive enzymes	Table 2.2

2.17 Thyroid

Anatomy

- Two lobes connected by an isthmus
- Lingual thyroid most common site for ectopic thyroid
- Microscopic (Figure 2.32)
- Follicle
  - Functional unit of the thyroid
  - Composed of follicular cells and colloid
  - Follicular cells
    - Produce thyroid hormone (T_3/T_4)
  - Colloid
    - Stores T_3/T_4
- Parafollicular cells

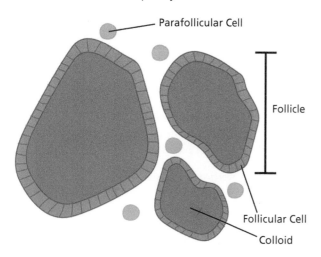

Microscopic Thyroid

Parafollicular Cell

Follicle

Follicular Cell

Colloid

Figure 2.32

Function

- Regulates metabolism
- Regulates Ca^{2+} levels

Blood Supply

- Superior thyroid artery
- Inferior thyroid artery

Innervation

- Parasympathetic
  - CN X
- Sympathetic
  - ~C_5–C_6

Endocrine/Exocrine

Thyroid hormone	*Production and secretion controlled by thyroid-stimulating hormone (TSH) from the anterior pituitary gland*
	↑ Metabolism
	↑ Beta adrenergic receptors
	Stimulates respiratory center
	↑ Bone and muscle growth
Calcitonin	*Secreted by parafollicular cells*
	↓ Serum Ca^{2+} by inhibiting osteoclasts

2.18　Parathyroid

Anatomy

- Four glands on the posterior thyroid
- Microscopic
  - Chief cells

Function

- Regulates serum calcium

Blood Supply

- Superior thyroid artery
- Inferior thyroid artery

Innervation

- Same as thyroid
- Parasympathetic
  - CN X
- Sympathetic
  - C_5–C_6

Endocrine/Exocrine (Figure 2.33)

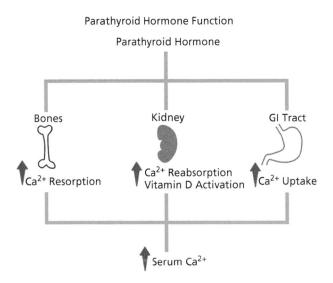

Figure 2.33

2.19   Adrenal Gland

Anatomy

- Superior pole of each kidney
- Cortex
- Medulla
- Microscopic (Figure 2.34)
  - Cortex
    - o Zona glomerulosa
    - o Zona fasciculata
    - o Zona reticularis
  - Medulla
    - o Chromaffin cells

Function

- Steroid secretion
- Catecholamine secretion

Blood Supply

- Adrenal arteries
- Adrenal veins

Innervation

- Parasympathetic
  - N/A

- Sympathetic
  - Celiac ganglion
  - Greater splanchnic nerve

Endocrine/Exocrine

Aldosterone	*Mineralocorticoid which is secreted by the zona glomerulosa* ↑ *Intravascular volume* ↑ *Renal Na$^+$ and H$_2$O absorption* ↑ *Renal K$^+$ excretion*
Cortisol	*Glucocorticoids which are secreted by the zona fasciculata* ↓ *Inflammation* *Immune system suppression* ↑ *Blood glucose* ↑ *Gluconeogenesis* ↓ *Peripheral glucose utilization* ↑ *Lipolysis* ↑ *Amino acid catabolism*
DHEA	*Androgen precursors for testosterone and estrogen, which is secreted by the zona reticularis*
Epinephrine norepinephrine	*Secreted by the adrenal medulla*

Adrenal Gland

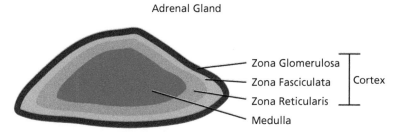

Figure 2.34

2.20   Vascular

Anatomy (Figure 2.35)

- Arteries
- Arterioles
- Venules
- Veins
- Microscopic
  - Capillaries
  - Endothelial cells
  - Smooth muscle

Function

- Blood reservoir
- Regulates blood pressure
- Transports nutrients and waste

Innervation

- Parasympathetic
  - N/A
- Sympathetic
  - α_1 and α_2
    - Smooth muscle walls of peripheral blood vessels
  - β_2
    - Predominantly in smooth muscle of blood vessels in skeletal muscle

Blood Supply

- N/A

Endocrine/Exocrine

- N/A

Blood Pressure Regulation

↑ Intravascular volume	Vasopressin
	Aldosterone
↓ Intravascular volume	Prostaglandins
	Atrial natriuretic peptide
Blood vessel contraction	Calcium
	Catecholamines
	Angiotensin II
	Vasopressin
Blood vessel dilation	Local factors
	K^+
	Acidosis[a]
	CO_2[a]
	Lactate
	Nitric oxide

[a] Vasoconstricts pulmonary vasculature.

Vascular Anatomy

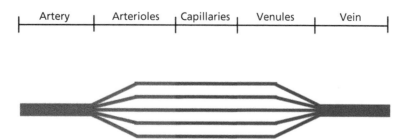

Figure 2.35

2.21 Hematology

Anatomy (Figure 2.36)

- Bone Marrow
  - Produces the below cell types and their precursors
- Microscopic
  - Hematopoietic stem cells
    - ○ Precursor to red blood cells, white blood cells, and platelets
    - ○ Erythrocytes
    - ○ Leukocytes
    - ○ Neutrophils
    - ○ Lymphocytes
    - ○ Eosinophils
    - ○ Monocytes
    - ○ Basophils
    - ○ Thrombocytes (Platelets)
  - Clotting factors (Formed in liver)
  - Coagulation factors (Formed in liver)

Blood Composition

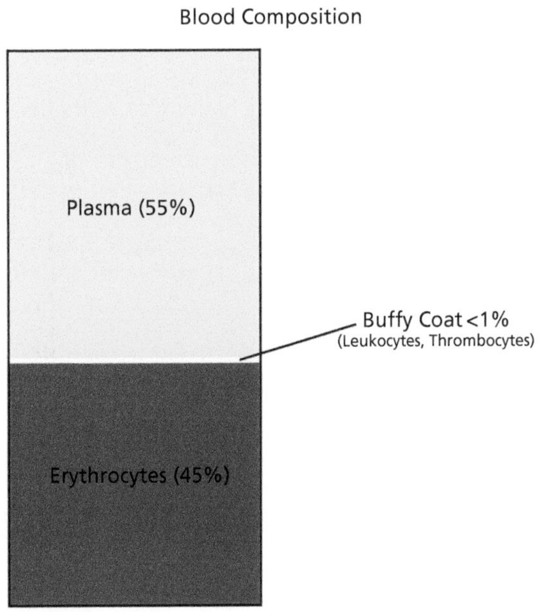

Figure 2.36

Function

- Immune system
- Oxygen and nutrient delivery
- Clotting and coagulation
- Acid–base balance
- Temperature regulation

Blood Supply

- N/A

Innervation

- N/A

Endocrine/Exocrine

- N/A

Platelet Plug and Coagulation Cascade

- Platelet Plug (Primary Hemostasis) (Figure 2.37)
  - Damaged epithelium exposes collagen
  - Von Willebrand factor facilitates collagen and glycoprotein-1 on the platelet to bind
  - Glycoprotein IIa/IIIb on the platelet further promotes platelet–platelet aggregation with fibrinogen
  - Temporary platelet plug forms and the coagulation cascade begins
- Coagulation Cascade (Secondary Hemostasis) (Figure 2.38)
  - Longer hemostasis by forming a fibrous clot

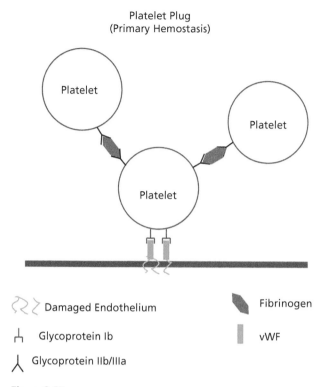

Platelet Plug
(Primary Hemostasis)

Damaged Endothelium

Glycoprotein Ib

Glycoprotein IIb/IIIa

Fibrinogen

vWF

Figure 2.37

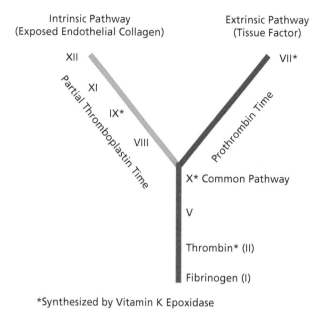

Coagulation Cascade
(Secondary Hemostasis)

Intrinsic Pathway
(Exposed Endothelial Collagen)

Extrinsic Pathway
(Tissue Factor)

XII

XI

IX*

VIII

Partial Thromboplastin Time

VII*

Prothrombin Time

X* Common Pathway

V

Thrombin* (II)

Fibrinogen (I)

*Synthesized by Vitamin K Epoxidase

Figure 2.38

Endogenous Anticoagulants

- *Oral anticoagulants covered on pages 90–91*

Protein S and C	*Degrade factors V and VIII*
Antithrombin	*Degrades thrombin*
Plasmin	*Activated by tissue plasminogen activator Cleaves fibrin*

References

1 Levac, B., Parlow, J.L., van Vlymen, J. et al. (2010). Ringer's lactate is compatible with saline-adenine-glucose-mannitol preserved packed red blood cells for rapid transfusion. *Can. J. Anaesth.* 57 (12): 1071–1077. https://doi.org/10.1007/s12630-010-9396-z.

2 Rodden, A.M., Spicer, L., Diaz, V.A., and Steyer, T.E. (2007). Does fingernail polish affect pulse oximeter readings? *Intensive Crit. Care Nurs.* 23 (1): 51–55. https://doi.org/10.1016/j.iccn.2006.08.006.

3 Hakverdioğlu Yönt, G., Akin Korhan, E., and Dizer, B. (2014). The effect of nail polish on pulse oximetry readings. *Intensive Crit. Care Nurs.* 30 (2): 111–115. https://doi.org/10.1016/j.iccn.2013.08.003.

4 Aravindhan, N. and Chisholm, D.G. (2000). Sulfhemoglobinemia presenting as pulse oximetry desaturation. *Anesthesiology* 93 (3): 883–884. https://doi.org/10.1097/00000542-200009000-00040.

5 London, M.J., Hollenberg, M., Wong, M.G. et al. (1988). Intraoperative myocardial ischemia: localization by continuous 12-lead electrocardiography. *Anesthesiology* 69 (2): 232–241.

6 Sessler, D.I. (2021). Perioperative temperature monitoring. *Anesthesiology* 134 (1): 111–118. https://doi.org/10.1097/ALN.0000000000003481.

Section 3
Preoperative Assessment

3.1 Psychology

Dental Fear and Anxiety

- Dental Anxiety
  - One of the most common phobias in society
  - Varying degrees of apprehension in anticipation of dental treatment
- Dental Fear
  - Relates to a specific threatening experience with physiological, behavioral, and emotional responses
- Dental Phobia
  - Extreme, irrational anxiety or fear of dental treatment that can hinder necessary care
- Risk Factors
  - Younger age [1]
  - Previous negative dental experience [2]

Nonpharmacologic Behavior Management [3]

- Tell-show-do
- Voice control
- Positive reinforcement
- Distraction
- Desensitization
- Morning appointment
- Calming background
- Animal-assisted therapy
- Protective stabilization

Anesthesia for Dental and Oral Maxillofacial Surgery, First Edition. Spencer D. Wade, Caroline M. Sawicki, Megann K. Smiley, Michael A. Cuddy, Steven Vukas, and Paul J. Schwartz.
© 2024 John Wiley & Sons, Inc. Published 2024 by John Wiley & Sons, Inc.

3.2 Sedation Levels

Minimal Sedation

- Normal response to verbal stimulation
- Airway reflexes unaffected
- Spontaneous ventilation unaffected
- Cardiovascular function unaffected

Moderate Sedation

- Purposeful response to verbal or tactile stimulation
  - Reflex withdrawal to painful stimulus is NOT purposeful movement
- Spontaneous ventilation is adequate
- Airway intervention is not required
- Cardiovascular function is maintained

Deep Sedation

- Purposeful response to repeated or painful stimulation
  - Reflex withdrawal to painful stimulus is NOT purposeful movement
- Spontaneous ventilation may be inadequate
- Airway intervention may be required
- Cardiovascular function is usually maintained

General Anesthesia

- Unable to arouse even with painful stimulation
- Spontaneous ventilation is frequently inadequate
- Airway intervention is often required
- Cardiovascular function may be impaired

3.3 ASA Physical Status Classification

- The American Society of Anesthesiologists (ASA) assigns a numerical score to help assess and communicate the overall health status and perioperative risk
- Examples from the ASA are listed below

ASA I

- Healthy individual
- No medical problems
- Normal BMI

ASA III

- Moderate-to-severe systemic disease
- Autism with severe limitations
- Substantive functional limitations
- Poorly controlled asthma
- COPD
- Poorly controlled hypertension
- Poorly controlled diabetes mellitus
- Insulin dependent diabetes mellitus (IDDM)
- Active hepatitis/alcohol dependence
- Morbid obesity (BMI ≥ 40)
- Previous myocardial infarction with or without CAD/stents (>3 months)
- Previous stroke/TIA (>3 months)
- Controlled CHF
- Implanted pacemaker
- ESRD undergoing regular dialysis
- Difficult airway
- Severe OSA

ASA V

- A moribund patient who is not expected to survive without the operation
- Trauma
- Ruptured TAAA
- Multiple organ system dysfunction

ASA II

- Mild systemic disease
- No substantive functional limitations
- Autism with mild limitations
- Current smoker
- Controlled asthma
- Controlled hypertension
- Controlled hypothyroidism
- Controlled diabetes
- Controlled hepatitis
- Controlled autoimmune disease
- Obesity (BMI 30–39)
- Mild/moderate obstructive sleep apnea (OSA)

ASA IV

- Severe systemic disease that is a constant threat to life
- Recent myocardial infarction with or without CAD/stents (<3 months)
- Recent stroke/TIA (<3 months)
- Myocardial infarction or stroke (<3 months)
- Significant cardiac dysfunction
- Significant pulmonary dysfunction
- ESRD not undergoing regular dialysis
- End-stage liver disease

ASA VI

- Organ donor

NPO

- Nil Per Os (NPO)
- Latin for "Nothing by mouth"
- These are only guidelines for NPO status. The anesthesia provider must also take into account medical history to determine the risk of aspiration
  - *Aspiration management covered on page 263*

NPO Guidelines [4]

2 h	Any liquid without particulates
	"Clears"
	Pedialyte
	Water
	Apple juice
	Soft drinks
	Medications
	Coffee without milk/nondairy creamer
4 h	Human breast milk
6 h	Light meal
	Nonhuman milk
	Infant formula
	Toast
	Crackers
	Tube feeds
	Orange juice with pulp
8 h	Fatty/protein rich meals

- Alcohol
  - Considered by some to be a clear liquid, but should be avoided preoperatively due to:
    - ↑ Risk of dehydration
    - Synergetic effects with anesthetic agents
    - ↑ Risk of electrolyte imbalances
    - Difficulty in obtaining informed consent
    - ↑ Gastric emptying time [5, 6]
  - Many practices discourage alcohol consumption the evening prior to procedure

Aspiration

- *Aspiration management covered on page 263*
- Gastric contents or foreign bodies enter the respiratory system
- Can be asymptomatic to life-threatening depending on volume, pH, and contents of aspirate
- Predisposing Factors
  - Violated NPO
    - Emergency
    - Trauma
    - Developmental delay
    - Children
  - ↑ Abdominal pressure
    - Pregnancy
    - Obesity
    - Ascites
  - Gastrointestinal pathology
    - GERD
    - Small bowel obstruction
    - Chronic aspiration
  - Previous gastrointestinal surgery
    - Bariatric surgery
    - Partial or total gastrectomy
    - Whipple
  - ↓ Gastric emptying
    - Diabetes mellitus
    - Vagus nerve dysfunction
    - Anxiety
    - Pain
    - Trauma

3.4 Preoperative Cardiac Testing

- The following chapter is a summation of the American College of Cardiologists and American Heart Association (ACC/AHA) guidelines (Figures 3.1–3.7)
- ACC/AHA guidelines, while thorough, do not address venue of surgery/general anesthesia, the level of anesthetic, and/or the capability of that venue to manage perioperative complications
- The individual anesthesia provider must determine if additional testing is prudent based on location of anesthesia and availability of resources
- Cardiac testing prior to noncardiac surgery is still a highly debated topic
- Decision-making for further needed cardiac testing is primarily dependent on
  - The procedure being performed
  - The metabolic equivalent of tasks (METs) completed without symptoms, such as chest pain, shortness of breath, and lightheadedness,

Procedure

- Dental/intraoral surgery is considered low-risk surgery
- Major maxillofacial, head and neck oncology, or reconstructive procedures are considered moderate risk surgery

Metabolic Equivalent of Tasks (METs)

- Estimates the cardiovascular capacity
- 1 MET is the physiologic consumption of $3.5\,\text{mlO}_2/\text{kg/min}$
- METs can be evaluated by Duke Activity Status Index (DASI) (Figure 3.8) [8]
- A DASI score of below than 34 correlates increased risk for a major adverse cardiac event (MACE), moderate-to-severe complications, and new disability [8]

Duke Activity Status Index

Take Care of Self	No: +0 Yes: +2.75	Do Heavy Work Around the House	No: +0 Yes: +8
Walk Indoors	No: +0 Yes: +1.75	Do Yardwork	No: +0 Yes: +4.5
Walk 1–2 Blocks	No: +0 Yes: +2.75	Have Sexual Relations	No: +0 Yes: +5.25
Climb a Flight of Stairs	No: +0 Yes: +5.5	Participate in Recreational Activities (Golf, Bowling, Dancing Doubles Tennis, Baseball, or Football)	No: +0 Yes: +6
Run a Short Distance	No: +0 Yes: +8		
Do Light Work Around the House	No: +0 Yes: +2.7	Participate in Strenuous Sports (Swimming, Singles Tennis Football, Basketball, Skiing)	No: +0 Yes: +7.5
Do Moderate Work Around the House	No: +0 Yes: +3.5		

Add up all the responses to get your DASI score

Figure 3.1 Adapted from Fleisher et al. [7]

Low Risk of MACE

"If the patient has a low risk of MACE (<1%), then no further testing is needed, and the patient may proceed to surgery."

Figure 3.2 Adapted from Fleisher et al. [7]

Elevated Risk of MACE, but Good Functional Capacity

"If the patient is at elevated risk of MACE, then determine functional capacity with an objective measure or scale such as the DASI. If the patient has moderate, good, or excellent functional capacity (≥4 METs), then proceed to surgery without further evaluation."

Figure 3.3 Adapted from Fleisher et al. [7]

The 12-Lead Electrocardiogram

"Preoperative resting 12-lead electrocardiogram (ECG) is reasonable for patients with known coronary heart disease, significant arrhythmia, peripheral arterial disease, cerebrovascular disease, or other significant structural heart disease, except for those undergoing low-risk surgery."

"Preoperative resting 12-lead ECG may be considered for asymptomatic patients without known coronary heart disease, except for those undergoing low-risk surgery."

"Routine preoperative resting 12-lead ECG is not useful for asymptomatic patients undergoing low-risk surgical procedures."

Figure 3.4 Adapted from Fleisher et al. [7]

Assessment of Left Ventricular Function

"It is reasonable for patients with dyspnea of unknown origin to undergo preoperative evaluation of left ventricular (LV) function."

It is reasonable for patients with heart failure (HF) with worsening dyspnea or other change in clinical status to undergo preoperative evaluation of LV function."

"Reassessment of LV function in clinically stable patients with previously documented LV dysfunction may be considered if there has been no assessment within a year."

"Routine preoperative evaluation of LV function is not recommended."

Figure 3.5 Adapted from Fleisher et al. [7]

Exercise Testing

"For patients with elevated risk and excellent functional capacity, it is reasonable to forgo further exercise testing with cardiac imaging and proceed to surgery."

"For patients with elevated risk and [poor or] unknown functional capacity, it may be reasonable to perform exercise testing to assess for functional capacity if it will change management."

"For patients with elevated risk and moderate to good functional capacity, it may be reasonable to forgo further exercise testing with cardiac imaging and proceed to surgery."

"Routine screening with noninvasive stress testing is not useful for patients at low risk for noncardiac surgery."

Figure 3.6 Adapted from Fleisher et al. [7]

Coronary Revascularization Before Noncardiac Surgery

"Coronary revascularization is not recommended before noncardiac surgery exclusively to reduce perioperative cardiac events."

"Revascularization before noncardiac surgery is recommended when indicated by existing practice guidelines."

Figure 3.7 Adapted from Fleisher et al. [7]

Timing of Elective Noncardiac Surgery in Patients
With Previous Percutaneous Coronary Intervention (PCI)

Many of the below recommendations discuss noncardiac surgery, but there is insufficient evidence on dental surgery. It would be prudent to continue antiplatelet and anticoagulants as necessary if the procedure allows. Insufficient evidence to dictate delay for mild elective oral surgical procedures (extraction(s), implant(s), biopsy(ies)).

"Elective noncardiac surgery should be delayed 14 days after balloon angioplasty and 30 days after bare metal stent (BMS) implantation."

"Elective noncardiac surgery should optimally be delayed 365 days after drug-eluting stent (DES) implantation."

"Elective noncardiac surgery after DES implantation may be considered after 180 days if the risk of further delay is greater than the expected risks of ischemia and stent thrombosis."

"Elective noncardiac surgery should not be performed within 30 days after BMS implantation or within 12 months after DES implantation in patients in whom dual antiplatelet therapy will need to be discontinued perioperatively."

"Elective noncardiac surgery should not be performed within 14 days of balloon angioplasty in patients in whom aspirin will need to be discontinued perioperatively."

Figure 3.8

3.5 Preoperative Pulmonary Testing

- Pulmonary preoperative testing is rarely indicated and is becoming increasingly less utilized for non-cardiothoracic procedures [9]
- Little to no guidelines on the following tests and their usefulness preoperatively prior to noncardiac surgery

Chest Radiography

- Function
  - Images the heart, lungs, airways, major vasculature, diaphragm, and pleural space of the chest
- Clinical Indications
  - Consider new preoperative chest radiograph if symptoms are significantly worsening or if they are diagnosed with poorly controlled
    o COPD
    o CHF

- Preoperative chest radiograph, if not available in clinically relevant timeframe, recommended
  o Radiation to chest
  o Chemotherapy with toxic pulmonary agents
  o Previous significant pulmonary infection
    - Tuberculosis
    - Histoplasmosis
    - Respiratory infection requiring ICU admission

Pulmonary Function Testing

- Function
  - Records volume, flow rates, and function of the lungs (Figure 3.9)
- Clinical Indications
  - Preoperative spirometry and chest radiography should not be used routinely for predicting postoperative pulmonary complications [10]

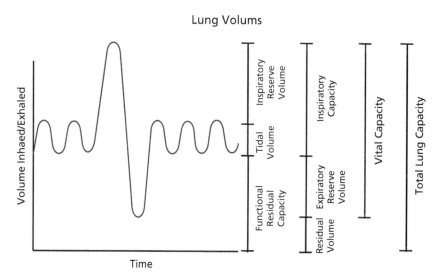

Figure 3.9

Tidal volume	*The volume inspired and expired during quiet breathing* *Normal ~6–8 ml/kg*
Inspiratory reserve volume	*The volume that can be inhaled after inspiring a normal tidal volume*
Inspiratory capacity	*Tidal volume + inspiratory reserve volume*
Expiratory reserve volume	*The volume that can be exhaled after an expiring a normal tidal volume*
Residual volume	*The volume remaining after complete forced exhalation*
Functional residual capacity	*The total volume remaining after passive exhalation of normal tidal volume* *Residual volume + expiratory reserve volume*
Vital capacity	*The total volume expired after maximal inhalation* *Inspiratory reserve volume + expiratory reserve volume + tidal volume*
Total lung capacity	*The volume at maximal inflation* *Vital capacity + residual volume*
Forced vital capacity	*The total volume forcefully exhaled*
Forced expiratory volume 1	*The volume forcefully exhaled in one second*
FEV$_1$/FVC	*The ratio of forceful exhalation in one second to the forced vital capacity* *Normal ~0.7–0.8*
Forced expiratory force	*The maximum flow rate achieved during forced exhalation capacity*

Flow-Volume Loops (Figure 3.10)

- Useful in detecting degree of obstruction or restriction

Diffusing Lung Capacity

- Function
  - Evaluates the diffusion efficiency of oxygen from the alveoli to capillaries
  - Utilizes carbon monoxide
  - Does not detect obstructive or restrictive disease

- Clinical Indications
  - Chronic inhalant exposure
  - Dyspnea of unknown origin
  - Low SpO$_2$
  - Interstitial lung disease

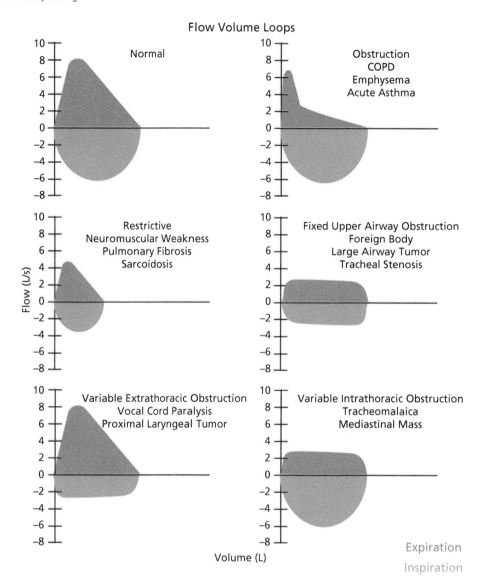

Figure 3.10

3.6 Preoperative Labs

- Preoperative testing is overused for those undergoing low-risk, ambulatory surgery [11]
- The below lab value ranges for "normal" can vary between institution and "ideal" lab values are patient and scenario specific

Blood Glucose

- Normal blood glucose (70–140 mg/dl)
- Depends on current fasting state and age
- Children, both with and without diabetes, will have higher blood glucose levels

Hypoglycemia	Prolonged fasting
	Malnourishment
	Insulinoma
	Exogenous insulin
	Oral hypoglycemics
Hyperglycemia	Diabetic/Prediabetic
	Morbid obesity
	Stress
	Surgery
	Illness
	Withholding hypoglycemic agents
	Glucocorticoids

Hemoglobin A1c (HbA1c)

- The percent of glucose bound (glycosylated) to hemoglobin
  - Results valid for ~3–4 months as that is the lifespan of the RBC
  - Recent blood transfusion can distort results
- Adults
  - Normal: <5.7%
  - Prediabetes: 5.7–6.4%
  - Diabetic: >6.5%

- Pediatrics
  - Normal: <5.7%
  - Target for NIIDM: <7%
  - Target for IDDM: <7.5%

HbA1c (%)	Average blood glucose (mg/dl)	Average blood glucose (mmol/l)
7	154	8.6
8	183	10.1
9	212	11.8
10	240	13.4

Basic Metabolic Panel (BMP) (Figure 3.11)

Sodium	Chloride	BUN	Glucose
135–145 mEq/L	98–108 mEq/L	7–24 mg/dL	70–140 mg/dL
Potassium	Carbon dioxide	Creatinine	
3.5–5 mEq/L	22–30 mEq/L	0.7–1.5 mg/dL	

Figure 3.11

Hypernatremia	Hypovolemia
	Diabetes insipidus
Hyponatremia	Hypovolemia
	Malnourishment
	Alcoholism
	Diuretics
	CHF
	CKD
	ESRD
Hyperkalemia	ESRD
	Addison's Disease
	Rhabdomyolysis
	Digoxin
	ACEi
	ARBs

Hypokalemia	*Sweating*
	Hypomagnesemia
	Emesis
	Diarrhea
	Antiretrovirals
	Loop diuretics
	Thiazide diuretics
	Insulin
	β₂ agonists
Hypercalcemia	*Hyperparathyroidism*
	Osteoblastic lesions
	Thiazide diuretics
	Immobility
Hypocalcemia	*CKD*
	Vitamin D deficiency
	Loop diuretics
↑ *Creatinine*	*Trauma*
	Dehydration
	CKD
	Renal obstructions
↓ *Creatinine*	*Malnourished*
	Female
	Low muscle mass
	Extremes of age
	Immobile

Arterial Blood Gas

↓ *pH*	*Lactic acidosis*
	Critically ill
	Hypercarbia
	CKD
	Diarrhea
	Ketoacidosis
	Laxatives
↑ *pH*	*Emesis*
	Dehydration
	Antacid consumption
	Hyperventilation

Complete Blood Count (Figure 3.12)

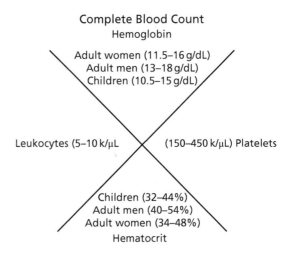

Figure 3.12

↑ *Hemoglobin/Hematocrit*	*Polycythemia vera*
	Smoking
	COPD
	High altitude exposure
	Exogenous EPO (Doping)
	Renal cancer
	Dehydration
↓ *Hemoglobin/Hematocrit*	↓ *Production*
	Iron deficiency anemia
	Porphyria
	CKD
	Aplastic anemia
	Leukemia
	Lymphoma
	B₁₂ deficiency
	Folate deficiency
	Medications
	↑ *Destruction*
	Thalassemia
	Sickle cell
	Splenomegaly
	Paroxysmal nocturnal hemoglobinuria
	G6PD deficiency
	Hereditary spherocytosis
	Blood loss
	Recent surgical procedure
	Trauma/bleeding
	Menstruation
	Hemodilution
↑ *Leukocytes*	*Certain cancers*
	Steroid use
	Infection

(Continued)

↓ Leukocytes	HIV
	AIDS
	Immunocompromised
	Radiation
	Chemotherapy
↑ Platelets	Asplenia
	Inflammatory states
	Recent surgery
	Cancer
↓ Platelets	↓ Production
	Aplastic anemia
	Chemotherapy
	↑ Breakdown/activation
	Thrombotic thrombocytopenic purpura
	Hemolytic uremic syndrome
	Idiopathic thrombocytopenic purpura
	Heparin induced thrombocytopenia
	Medications [12]
	Abciximab
	Procainamide
	Heparin
	Quinine
	Anticonvulsants

Coagulation Study (Figure 3.13)

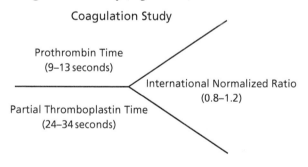

Coagulation Study

Prothrombin Time
(9–13 seconds)

Partial Thromboplastin Time
(24–34 seconds)

International Normalized Ratio
(0.8–1.2)

Figure 3.13

↑ Prothrombin time/INR	Warfarin
	Vitamin K deficiency
	Hepatic disease
↑ Partial thromboplastin time	Warfarin
	Vitamin K deficiency
	von Willebrand Disease [13]
	Hepatic disease
	Hemophilia

Liver Function Tests

↑ Liver enzymes	Hepatic disease
	Hepatitis
	Drug/alcohol abuse
	Malnourishment
	Obesity
	High acetaminophen usage
	Antiepileptics
	Antiretrovirals

Thyroid Testing

↑ TSH and ↑ T_3/T_4	Pituitary adenoma
↑ TSH and Normal T_3/T_4	Subclinical hypothyroidism
↑ TSH and ↓ T_3/T_4	Radiation to head and neck
	Hypothyroidism
	Surgical removal of thyroid
	Iodine deficiency
	Hashimoto's thyroiditis
↓ TSH and ↑ T_3/T_4	Hyperthyroidism
	Excessive exogenous levothyroxine
	Graves' disease
	Thyroid adenoma
↓ TSH and Normal T_3/T_4	Subclinical hyperthyroidism

Pregnancy Testing

- Clinical Indications
  - Menstruating female
  - Positive sex history
  - No common consensus on necessity or minimum age
  - It is very important to have a conversation about the risks that anesthesia could pose to a fetus if a pregnancy test is not warranted
  - For non-emancipated minors, they may have some privacy protection from their parents knowing in some states
  - Important to check with hospital and institutional guidelines

Type and Screen

- Function
  - ABO/Rh antigens on the RBCs

- Clinical Indications
  - Chance that a blood transfusion will be required
  - Blood may be returned to blood bank

Type and Cross

- Function
  - Crossmatches the patient's blood with a donor unit
  - ↓ Risk of an adverse transfusion reaction

- Clinical Indications
  - Higher risk procedure
  - Transfusion is likely/expected
  - Bleeding disorder
  - Blood loss suspected
  - Blood may not be returned to blood bank

3.7 Airway Evaluation

- There is not a single factor in airway assessment that can predict difficult airway
- *Anticipated difficult airway covered in section IX*
- *Difficult airway covered on page 258*

Previous Airway/Intubations History

- Airway type
- Attempts
- Blade size
- Laryngeal view classification (Figure 3.14)
- Final airway size

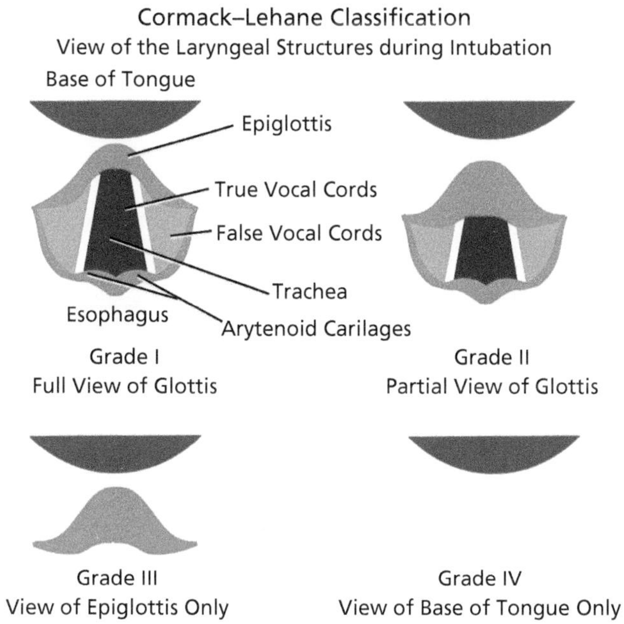
Cormack–Lehane Classification
View of the Laryngeal Structures during Intubation
Base of Tongue
Epiglottis
True Vocal Cords
False Vocal Cords
Trachea
Esophagus
Arytenoid Carilages
Grade I
Full View of Glottis
Grade II
Partial View of Glottis
Grade III
View of Epiglottis Only
Grade IV
View of Base of Tongue Only

Figure 3.14

Presence/Suspicion of Obstructive Sleep Apnea (OSA) (Figure 3.15)

- *OSA clinical management covered on pages 315–317*
- *Pediatric OSA covered on page 233*
- Apnea Hypopnea Index (AHI)
  - The AHI is the average number of apneic or hypopneic events lasting a minimum of 10 seconds per hour of sleep recorded during polysomnography
  - Severity of OSA is dependent on their AHI

Severity	Apnea hypopnea events (per hour)
Normal	*<5*
Mild OSA	*5–15*
Moderate OSA	*15–30*
Severe OSA	*>30*

STOPBANG Questionnaire
Screening Tool for OSA

S - Snoring	Snore Loud Enough to Hear through a Door?
T - Tiredness	Often Feel Tired throughout the Day?
O – Observed Apnea	Observed to Stop Breathing during Sleep?
P - Pressure	Presence of Hypertension?
B - BMI	> BMI 35?
A - Age	> Age 50
N – Neck Circumference	> 17 inches (Male); > 16 inches (Female)
G - Gender	Male

STOPBANG Score (1 Point for Each Yes)	Probability of Severe OSA (%)
3	25
4	35
5	45
6	55
7/8	75

Figure 3.15 Adapted from Nagappa et al. [14]

Clinical Airway Evaluation

- Radiographically
  - Performed only under specific indications
    - Major head and neck surgery
    - Airway compromise
    - Swelling
  - Lateral cephalogram
  - Head/neck CT
  - Head/neck MRI
- Extraoral
  - Significant facial deformity/asymmetry
  - Significant maxillary/mandibular discrepancy
    - Upper lip bite test
  - Previous head and neck radiation
  - Limited mouth opening
  - Facial burns
  - Infection/swelling
  - Obesity
  - Facial hair
  - Cervical considerations
    - Neck circumference
    - Short neck
    - Neck flexion/extension
    - Thyromental distance
- Intraoral
  - Loose/missing teeth
  - Infection/swelling
  - Central incisor prominence
  - Maximal interincisal distance on opening
  - Removable devices
  - Mallampati Score (Figure 3.16)
  - Brodsky Score (Figure 3.17)

Nasal Intubation Specifics

- Previous nasal intubation history/notes
- Previous nasal endoscopy
- Midface/nasal anatomy
  - Presence of mouth breathing
  - Deviated septum
  - Certain syndromes
  - Previous nasal/maxillary trauma
  - Previous nasal/pharyngeal surgeries
    - Cleft palate repair
    - Adenoidectomy
    - Rhinoplasty
- Presence/history of epistaxis
- Coagulopathy concerns

Mallampati Score

The Visibility of Soft Tissue Structures of the Pharynx

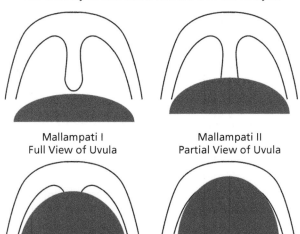

Mallampati I
Full View of Uvula

Mallampati II
Partial View of Uvula

Mallampati III
View of Soft Palate and Base
of Uvula

Mallampati IV
View of Hard Palate Only

Figure 3.16

Brodsky Score

The Proportion of Oropharyngeal Width
Occupied by the Tonsils

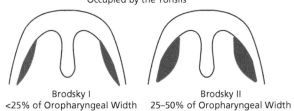

Brodsky I
<25% of Oropharyngeal Width

Brodsky II
25–50% of Oropharyngeal Width

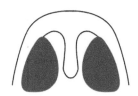
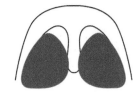

Brodsky III
50–75% of Oropharyngeal Width

Brodsky IV
>75% of Oropharyngeal Width

Figure 3.17

- Nostril patency
  - "Blow" test
  - Endoscope
  - MRI
  - CT [15]

Predictors of Difficult Airway

- Difficult Intubation
  - History of difficult intubation
  - Mallampati III/IV
  - Male
  - ↑ BMI
  - ↑ Neck circumference
  - ↓ Neck height
  - ↓ Thyromental distance
  - ↓ Maximal interincisal distance on opening
  - ↓ Upper lip bite test
  - ↓ Neck flexion/extension [16]
  - Obstructive sleep apnea
  - STOP-Bang score >3 [17]
- Difficult Mask Ventilation [18]
  - History of difficult intubation
  - Significant facial deformities/asymmetries
  - ↑ Age
  - ↑ BMI
  - ↑ Neck circumference
  - Facial hair
  - ↓ Neck height
  - Obstructive sleep apnea
  - Edentulous

References

1 Townsend, J.A. and Randall, C.L. (2021). Adolescent dental fear and anxiety: background, assessment, and nonpharmacologic behavior guidance. *Dent. Clin. North Am.* 65 (4): 731–751. https://doi.org/10.1016/j.cden.2021.07.002.

2 Appukuttan, D.P., Tadepalli, A., Cholan, P.K. et al. (2013). Prevalence of dental anxiety among patients attending a dental educational institution in Chennai, India—a questionnaire based study. *Oral Health Dent. Manag.* 12 (4): 289–294.

3 Clinical Affairs Committee-Behavior Management Subcommittee AAoPD (2015). Guideline on behavior guidance for the pediatric dental patient. *Pediatr. Dent.* 37 (5): 57–70.

4 Joshi, G.P., Abdelmalak, B.B., Weigel, W.A. et al. (2023). American Society of Anesthesiologists Practice Guidelines for preoperative fasting: carbohydrate-containing clear liquids with or without protein, chewing gum, and pediatric fasting duration-a modular update of the 2017 American Society of Anesthesiologists Practice Guidelines for preoperative fasting. *Anesthesiology* 138 (2): 132–151. https://doi.org/10.1097/ALN.0000000000004381.

5 Barboriak, J.J. and Meade, R.C. (1970). Effect of alcohol on gastric emptying in man. *Am. J. Clin. Nutr.* 23 (9): 1151–1153. https://doi.org/10.1093/ajcn/23.9.1151.

6 Mushambi, M.C., Bailey, S.M., Trotter, T.N. et al. (1993). Effect of alcohol on gastric emptying in volunteers. *Br. J. Anaesth.* 71 (5): 674–676. https://doi.org/10.1093/bja/71.5.674.

7 Fleisher, L.A., Fleischmann, K.E., Auerbach, A.D. et al. (2014). ACC/AHA guideline on perioperative cardiovascular evaluation and management of patients undergoing noncardiac surgery: executive summary: a report of the American College of Cardiology/American Heart Association Task Force on practice guidelines. Developed in collaboration with the American College of Surgeons, American Society of Anesthesiologists, American Society of Echocardiography, American Society of Nuclear Cardiology, Heart Rhythm Society, Society for Cardiovascular Angiography and Interventions, Society of Cardiovascular Anesthesiologists, and Society of Vascular Medicine Endorsed by the Society of Hospital Medicine. *J. Nucl. Cardiol.* 22 (1): 162–215. https://doi.org/10.1007/s12350-014-0025-z.

8 Hlatky, M.A., Boineau, R.E., Higginbotham, M.B. et al. (1989). A brief self-administered questionnaire to determine functional capacity (the Duke activity status index). *Am. J. Cardiol.* 64 (10): 651–654. https://doi.org/10.1016/0002-9149(89)90496-7.

9 Sun, L.Y., Gershon, A.S., Ko, D.T. et al. (2015). Trends in pulmonary function testing before noncardiothoracic surgery. *JAMA Intern. Med.* 175 (8): 1410–1412. https://doi.org/10.1001/jamainternmed.2015.2087.

10 Dankert, A., Neumann-Schirmbeck, B., Dohrmann, T. et al. (2022). Preoperative spirometry in patients with known or suspected chronic obstructive pulmonary disease undergoing major surgery: the prospective observational PREDICT study. *Anesth. Analg.* https://doi.org/10.1213/ANE.0000000000006235.

11 Benarroch-Gampel, J., Sheffield, K.M., Duncan, C.B. et al. (2012). Preoperative laboratory testing in patients undergoing elective, low-risk ambulatory surgery. *Ann. Surg.* 256 (3): 518–528. https://doi.org/10.1097/SLA.0b013e318265bcdb.

12 Danese, E., Montagnana, M., Favaloro, E.J., and Lippi, G. (2020). Drug-induced thrombocytopenia: mechanisms and laboratory diagnostics. *Semin. Thromb. Hemost.* 46 (3): 264–274. https://doi.org/10.1055/s-0039-1697930.

13 Totonchi, A., Eshraghi, Y., Beck, D. et al. (2008). Von Willebrand disease: screening, diagnosis, and management. *Aesthet. Surg. J.* 28 (2): 189–194. https://doi.org/10.1016/j.asj.2007.12.002.

14 Nagappa, M., Liao, P., Wong, J. et al. (2015). Validation of the STOP-bang questionnaire as a screening tool for obstructive sleep apnea among different populations: a systematic review and meta-analysis. *PLoS One* 10 (12): e0143697. https://doi.org/10.1371/journal.pone.0143697.

15 Grimes, D., MacLeod, I., Taylor, T. et al. (2016). Computed tomography as an aid to planning intubation in the difficult airway. *Br. J. Oral Maxillofac. Surg.* 54 (1): 80–82. https://doi.org/10.1016/j.bjoms.2015.09.034.

16 Shah, P.N. and Sundaram, V. (2012). Incidence and predictors of difficult mask ventilation and intubation. *J. Anaesthesiol. Clin. Pharmacol.* 28 (4): 451–455. https://doi.org/10.4103/0970-9185.101901.

17 Toshniwal, G., McKelvey, G.M., and Wang, H. (2014). STOP-bang and prediction of difficult airway in obese patients. *J. Clin. Anesth.* 26 (5): 360–367. https://doi.org/10.1016/j.jclinane.2014.01.010.

18 Cattano, D., Killoran, P.V., Cai, C. et al. (2014). Difficult mask ventilation in general surgical population: observation of risk factors and predictors. *F1000Res* 3: 204. https://doi.org/10.12688/f1000research.5131.1.

Section 4
Outpatient Medications

4.1 Antibiotic Prophylaxis (Figures 4.1–4.6)

Infective Endocarditis

- Endocardium colonized by microorganisms introduced via procedure, trauma, infection, etc.
- Infective agents [1]:
  - *Staphylococcus aureus* (Most common)
  - Streptococci (oral viridans group streptococci)
  - Coagulase-negative staphylococci
  - Enterococcus
  - *Streptococcus bovis*

Infective Endocarditis Risk Factors

"We continue to recommend viridans group streptococci infective endocarditis prophylaxis only for categories of patients at highest risk for adverse outcome while emphasizing the critical role of good oral health and regular access to dental care for all."

Figure 4.1 *Source:* Adapted from Wilson et al. [2].

Underlying Conditions for Which Antibiotic Prophylaxis Is Suggested

Previous, relapse, or recurrent IE
Prosthetic cardiac valve or material including transcatheter also including pulmonary artery valve or conduit placement such as Melody valve and Contegra conduit
Cardiac valve repair with devices, including annuloplasty, rings, or clips
Left ventricular assist devices
Implantable artificial heart
Unrepaired cyanotic CHD
Repaired congenital heart defect with prosthetic material or device during the first 6 months
Repaired CHD with residual defects
Cardiac transplant recipients who develop cardiac valvulopathy

Figure 4.2 *Source:* Adapted from Wilson et al. [2].

Anesthesia for Dental and Oral Maxillofacial Surgery, First Edition. Spencer D. Wade, Caroline M. Sawicki, Megann K. Smiley, Michael A. Cuddy, Steven Vukas, and Paul J. Schwartz.
© 2024 John Wiley & Sons, Inc. Published 2024 by John Wiley & Sons, Inc.

Dental Procedures and Antibiotic Prophylaxis

"All dental procedures that involve manipulation of gingival tissue or the periapical region of teeth or perforation of the oral mucosa."

Figure 4.3 *Source:* Adapted from Wilson et al. [2].

Antibiotic Prophylaxis Timing

"An antibiotic for prophylaxis should be administered in a single dose before the procedure. If the dosage of antibiotic is inadvertently not administered before the procedure, the dosage may be administered up to two hours after the procedure."

Figure 4.4 *Source:* Adapted from Wilson et al. [3].

Antibiotic Prophylaxis Dosing

Drug	Dose	Route
Amoxicillin	PO	50 mg/kg (Max 2000 mg)
Ampicillin	IM/IV	50 mg/kg (Max 2000 mg)
Cefazolin/Ceftriaxone	IM/IV	50 mg/kg (Max 1000 mg)
Azithromycin/Clarithromycin	PO	15 mg/kg (Max 500 mg)

Clindamycin is no longer recommended for antibiotic prophylaxis even in amoxicillin allergic patients.

Figure 4.5 *Source:* Adapted from Wilson et al. [2].

Prosthetic Joint Replacement and Antibiotic Prophylaxis

"Evidence fails to demonstrate an association between dental procedures and prosthetic joint infection or any effectiveness for antibiotic prophylaxis."

"For patients with serious health conditions, such as immunocompromising diseases, it may be appropriate for the orthopedic surgeon to recommend an antibiotic regimen."

A few orthopedic surgeons may demand that their patients receive antibiotic prophylaxis. The political challenge may make it difficult for the anesthesia provider to provide such prophylaxis placing the patient in the middle of the discussion.

Figure 4.6 *Source:* Adapted from Meyer [4]; Sollecito et al. [5].

4.2 Smoking

- Smoking is associated with an increased risk of perioperative complications [6]
- Should encourage smoking cessation as much and as early as possible prior to the procedure. Past clinical practice posed that short-term smoking cessation may increase perioperative cardiopulmonary complications, but this has been debunked [7, 8]

Effects of Smoking

- Mechanism of Action
  - Nicotine increases cholinergic and dopaminergic stimulation
- Clinical Implications
  - Induces P_{450}
  - ↑ Postoperative opioid requirement [9–11]
  - ↓ Wound healing
  - Neurologic
    o Stimulant
    o Anxiolytic
  - Cardiovascular
    o ↑ BP
    o ↑ HR
    o ↑ Risk of coronary artery disease
  - Pulmonary
    o ↑ Destruction of alveoli
    o ↑ Risk of COPD
    o ↑ Carboxyhemoglobin
    o ↓ Cilia function

Smoking Cessation [6]

30 min	↓ Sympathetic effects
4 h	↓ Carboxyhemoglobin
1 wk	Normalized secretions
>4 wk	Improved pulmonary outcomes

4.3   Substance Use Disorder Treatment

- Consider coordinating with the pain and/or rehabilitation doctor and surgeon to establish a plan regarding adjusting substance use disorder medications for an elective procedure, balancing the risk between relapse, perioperative complications, and/or pain control in the perioperative period
- Among medical specialties, anesthesiologists tend to have a higher rate of substance abuse likely related to a stressful environment and ease of diversion [12]

Varenicline

- Treatment for nicotine abuse
- Mechanism of Action
  - Partial nicotinic receptor agonist
- Clinical Implications
  - Continue drug perioperatively
  - Chronic exposure may lead to negative cardiovascular effects [13]

Acamprosate

- Treatment for alcohol abuse
- Mechanism of Action
  - Not well established
- Clinical Implications
  - Continue drug perioperatively

Disulfiram

- Treatment for alcohol abuse
- Mechanism of Action (Figure 4.7)

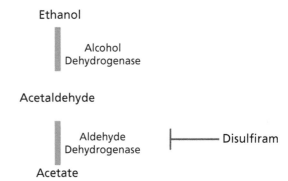

Figure 4.7

- Inhibits aldehyde dehydrogenase which causes an unpleasant reaction with concomitant use of alcohol
- Clinical Implications
  - Discontinue drug 10 days prior to procedure
  - If continued, increased risk of intraoperative hypotension [14]
  - Reduces clearance of warfarin
  - Important to encourage continued alcohol cessation while this medication is held

Naltrexone

- Treatment for alcohol and opioid abuse
- Mechanism of Action
  - Opioid receptor antagonist
- Clinical Implications
  - If continued
    - o Opioids may be less effective
    - o Use opioid sparing techniques
    - o Attempt to using local measures

- Moderate/high invasive procedures
  - Oral
    - Discontinue naltrexone for 72 hours prior to procedure [15]
  - Intramuscular
    - Discontinue naltrexone for 4 weeks prior to procedure [15, 16]

Methadone

- Treatment for opioid abuse and chronic pain
- Mechanism of Action
  - Opioid receptor agonist
- Clinical Implications
  - Continue drug perioperatively [15, 17]
  - May require increased opioids perioperatively
  - Use opioid sparing techniques
  - Methadone may have synergistic effects with anesthetic agents

Buprenorphine [18]

- Treatment for opioid abuse and chronic pain
- Practice Guidelines for the Administration of Buprenorphine for Treating Opioid Use Disorder. From Human Health Services. Effective: 28 April 2021.
  - The prescribing of buprenorphine is no longer restricted to substance abuse physicians only. Eligible individuals must also have a DEA license
  - Eligible Individuals
    - Primary care providers
    - Physicians
    - Physician assistants, nurse practitioners
    - Clinical nurse specialists
    - Certified registered nurse anesthetists
    - Certified nurse midwives
    - Dentists are not included
- Clinical Implications
  - Consider continuing drug perioperatively [15, 17]
  - Use opioid sparing techniques
  - May have increased opioid requirement postoperatively [19]

4.4 Antiplatelets

- Consider coordinating with physician and surgeon to establish a plan regarding adjusting antiplatelets for an elective procedure, balancing the risk between re-thrombosis and perioperative hemostasis
- If antiplatelets and/or anticoagulants are to be continued perioperatively, consider the following local hemostasis techniques:
  - Local anesthetics with vasoconstrictors
  - Hemostatic agents
    - o Topical thrombin
    - o Oxidized cellulose (Surgicel®)
    - o Absorbable gelatin (GelFoam®)
    - o Absorbable collagen (CollaTape®)
  - Primary closure
  - Cautery
  - Staging the procedure

Cyclooxygenase (COX) Inhibitors (NSAIDs)

- Mechanism of Action (Figure 4.8)

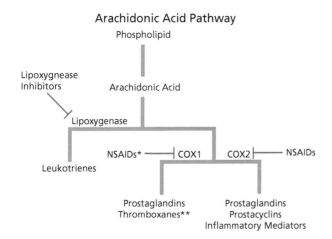

Arachidonic Acid Pathway

*Does not include celecoxib or other COX2 inhibitors
**Involved with platelet aggregation

Figure 4.8

Aspirin	*Irreversibly inhibits COX_1 and COX_2 for the platelet's lifespan (10 days)*
Ibuprofen Naproxen	*Reversibly inhibits COX_1 and COX_2*
Celecoxib	*Reversibly inhibits COX_2 Minimal platelet effects*

- Clinical Implications
  - Local hemostasis techniques
  - Minimally invasive procedure
    - o Continue drug perioperatively
  - Moderate/high bleeding expected
    - o Aspirin
      - Discuss with surgeon and physician
      - Can likely continue low-dose aspirin (75–100 mg) if for cardiovascular/DAPT benefit [20]
      - Discontinue high-dose aspirin for 10 days
    - o Ibuprofen
      - Discontinue 1 day
      - Half-life ~2 hours
    - o Naproxen
      - Discontinue 3–4 days
      - Half-life ~15 hours
    - o Celecoxib
      - Continue [21]
  - Reversal
    - o No specific reversal
    - o Platelet transfusion

Thienopyridines

- Clopidogrel
- Prasugrel
- Ticagrelor
- Commonly used in conjunction with aspirin for DAPT

- Mechanism of Action
  - P2Y12 receptor antagonist
- Clinical Implications
  - Local hemostasis techniques
  - Minimally invasive procedure
    o Continue single or dual antiplatelet therapy [22]
  - Moderate/high bleeding expected
    o Discuss with surgeon and physician if procedure necessary and if able to continue DAPT

o Consider delaying elective cases until patient no longer requires DAPT therapy
o Consider heparin bridge therapy for high-risk patients
  - Reversal
    o No specific reversal
    o Platelet transfusion

4.5 Anticoagulants (Figure 4.9)

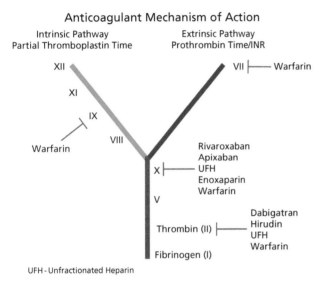

Anticoagulant Mechanism of Action

Intrinsic Pathway
Partial Thromboplastin Time

Extrinsic Pathway
Prothrombin Time/INR

XII   VII ├── Warfarin

XI

IX

VIII

Warfarin

X ├── Rivaroxaban
Apixaban
UFH
Enoxaparin
Warfarin

V

Thrombin (II) ├── Dabigatran
Hirudin
UFH
Warfarin

Fibrinogen (I)

UFH - Unfractionated Heparin

Figure 4.9

- Consider coordinating with physician and surgeon to establish a plan regarding adjusting anticoagulants for an elective procedure, balancing the risk between re-thrombosis and postoperative hemostasis

Direct Thrombin Inhibitors

- Dabigatran
- Hirudin
- Mechanism of Action
  - Directly binds and inhibits thrombin
- Clinical Implications
  - Local hemostasis techniques
  - Minimally invasive procedure
    - Continue drug perioperatively [23]
  - Moderate/high bleeding expected
    - Discuss with surgeon and physician
    - Consider delaying elective cases until patient no longer requires anticoagulant therapy

- Consider heparin bridge therapy for high-risk patients
- Discontinuation time depends on renal function [24]
- Reversal
  - Dabigatran
    - Idarucizumab
  - Hirudin
    - No specific reversal
    - Transfusion

Heparin

Unfractionated heparin	Indirectly inhibits factor Xa and thrombin
Enoxaparin	Indirectly inhibits factor Xa

- Clinical Implications
  - Local hemostasis techniques
  - Consider coagulation studies
  - Minimally invasive procedure
    - Continue drug perioperatively [25]
  - Moderate/high invasive bleeding expected
    - Discuss with surgeon and physician
    - Consider delaying elective cases until the patient no longer requires heparin
    - Unfractionated heparin
      - Consider discontinuing 6 hours before procedure with physician approval
      - Resume once hemostasis achieved
    - LMWH
      - Consider discontinuing 24 hours before procedure with physician approval
      - Resume once hemostasis achieved
- Reversal
  - Protamine sulfate

Warfarin

- Being phased out in lieu of direct factor Xa inhibitors which require less monitoring, more predictable pharmacokinetics, and minimal food interactions [26]

- Mechanism of Action
  - Vitamin K epoxidase antagonist
    - Decreases factors II, VII, IX, and X
- Clinical Implications
  - Local hemostasis techniques
  - Recent PT/INR within 24 hours of surgery to assess coagulation status
  - Minimally invasive procedure
    - Discuss with surgeon and physician for desired INR, but can likely continue drug perioperatively [27]
  - Moderate/high bleeding expected
    - Discuss with surgeon and physician regarding desired INR
    - Consider delaying elective cases until the patient no longer requires anticoagulation
    - Consider heparin bridge therapy for high-risk patients
  - Reversal
    - Vitamin K
    - Fresh frozen plasma
    - Plasma

Direct Factor Xa Inhibitors

- Rivaroxaban
- Apixaban
- Mechanism of Action
  - Inhibits coagulation factor Xa
- Clinical Implications
  - Local hemostasis techniques
  - Consider coagulation studies
  - Minimally invasive procedure
    - Continue drug perioperatively, but consider timing procedure right before next dose [28]
  - Moderate/high bleeding expected
    - Discuss with surgeon and physician
    - Consider delaying elective cases until the patient no longer requires anticoagulation
    - Consider heparin bridge therapy for high-risk patients
    - Discontinuation time depends on renal function
  - Reversal
    - Andexanet alfa
    - Prothrombin complex
    - Recombinant factor X

4.6 Antihypertensives

Angiotensin-Converting Enzyme Inhibitors

- Benazepril
- Enalapril
- Fosinopril
- Lisinopril
- Moexipril
- Perindopril
- Quinapril
- Trandolapril
- Other "-pril" drugs
- Mechanism of Action
  - Angiotensin converting enzyme inhibitor (Figure 4.10)
- Clinical Implications
  - Consider continuing for moderate and deep sedation based on patient and surgical risk factors
  - Discontinue day of surgery for general anesthesia
  - If continued, may have increased risk of intraoperative hypotension, but an increase in perioperative cardiac events or mortality has not been demonstrated [29]
    - If epinephrine is ineffective in managing hypotension, consider vasopressin
  - Consider electrolyte panel for patients in new/recently adjusted medication
    - Increased risk of hyperkalemia

Angiotensin Receptor Blockers

- Losartan
- Valsartan
- Other "-sartan" drugs
- Mechanism of Action
  - Angiotensin II receptor antagonist (Figure 4.10)
- Clinical Implications
  - Consider continuing for moderate and deep sedation based on patient and surgical risk factors
  - Discontinue day of surgery for general anesthesia
  - If continued, may have increased risk of intraoperative hypotension, but an increase in perioperative cardiac events or mortality has not been demonstrated [29]
  - Consider electrolyte panel for patients in new/recently adjusted medication
    - ↑ Risk of hyperkalemia

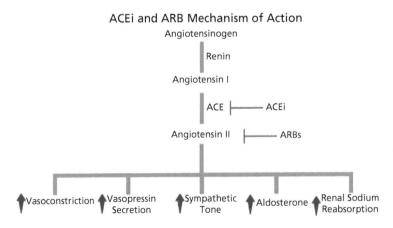

Figure 4.10

Calcium Channel Blockers (Dihydropyridines)

- *Non-dihydropyridines (verapamil and diltiazem) covered on page 96*
- Amlodipine
- Felodipine
- Isradipine
- Nicardipine
- Nifedipine
- Nisoldipine
- Other "-ipine" drugs
- Mechanism of Action
  - Dihydropyridine calcium channel antagonist on blood vessels

- Clinical Implications
  - Continue drug perioperatively [30, 31]

Nitrates

- Isosorbide dinitrate
- Isosorbide mononitrate
- Mechanism of Action
  - Converts to nitric oxide in vivo
- Clinical Implications
  - Continue drug perioperatively
  - ↑ Risk of methemoglobinemia
    - *Methemoglobinemia further covered on page 285*

4.7   Diuretics

- Consider discontinuing diuretics day of surgery to avoid volume depletion augmented by NPO and possible electrolyte derangement

Thiazides

- Chlorthalidone
- Hydrochlorothiazide
- Indapamide
- Metolazone
- Quinethazone
- Mechanism of Action
  - Inhibits Na^+–Cl^- cotransporter at the distal convoluted tubule (Figure 4.11)
- Clinical Implications
  - Consider continuing for moderate and deep sedation based on patient and surgical risk factors
  - Discontinue day of surgery for general anesthesia
  - If continued, there is an increased risk of intraoperative hypotension, but this can likely be conservatively managed
  - Consider electrolyte panel for patients in new/recently adjusted medication
    - o Increased risk of hypokalemia and hypercalcemia

Loop Diuretics

- Bumetanide
- Ethacrynic acid
- Furosemide
- Torsemide
- Mechanism of Action
  - Inhibits Na^+–K^+–Cl^- cotransporter at the ascending loop of Henle (Figure 4.11)
- Clinical Implications
  - Consider continuing for moderate and deep sedation based on patient and surgical risk factors
  - Discontinue day of surgery for general anesthesia
    - o If continued, there is an increased risk of intraoperative hypotension, but this can likely be conservatively managed
  - Consider electrolyte panel for patients in new/recently adjusted medication
    - o ↑ Risk of hypokalemia, hyponatremia, hypomagnesemia, and hypocalcemia

Potassium Sparing Diuretics

- Mechanism of Action (Figure 4.11)

Eplerenone Spironolactone	Aldosterone receptor antagonist at the collecting duct
Amiloride Triamterene	Inhibits Na^+ channels at the collecting duct

- Clinical Implications
  - Consider continuing for moderate and deep sedation based on patient and surgical risk factors
  - Discontinue day of surgery for general anesthesia
  - If continued, there is an increased risk of intraoperative hypotension, but this can likely be conservatively managed
  - Consider electrolyte panel for patients in new/recently adjusted medication
    - o ↑ Risk of hyperkalemia

Diuretic Mechanism of Action

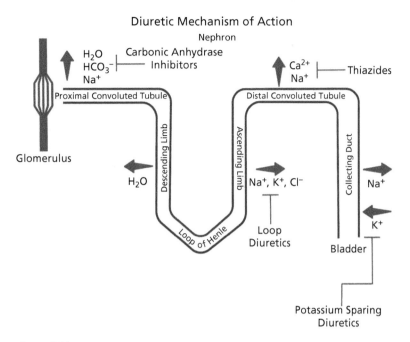

Figure 4.11

4.8 Antidysrhythmics

- Continue all antidysrhythmics the day of surgery

β-Blockers (Figures 4.12 & 4.13)

- Clinical Implications
  - Continue drug perioperatively
  - If discontinued, increased risk of rebound hypertension and tachycardia
    - Consider supplementing IV beta blocker for patients who did not take their β-Blockers prior to procedure
    - Metoprolol PO : IV conversion is 2.5:1; 5 mg q 5 minutes until desired effect/titration

Digoxin

- Being phased out by newer medications with fewer side effects
- Mechanism of Action
  - Inhibits Na^+/K^+ ATPase on the myocardium
- Clinical Implications
  - Continue drug perioperatively
  - Consider electrolyte panel
  - Consider digoxin level
    - Narrow therapeutic index
    - ↑ Risk of hyperkalemia
    - Digoxin effects exacerbated by hypokalemia
  - Avoid hyperventilation as it may lead to hypokalemia and exaggerated digoxin effects
  - Can have significant cardiac effects with local anesthetics [32]
  - Reversal
    - Digoxin-specific antibody

Calcium Channel Blockers (Non-dihydropyridines)

- Diltiazem
- Verapamil
- Mechanism of Action
  - Non-dihydropyridine calcium channel antagonist (Figure 4.12)
- Clinical Implications
  - Continue drug perioperatively

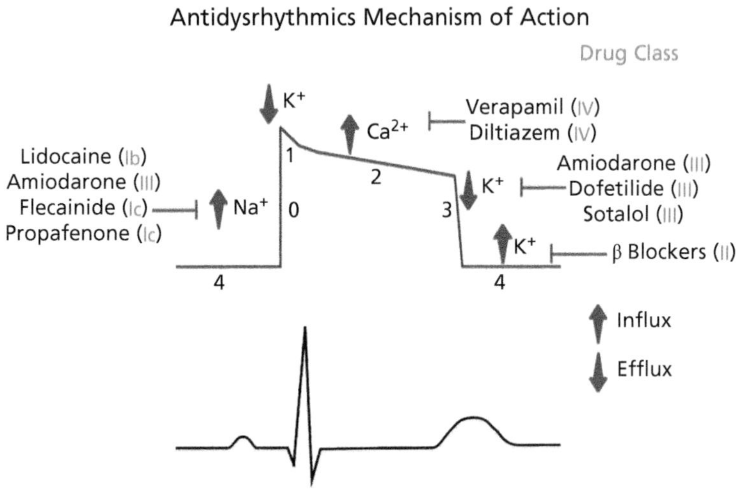

Figure 4.12

Carvedilol* Labetalol* Nadolol Propranolol Sotalol**	Nonselective β Adrenergic Receptor Antagonist
Atenolol Acebutolol Metoprolol Nebivolol	Selective β_1 Adrenergic Receptor Antagonist

*Also have α_1 adrenergic antagonistic properties
**Also has potassium channel blocking effects

Figure 4.13

4.9 Pulmonary

- Beneficial to continue all pulmonary medications on day of surgery except methylxanthines (rarely prescribed now)
- Inhaled medications offer a greater benefit over oral medications as they are delivered directly to the lungs, have less systemic side effects, and are quicker acting
- Mechanism of Action (Figure 4.14)

β₂ Receptor Agonists

Albuterol	*Short-acting β₂ agonists*
Levalbuterol	
Formoterol	*Long-acting β₂ agonists*
Salbutamol	
Salmeterol	

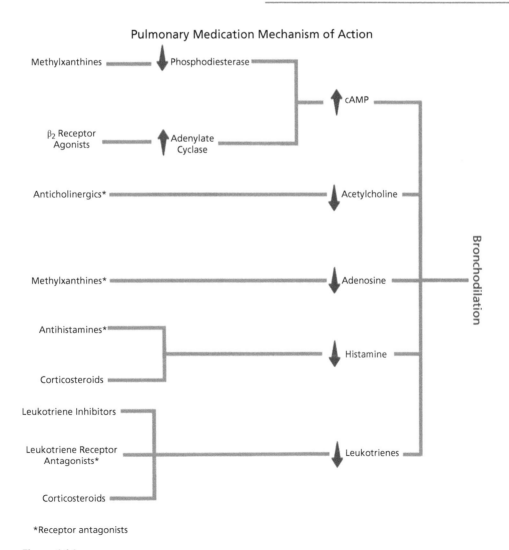

Figure 4.14

- Clinical Implications
  - Continue drug perioperatively
  - Mixed data if using β_2 agonist, specifically salbutamol, preoperatively decreases risk of adverse respiratory events whether patient is asymptomatic, has had recent URI, and/or a current diagnosis of reactive airway disease [33–35]
  - More frequent than usually use may contribute to hypokalemia and tachycardia, but stable therapy likely does not require metabolic panel

Corticosteroids

- Budesonide
- Fluticasone
- Triamcinolone
- Mechanism of Action
  - Anti-inflammatory, mast cell stabilizers (Figure 4.14)
- Clinical Implications
  - Continue drug perioperatively
  - If discontinued, consider supplementation or delaying elective procedure especially with more invasive procedures
  - Adrenal suppression is possible but more common with oral administration consider steroid supplementation
    - *Adrenal suppression covered on page 108*

Anticholinergics

- Ipratropium
- Tiotropium
- Other "-tropium" drugs
- Mechanism of Action
  - Muscarinic receptor antagonist (Figure 4.14)
- Clinical Implications
  - Continue drug perioperatively
  - If discontinued, consider supplementation or delaying elective procedure
  - Less tachycardia than β_2 agonists

Methylxanthines

- Theophylline
- Rarely used now due to unwanted side effects
- Mechanism of Action (Figure 4.14)

- Phosphodiesterase inhibitor
- Adenosine receptor antagonist
- Clinical Implications
  - Discontinue day of surgery [36]
  - Consider electrolyte panel
  - Consider theophylline levels
    - Narrow therapeutic index
  - ↑ Adenosine dosing required
  - ↑ Risk of hypokalemia [37]

Histamine-1 Receptor Antagonists

Diphenhydramine	*First generation*
Promethazine	
Cetirizine	*Second generation*
Loratadine	
Desloratadine	*Third generation*
Fexofenadine	

- Mechanism of Action
  - Histamine receptor antagonist (Figure 4.14)
- Clinical Implications
  - Continue drug perioperatively
  - First generation drugs may have synergistic sedative effects

Leukotriene Receptor Antagonists

- Montelukast
- Zafirlukast
- Other "-lukast" drugs
- Mechanism of Action
  - Leukotriene receptor antagonist (Figure 4.14)
- Clinical Implications
  - Continue drug perioperatively

5-Lipoxygenase Inhibitors

- Zileuton
- Other "-leuton" drugs
- Mechanism of Action
  - Inhibit 5-lipoxygenase (Figure 4.8)
- Clinical Implications
  - Continue drug perioperatively

4.10   Non-Insulin Hypoglycemics

- The anesthesia provider must balance the risk of hypoglycemia and hyperglycemia. Previous practice patterns involved discontinuing all non-insulin hypoglycemic agents day of surgery (and multiple doses of metformin), but this practice is evolving
- For medications held/discontinued, many can be restarted postoperatively once the patient is eating/drinking
- Strongly consider checking preoperative blood glucose
- Consider HbA1c
- *Perioperative management of Type II covered on pages 191–192*
- *Perioperative management of Type I covered on pages 231–232*
- *Insulin management covered on pages 101–102*

Biguanides

- Metformin
- Mechanism of Action (Figure 4.15)
  - ↓ Hepatic gluconeogenesis
  - ↑ Glucose utilization by skeletal muscles
- Clinical Implications
  - Continue drug perioperatively [38]
  - If discontinued, able to proceed without supplementation
  - Previous anesthetic concerns were that metformin and NPO coupled with decreased renal excretion could increase risk of lactic acidosis, but this is no longer as extensive as a threat as once thought [39]

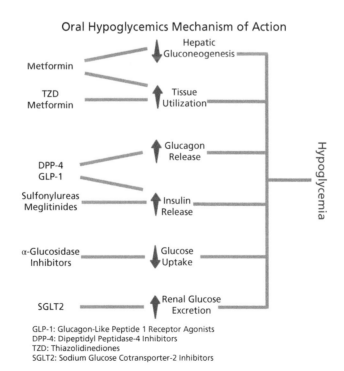

Figure 4.15

Sulfonylureas

- Glimepiride
- Glipizide
- Glyburide
- Mechanism of Action
  - ↑ Insulin secretion from β islet cells (Figure 4.15)
- Clinical Implications
  - Hold day of surgery
  - If continued, consider more frequent perioperative blood glucose monitoring due to increased risk of hypoglycemia [38]

Meglitinides

- Repaglinide
- Nateglinide
- Mechanism of Action
  - ↑ Insulin secretion from β islet cells (Figure 4.15)
- Clinical Implications
  - Hold day of surgery
  - If continued, consider more frequent perioperative blood glucose monitoring due to increased risk of hypoglycemia [40]

Thiazolidinediones (TZDs)

- Pioglitazone
- Rosiglitazone
- Other "-glitazone" drugs
- Mechanism of Action (Figure 4.15)
  - Peroxisome proliferator-activated receptor (PPAR) agonist
    - ↓ Insulin resistance of tissues
    - ↑ Tissue glucose utilization
- Clinical Implications
  - Continue drug perioperatively [41]
  - If discontinued, able to proceed without supplementation

Sodium Glucose Cotransporter-2 Inhibitors (SGLT2)

- Canagliflozin
- Dapagliflozin
- Empagliflozin
- Other "-gliflozin" drugs
- Mechanism of Action (Figure 4.15)
  - Inhibits Na^+/glucose cotransporter in the kidney
    - ↓ Renal glucose reabsorption
    - ↑ Glucose excretion
- Clinical Implications
  - Discontinue 24–72 hours prior to surgery
  - If continued, increased risk of euglycemic ketoacidosis [38]
  - ↑ Risk of UTI

α-Glucosidase Inhibitors

- Acarbose
- Miglitol
- Mechanism of Action (Figure 4.15)
  - Inhibits brush border enzymes of the small intestines
    - ↓ Glucose uptake
- Clinical Implications
  - Only continue DOS if patient eats in AM [41]

Dipeptidyl Peptidase-4 Inhibitors (DPP-4)

- Linagliptin
- Sitagliptin
- Saxagliptin
- Other "-gliptin" drugs
- Mechanism of Action (Figure 4.15)
  - Dipeptidyl peptidase-4 inhibitor
    - ↑ Insulin release
    - ↓ Glucagon release
- Clinical Implications
  - Continue or discontinue are both reasonable [38]

Glucagon-Like Peptide 1 Receptor Agonists (GLP-1)

- Dulaglutide
- Exenatide
- Liraglutide
- Semaglutide
- Mechanism of Action (Figure 4.15)
  - Glucagon-like peptide 1 receptor agonist
    - ↑ Insulin release
    - ↓ Glucagon release
- Clinical Implications
  - IM injection
  - Continue or discontinue are both reasonable [38]

4.11 Insulin

- A glucometer must be available when managing IDDM
- Consider coordinating with physician to establish a plan regarding discontinuing/adjusting insulin (especially for complicated diabetic patients) for an elective procedure, balancing the risk between hypoglycemia and hyperglycemia
  - *Perioperative management of Type II covered on pages 191–192*
  - *Perioperative management of Type I covered on pages 231–232*
- Clinical Implications of Insulin
  - Always check blood glucose pre, intra, and post-operatively
  - Consider HbA1c
  - Consider BMP for patients on new/recently adjusted insulin dose
    - ↑ Risk of hypokalemia
- While no specific literature states what an optimal intra-operative blood glucose level is, current consensus states an adequate target is <180 mg/dl [42]

Rapid-Acting Insulin

- Aspart
- Lispro
- Rapid-acting inhaled
- Duration of Action (Figure 4.16)
  - Onset 15 minutes
  - Peak 1 hour
  - Duration 2–4 hours
- Clinical Implications
  - Discontinue day of surgery, especially if patient is NPO
  - If required, useful for correcting perioperative hyperglycemia
  - Ask the patient for personal correction factor, i.e. how much does one unit of rapid-acting insulin lower their BG

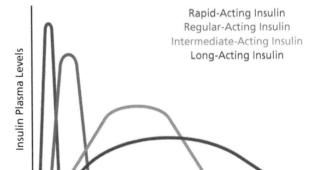

Insulin Duration of Action

Rapid-Acting Insulin
Regular-Acting Insulin
Intermediate-Acting Insulin
Long-Acting Insulin

Insulin Plasma Levels

Duration (Hours) 4 8 12 16 20

Figure 4.16

- If personal correction factor is not known, there are two "rule-of-thumb":
  - One unit of insulin will on average decrease BG by 30–40 mg/dl
  - "1800 Rule" – Dividing 1800 by the amount of daily fast-acting insulin use. The total will give you an approximation of expected decreased of BG per unit [42]

Regular-Acting Insulin

- Regular insulin
- Duration of Action (Figure 4.16)
  - Onset 30 minutes
  - Peak 2–3 hours
  - Duration 3–6 hours
- Clinical Implications
  - Discontinue day of surgery [43]

Intermediate-Acting Insulin

- Lente
- Neutral Protamine Hagedorn (NPH)
- Duration of Action (Figure 4.16)
  - Onset 2–4 hours
  - Peak 4–12 hours
  - Duration 12–18 hours
- Clinical Implications
  - Continue 50% of dose morning of surgery [44]

Long-Acting Insulin

- Detemir
- Glargine
- Duration of Action (Figure 4.16)
  - Onset 2 hours
  - No Peak
  - Duration up to 24 hours
- Clinical Implications
  - Once daily dosing
    - o Consider no reduction in evening dose if patient does not experience episodes of nighttime or morning hypoglycemia
  - AM and PM dosing
    - o Consider continuing 75–100% of dose day of surgery

Insulin Pumps

- Typically use rapid-acting insulin
- Consider sleep basal rates perioperatively
- In general, try not to alter the insulin pump due to postoperative challenges

4.12   Antidepressants

- All antidepressants should be continued day of surgery. The risk of the patient being discontinued, especially for prolonged periods, may contribute to symptoms of depression, delirium, and/or confusion [45]

Tricyclics (TCAs)

- Amitriptyline
- Desipramine
- Imipramine
- Nortriptyline
- Other "-triptyline" or "-ipramine" drugs
- Being phased out due to their many side effects and drug interactions
- Mechanism of Action
  - ↓ Reuptake of norepinephrine and serotonin in the synapse
- Clinical Implications
  - Continue drug perioperatively
  - If discontinued, have patient continue when surgery completed
  - Can have synergistic sedation effects
  - Drug interactions that can increase risk of tachycardia and hypertension [46, 47]
    - ○ Anticholinergics
    - ○ Ephedrine
    - ○ Epinephrine
    - ○ Meperidine
    - ○ Norepinephrine
    - ○ Phenylephrine
    - ○ Tramadol

Monoamine Oxidase Inhibitors (MAOIs)

- Isocarboxazid
- Phenelzine
- Selegiline
- Tranylcypromine
- Being phased out due to their many side effects and drug interactions
- Mechanism of Action
  - Inhibits monoamine oxidase
    - ○ ↑ Serotonin, dopamine, norepinephrine in the synapse
- Clinical Implications
  - Continue drug perioperatively
  - If discontinued, have patient continue when surgery completed
  - Pain may lead to exaggerated sympathetic response
  - Drug interactions that can increase risk of tachycardia and hypertension [48]
    - ○ Anticholinergics
    - ○ Ephedrine
    - ○ Meperidine
    - ○ Stimulants
    - ○ Tramadol
    - ○ Tyramine-rich foods

Atypical Antidepressants

- Bupropion
- Mirtazapine
- Nefazodone
- Trazodone
- Mechanism of Action
  - Multiple and variable, but overall predominately serotonin effects
- Clinical Implications
  - Continue drug perioperatively
  - If discontinued, have patient continue when surgery completed
  - Does not have the same drug-interaction concerns as TCAs, SNRIs, or MAOIs [49]

Serotonin Norepinephrine Reuptake Inhibitors (SNRIs)

- Duloxetine
- Venlafaxine/desvenlafaxine
- Levomilnacipran
- Less commonly used than the SSRI class of medication
- Mechanism of Action
  - ↓ Reuptake of norepinephrine and serotonin in the synapse
- Clinical Implications
  - Continue drug perioperatively
  - If discontinued, have patient continue when surgery completed
  - Drug interactions that can increase risk of tachycardia and hypertension [50]
    - o Ephedrine
    - o Epinephrine
    - o Meperidine
    - o Stimulants
    - o Tramadol
    - o Tyramine-rich foods

Selective Serotonin Reuptake Inhibitors (SSRIs)

- Citalopram
- Escitalopram
- Fluoxetine
- Paroxetine
- Sertraline
- Mechanism of Action
  - ↓ Reuptake of serotonin from the synapse
- Clinical Implications
  - Continue drug perioperatively
  - If discontinued, have patient continue when surgery completed
  - Does not have the same drug-interaction concerns as TCAs, SNRIs, or MAOIs [49]

4.13 Psychiatric

Antipsychotics

- Aripiprazole
- Chlorpromazine
- Haloperidol
- Olanzapine
- Quetiapine
- Risperidone
- -azine
- -apine
- -idone
- Mechanism of Action
  - Central dopamine receptor antagonist
- Clinical Implications
  - Continue drug perioperatively
  - If discontinued, have patient continue when surgery completed
  - Extrapyramidal side effects
    - Involuntary muscle contractions, tremors, and movement
    - More common with older agents (Haloperidol, chlorpromazine) and after recent medication change/increase
  - These medications can lead to neuroleptic malignant syndrome
    - *Neuroleptic malignant syndrome management covered on page 275*

α₂ Adrenergic Agonists

- Clonidine
- Guanfacine
- Tizanidine
- Mechanism of Action
  - α₂ adrenergic receptor agonist
- Clinical Implications
  - Continue drug perioperatively
  - If discontinued, acute withdrawal may increase risk for tachycardia, hypertension, and unwanted behavioral side effects
    - Consider IV supplementation with α_2 agonist dexmedetomidine

Lithium

- Mechanism of Action
  - Not well established
- Clinical Implications
  - Ensure lithium levels checked recently
  - Narrow therapeutic index
  - Prolongs neuromuscular blockade
  - Renally excreted so plasma levels could increase if renal function is compromised
    - Reasonable to continue drug for less invasive/lengthy procedures/anesthetics [49]
  - Consider discontinuing 72 hours prior with invasive/deeper anesthetics
    - No significant withdrawal effects reported [49]

Amphetamines

- Dextroamphetamine
- Lisdexamfetamine
- Methylphenidate
- Mechanism of Action
  - ↓ Catecholamines reuptake from synapse
- Clinical Implications
  - Reasonable to continue drug perioperatively, especially if helpful with behavior/cooperation

Sleep Aids

- Eszopiclone
- Zaleplon
- Zolpidem
- Mechanism of Action
  - GABA$_A$ receptor allosteric modulators
- Clinical Implications
  - May continue evening before procedure

4.14   Neurologic

Antiepileptics [51]

Benzodiazepines *Phenobarbital*	*GABA$_A$ receptor agonist*
Carbamazepine *Lacosamide* *Lamotrigine* *Phenytoin* *Valproic Acid* *Zonisamide*	*Voltage-gated sodium channels antagonist*
Ethosuximide	*Calcium channel antagonist*
Levetiracetam	*Binding of synaptic vesicle protein 2a [52]*

- Clinical Implications
  - Continue drug perioperatively
  - If discontinued, increase risk of perioperative seizure

Carbamazepine	*P$_{450}$ Inducer [53]* *Resistant to neuromuscular blockade [54]*
Phenobarbital	*P$_{450}$ inducer*
Phenytoin	*Gingival hyperplasia [55]* *P$_{450}$ inducer* *Resistant to neuromuscular blockade [54]*
Valproic acid	*Liver damage* *Surgical bleeding [56, 57]*

Dopaminergics

Amantadine	*↑ Dopamine release*
Carbidopa- *Levodopa*	*Dopamine precursor with decarboxylase inhibitor*
Entacapone *Tolcapone*	*COMT inhibitor*
Pramipexole *Ropinirole*	*Dopamine receptor agonist*

- Clinical Implications
  - Continue drug perioperatively
  - If discontinued, abrupt withdrawal can lead to neuroleptic malignant syndrome
    - Dopamine antagonist administration can also precipitate neuroleptic malignant syndrome
    - *Neuroleptic malignant syndrome management covered on page 275*
  - Avoid/reduce dose of additional catecholamines (including epinephrine in local anesthetics) as can have synergistic effects, especially COMT inhibitors

Cholinesterase Inhibitors

- Donepezil
- Galantamine
- Pyridostigmine
- Rivastigmine
- Tacrine
- -stigmine
- Mechanism of Action
  - Inhibits acetylcholinesterase
    - ↑ Acetylcholine in the synapse
- Clinical Implications
  - Continue drug perioperatively
  - If discontinued, may contribute to postanesthetic neurocognitive decline
  - May cause prolonged depolarizing NMB and resistance to nondepolarizing NMB [58]
  - Avoid centrally acting anticholinergics perioperatively
    - Atropine
    - Scopolamine

4.15   Gastrointestinal

H₂ Receptor Antagonists

- Cimetidine
- Famotidine
- Mechanism of Action
  - Histamine-2 receptor antagonist (Figure 4.17)
- Clinical Implications
  - Continue drug perioperatively
  - If discontinued, consider delaying procedure or IV supplementation as there may be an increased risk of GERD and associated comorbidities

Proton Pump Inhibitors (PPI)

- Esomeprazole
- Omeprazole
- Pantoprazole
- -prazole
- Mechanism of Action
  - Inhibits the gastric H^+/K^+ ATPase to reduce stomach acid (HCL) formation (Figure 4.17)

- Clinical Implications
  - Continue drug perioperatively
  - If taken in AM, consider bedtime dosing preoperatively
  - If discontinued, consider delaying procedure or IV supplementation as there may be an increased risk of GERD and associated comorbidities

Antacids

- Mechanism of Action (Figure 4.17)
  - Directly neutralize stomach acid

Magnesium trisilicate	Particulate
Aluminum hydroxide	
Sodium citrate	Non-particulate

- Clinical Implications
  - Discontinue day of surgery
  - If continued, consider delaying elective procedure
  - Debate if sodium citrate decreases risk of aspiration pneumonia as it decreases stomach acid pH, but increases overall volume

Site of Action for Gastrointestinal Medications

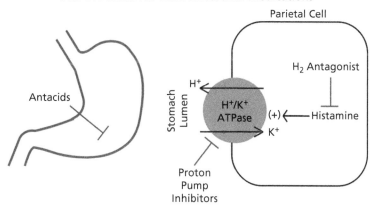

Figure 4.17

4.16   Glucocorticosteroids

- Patients on chronic steroids may develop adrenal suppression presenting as refractory intraoperative hypotension [59]
- There is a lack of evidence on the dose and duration of systemic steroids required to induce adrenal suppression. However, practitioners are generally supportive of at least 20 mg daily of prednisone (or equivalent) for more than two weeks in the past two months may suppress adrenal function

- If discontinued, strongly consider IV supplementation in addition to "stress dose"
- A typical "stress dose" of steroids is ~75–125 mg hydrocortisone given at induction if concerns of adrenal suppression, but recent evidence suggestions that a lower dose of 25 mg on induction is sufficient regardless of invasiveness of procedure [60]
- Dexamethasone is the only steroid without mineralocorticoid effects

Glucocorticosteroids

- Cortisone
- Dexamethasone
- Fludrocortisone
- Hydrocortisone
- Methylprednisolone
- Prednisone
- Prednisolone
- Mechanism of Action
  - Not well established
- Clinical Implications
  - Continue normal dose of steroids perioperatively

Steroid Equivalency Chart

	Equivalent dose (mg)
Hydrocortisone	20
Cortisone	25
Dexamethasone	0.75
Prednisone	5
Prednisolone	5
Methylprednisolone	4
Fludrocortisone	2

4.17 Other Medications

Statins

- Atorvastatin
- Fluvastatin
- Lovastatin
- Pitavastatin
- Rosuvastatin
- Simvastatin
- -statin
- Mechanism of Action
  - Inhibit HMG-CoA reductase
- Clinical Implications
  - Continue the drug as acute withdrawal of the statin may decrease the levels of nitric oxide and increase the risk of myocardial infarction
  - If discontinued, have patient restart when surgery completed

Thyroid

Levothyroxine	*Thyroid hormone replacement*
Liothyronine	*(Hypothyroidism)*
Methimazole	*Thyroid hormone inhibitors*
Propylthiouracil	*Variety of mechanisms*
Potassium iodide	*(Hyperthyroidism)*
Sodium iodide i-131	

- Clinical Implications
  - Continue thyroid hormone substitutes perioperatively
  - If discontinued, have the patient restart when surgery completed as they have a long half-life
  - Delay elective surgery if thyroid hormone inhibitors are being taken for active hyperthyroid treatment

Antiretrovirals

- Many different classes, drugs, and combinations of drugs

Efavirenz	*Nonnucleoside reverse transcriptase inhibitors*
Ibalizumab	*Entry inhibitors*
Raltegravir	*Integrase strand transfer inhibitors*
Ritonavir	*Protease inhibitors*
Tenofovir	*Nucleoside reverse transcriptase inhibitors*

- Clinical Implications
  - Continue drug perioperatively
  - Consider CBC
  - Consider BMP
  - Consider LFT
  - Many are P450 inhibitors

Ophthalmic

- Class of drug based on the color of the eye drop cap (Figure 4.18)
- Clinical Implications
  - Continue drug perioperatively

Color of Eye Drop Bottle Cap

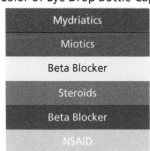

Mydriatics
Miotics
Beta Blocker
Steroids
Beta Blocker
NSAID

Figure 4.18

- Systemic effects can occur at abnormally high doses
- For echothiophate iodide drops (miotics), it is a potent long-acting pseudocholinesterase inhibitor
  - Suggest discontinuation of echothiophate for three months before administration of succinylcholine or use nondepolarizing NMB

Herbal Medications

- Mechanism of Action
  - Variable
- Clinical Implications
  - Recommend discontinuing for at least two weeks prior to procedure [61]

Aloe *Ginger* *Gingko* *Vitamin E Chamomile Ginseng* *Grapefruit*	*Increase risk of bleeding [62]*
Ginseng *Ephedra*	*Increase heart rate and blood pressure*
Kava *Valerian root* *St John's Wort*	*Increase sedative effects*
St John's Wort	P_{450} *inducer*

α_1 Adrenergic Antagonists

- Alfuzosin
- Doxazosin
- Prazosin
- Silodosin
- Tamsulosin
- Terazosin
- -osin
- Mechanism of Action
  - α_1 adrenergic receptor antagonist
- Clinical Implications
  - Continue drug perioperatively
  - May contribute to perioperative hypotension

References

1 Vogkou, C.T., Vlachogiannis, N.I., Palaiodimos, L., and Kousoulis, A.A. (2016). The causative agents in infective endocarditis: a systematic review comprising 33,214 cases. *Eur. J. Clin. Microbiol. Infect. Dis.* 35 (8): 1227–1245. https://doi.org/10.1007/s10096-016-2660-6.

2 Wilson, W.R., Gewitz, M., Lockhart, P.B. et al. (2021). Prevention of viridans group streptococcal infective endocarditis: a scientific statement from the American Heart Association. *Circulation* 143 (20): e963–e978. https://doi.org/10.1161/CIR.0000000000000969.

3 Wilson, W., Taubert, K.A., Gewitz, M. et al. (2007). Prevention of infective endocarditis: guidelines from the American Heart Association: a guideline from the American Heart Association Rheumatic Fever, Endocarditis and Kawasaki Disease Committee, Council on Cardiovascular Disease in the Young, and the Council on Clinical Cardiology, Council on Cardiovascular Surgery and Anesthesia, and the Quality of Care and Outcomes Research Interdisciplinary Working Group. *J. Am. Dent.* *Assoc.* 138 (6): 739–745, 747–760. https://doi.org/10.14219/jada.archive.2007.0262.

4 Meyer, D.M. (2015). Providing clarity on evidence-based prophylactic guidelines for prosthetic joint infections. *J. Am. Dent. Assoc.* 146 (1): 3–5. https://doi.org/10.1016/j.adaj.2014.11.009.

5 Sollecito, T.P., Abt, E., Lockhart, P.B. et al. (2015). The use of prophylactic antibiotics prior to dental procedures in patients with prosthetic joints: evidence-based clinical practice guideline for dental practitioners--a report of the American Dental Association Council on Scientific Affairs. *J. Am. Dent. Assoc.* 146 (1): 11–16.e8. https://doi.org/10.1016/j.adaj.2014.11.012.

6 Carrick, M.A., Robson, J.M., and Thomas, C. (2019). Smoking and anaesthesia. *BJA Educ.* 19 (1): 1–6. https://doi.org/10.1016/j.bjae.2018.09.005.

7 Wong, J., Lam, D.P., Abrishami, A. et al. (2012). Short-term preoperative smoking cessation and postoperative complications: a systematic review and meta-analysis.

Can. J. Anaesth. 59 (3): 268–279. https://doi.org/10.1007/s12630-011-9652-x.

8 Lee, S.M., Landry, J., Jones, P.M. et al. (2013). The effectiveness of a perioperative smoking cessation program: a randomized clinical trial. *Anesth. Analg.* 117 (3): 605–613. https://doi.org/10.1213/ANE.0b013e318298a6b0.

9 Chiang, H.L., Chia, Y.Y., Lin, H.S., and Chen, C.H. (2016). The implications of tobacco smoking on acute postoperative pain: a prospective observational study. *Pain Res. Manag.* 2016: 9432493. https://doi.org/10.1155/2016/9432493.

10 Woodside, J.R. (2000). Female smokers have increased postoperative narcotic requirements. *J. Addict. Dis.* 19 (4): 1–10. https://doi.org/10.1300/J069v19n04_01.

11 Karlsdottir, B.R., Zhou, P.P., Wahba, J. et al. (2022). Male gender, smoking, younger age, and preoperative pain found to increase postoperative opioid requirements in 592 elective colorectal resections. *Int. J. Color. Dis.* 37 (8): 1799–1806. https://doi.org/10.1007/s00384-022-04208-5.

12 Gold, M.S., Byars, J.A., and Frost-Pineda, K. (2004). Occupational exposure and addictions for physicians: case studies and theoretical implications. *Psychiatr. Clin. North Am.* 27 (4): 745–753. https://doi.org/10.1016/j.psc.2004.07.006.

13 Selçuk, E.B., Sungu, M., Parlakpinar, H. et al. (2015). Evaluation of the cardiovascular effects of varenicline in rats. *Drug Des. Devel. Ther.* 9: 5705–5717. https://doi.org/10.2147/DDDT.S92268.

14 May, J.A., White, H.C., Leonard-White, A. et al. (2001). The patient recovering from alcohol or drug addiction: special issues for the anesthesiologist. *Anesth. Analg.* 92 (6): 1601–1608. https://doi.org/10.1097/00000539-200106000-00050.

15 Ward, E.N., Quaye, A.N., and Wilens, T.E. (2018). Opioid use disorders: perioperative management of a special population. *Anesth. Analg.* 127 (2): 539–547. https://doi.org/10.1213/ANE.0000000000003477.

16 Curatolo, C. and Trinh, M. (2014). Challenges in the perioperative management of the patient receiving extended-release naltrexone. *A. A. Case Rep.* 3 (11): 142–144. https://doi.org/10.1213/XAA.0000000000000069.

17 Macintyre, P.E., Russell, R.A., Usher, K.A. et al. (2013). Pain relief and opioid requirements in the first 24 hours after surgery in patients taking buprenorphine and methadone opioid substitution therapy. *Anaesth. Intensive Care* 41 (2): 222–230. https://doi.org/10.1177/0310057X1304100212.

18 Coluzzi, F., Bifulco, F., Cuomo, A. et al. (2017). The challenge of perioperative pain management in opioid-tolerant patients. *Ther. Clin. Risk Manag.* 13: 1163–1173. https://doi.org/10.2147/TCRM.S141332.

19 Jones, H.E., Johnson, R.E., and Milio, L. (2006). Post-cesarean pain management of patients maintained on methadone or buprenorphine. *Am. J. Addict.* 15 (3): 258–259. https://doi.org/10.1080/10550490600626721.

20 Levine, G.N., Bates, E.R., Bittl, J.A. et al. (2016). 2016 ACC/AHA guideline focused update on duration of dual antiplatelet therapy in patients with coronary artery disease: a report of the American College of Cardiology/American Heart Association Task Force on Clinical Practice Guidelines. *J. Thorac. Cardiovasc. Surg.* 152 (5): 1243–1275. https://doi.org/10.1016/j.jtcvs.2016.07.044.

21 Straube, S., Derry, S., McQuay, H.J., and Moore, R.A. (2005). Effect of preoperative Cox-II-selective NSAIDs (coxibs) on postoperative outcomes: a systematic review of randomized studies. *Acta Anaesthesiol. Scand.* 49 (5): 601–613. https://doi.org/10.1111/j.1399-6576.2005.00666.x.

22 Lillis, T., Ziakas, A., Koskinas, K. et al. (2011). Safety of dental extractions during uninterrupted single or dual antiplatelet treatment. *Am. J. Cardiol.* 108 (7): 964–967. https://doi.org/10.1016/j.amjcard.2011.05.029.

23 Breik, O., Cheng, A., Sambrook, P., and Goss, A. (2014). Protocol in managing oral surgical patients taking dabigatran. *Aust. Dent. J.* 59 (3): 296–301; quiz 401. https://doi.org/10.1111/adj.12199.

24 Nagarakanti, R. and Ellis, C.R. (2012). Dabigatran in clinical practice. *Clin. Ther.* 34 (10): 2051–2060. https://doi.org/10.1016/j.clinthera.2012.09.008.

25 Bajkin, B.V., Popovic, S.L., and Selakovic, S.D. (2009). Randomized, prospective trial comparing bridging therapy using low-molecular-weight heparin with maintenance of oral anticoagulation during extraction of teeth. *J. Oral Maxillofac. Surg.* 67 (5): 990–995. https://doi.org/10.1016/j.joms.2008.12.027.

26 Curto, A. and Albaladejo, A. (2016). Implications of apixaban for dental treatments. *J. Clin. Exp. Dent.* 8 (5): e611–e614. https://doi.org/10.4317/jced.53004.

27 Blinder, D., Manor, Y., Martinowitz, U., and Taicher, S. (2001). Dental extractions in patients maintained on oral anticoagulant therapy: comparison of INR value with occurrence of postoperative bleeding. *Int. J. Oral Maxillofac. Surg.* 30 (6): 518–521. https://doi.org/10.1054/ijom.2001.0172.

28 Curto, A., Curto, D., and Sanchez, J. (2017). Managing patients taking edoxaban in dentistry. *J. Clin. Exp. Dent.* 9 (2): e308–e311. https://doi.org/10.4317/jced.53431.

29 Hollmann, C., Fernandes, N.L., and Biccard, B.M. (2018). A systematic review of outcomes associated with withholding or continuing angiotensin-converting enzyme inhibitors and angiotensin receptor blockers before noncardiac surgery. *Anesth. Analg.* 127 (3):

678–687. https://doi.org/10.1213/ANE.0000000000002837.

30 Smith, I. and Jackson, I. (2010). Beta-blockers, calcium channel blockers, angiotensin converting enzyme inhibitors and angiotensin receptor blockers: should they be stopped or not before ambulatory anaesthesia? *Curr. Opin. Anaesthesiol.* 23 (6): 687–690. https://doi.org/10.1097/ACO.0b013e32833eeb19.

31 Takeuchi, K., Hayashida, M., Kudoh, O. et al. (2022). Continuing versus withholding angiotensin receptor blocker (ARB)/calcium channel blocker (CCB) combination tablets during perioperative periods in patients undergoing minor surgery: a single-blinded randomized controlled trial. *J. Anesth.* 36 (3): 374–382. https://doi.org/10.1007/s00540-022-03053-8.

32 Blinder, D., Shemesh, J., and Taicher, S. (1996). Electrocardiographic changes in cardiac patients undergoing dental extractions under local anesthesia. *J. Oral Maxillofac. Surg.* 54 (2): 162–165; discussion 165–166. https://doi.org/10.1016/s0278-2391(96)90438-3.

33 von Ungern-Sternberg, B.S., Habre, W., Erb, T.O., and Heaney, M. (2009). Salbutamol premedication in children with a recent respiratory tract infection. *Paediatr. Anaesth.* 19 (11): 1064–1069. https://doi.org/10.1111/j.1460-9592.2009.03130.x.

34 Ramgolam, A., Hall, G.L., Sommerfield, D. et al. (2017). Premedication with salbutamol prior to surgery does not decrease the risk of perioperative respiratory adverse events in school-aged children. *Br. J. Anaesth.* 119 (1): 150–157. https://doi.org/10.1093/bja/aex139.

35 Silvanus, M.T., Groeben, H., and Peters, J. (2004). Corticosteroids and inhaled salbutamol in patients with reversible airway obstruction markedly decrease the incidence of bronchospasm after tracheal intubation. *Anesthesiology* 100 (5): 1052–1057. https://doi.org/10.1097/00000542-200405000-00004.

36 Redden, R.J. (1996). Possible theophylline toxicity during anesthesia. *Anesth. Prog.* 43 (2): 67–72.

37 Shannon, M. and Lovejoy, F.H. (1989). Hypokalemia after theophylline intoxication. The effects of acute vs chronic poisoning. *Arch. Intern. Med.* 149 (12): 2725–2729. https://doi.org/10.1001/archinte.149.12.2725.

38 Kuzulugil, D., Papeix, G., Luu, J., and Kerridge, R.K. (2019). Recent advances in diabetes treatments and their perioperative implications. *Curr. Opin. Anaesthesiol.* 32 (3): 398–404. https://doi.org/10.1097/ACO.0000000000000735.

39 Duncan, A.I., Koch, C.G., Xu, M. et al. (2007). Recent metformin ingestion does not increase in-hospital morbidity or mortality after cardiac surgery. *Anesth. Analg.* 104 (1): 42–50. https://doi.org/10.1213/01.ane.0000242532.42656.e7.

40 Preiser, J.C., Provenzano, B., Mongkolpun, W. et al. (2020). Perioperative management of oral glucose-lowering drugs in the patient with type 2 diabetes. *Anesthesiology* 133 (2): 430–438. https://doi.org/10.1097/ALN.0000000000003237.

41 Barker, P., Creasey, P.E., Dhatariya, K. et al. (2015). Peri-operative management of the surgical patient with diabetes 2015: Association of Anaesthetists of Great Britain and Ireland. *Anaesthesia* 70 (12): 1427–1440. https://doi.org/10.1111/anae.13233.

42 Joshi, G.P., Chung, F., Vann, M.A. et al. (2010). Society for Ambulatory Anesthesia consensus statement on perioperative blood glucose management in diabetic patients undergoing ambulatory surgery. *Anesth. Analg.* 111 (6): 1378–1387. https://doi.org/10.1213/ANE.0b013e3181f9c288.

43 Duggan, E.W., Carlson, K., and Umpierrez, G.E. (2017). Perioperative hyperglycemia management: an update. *Anesthesiology* 126 (3): 547–560. https://doi.org/10.1097/ALN.0000000000001515.

44 Simha, V. and Shah, P. (2019). Perioperative glucose control in patients with diabetes undergoing elective surgery. *JAMA* 321 (4): 399–400. https://doi.org/10.1001/jama.2018.20922.

45 Kudoh, A., Katagai, H., and Takazawa, T. (2002). Antidepressant treatment for chronic depressed patients should not be discontinued prior to anesthesia. *Can. J. Anaesth.* 49 (2): 132–136. https://doi.org/10.1007/BF03020484.

46 Saraghi, M., Golden, L.R., and Hersh, E.V. (2017). Anesthetic considerations for patients on antidepressant therapy-part I. *Anesth. Prog.* 64 (4): 253–261. https://doi.org/10.2344/anpr-64-04-14.

47 Boakes, A.J., Laurence, D.R., Teoh, P.C. et al. (1973). Interactions between sympathomimetic amines and antidepressant agents in man. *Br. Med. J.* 1 (5849): 311–315. https://doi.org/10.1136/bmj.1.5849.311.

48 Ebrahim, Z.Y., O'Hara, J., Borden, L., and Tetzlaff, J. (1993). Monoamine oxidase inhibitors and elective surgery. *Cleve. Clin. J. Med.* 60 (2): 129–130. https://doi.org/10.3949/ccjm.60.2.129.

49 Attri, J.P., Bala, N., and Chatrath, V. (2012). Psychiatric patient and anaesthesia. *Indian J. Anaesth.* 56 (1): 8–13. https://doi.org/10.4103/0019-5049.93337.

50 Gillman, P.K. (2007). Tricyclic antidepressant pharmacology and therapeutic drug interactions updated. *Br. J. Pharmacol.* 151 (6): 737–748. https://doi.org/10.1038/sj.bjp.0707253.

51 Sills, G.J. and Brodie, M.J. (2001). Update on the mechanisms of action of antiepileptic drugs. *Epileptic Disord.* 3 (4): 165–172.

52 Abou-Khalil, B. (2008). Levetiracetam in the treatment of epilepsy. *Neuropsychiatr. Dis. Treat.* 4 (3): 507–523. https://doi.org/10.2147/ndt.s2937.

53 Tateishi, T., Asoh, M., Nakura, H. et al. (1999). Carbamazepine induces multiple cytochrome P450 subfamilies in rats. *Chem. Biol. Interact.* 117 (3): 257–268. https://doi.org/10.1016/s0009-2797(98)00110-0.

54 Kawamura, G., Inoue, R., Araki, Y. et al. (2014). Effects of preoperatively administered carbamazepine and phenytoin on rocuronium-induced neuromuscular block under sevoflurane anesthesia: a retrospective clinical study. *Masui* 63 (8): 877–880.

55 Scheinfeld, N. (2003). Phenytoin in cutaneous medicine: its uses, mechanisms and side effects. *Dermatol. Online J.* 9 (3): 6.

56 Cannizzaro, E., Albisetti, M., Wohlrab, G., and Schmugge, M. (2007). Severe bleeding complications during antiepileptic treatment with valproic acid in children. *Neuropediatrics* 38 (1): 42–45. https://doi.org/10.1055/s-2007-981448.

57 Abdallah, C. (2014). Considerations in perioperative assessment of valproic acid coagulopathy. *J. Anaesthesiol. Clin. Pharmacol.* 30 (1): 7–9. https://doi.org/10.4103/0970-9185.125685.

58 Crowe, S. and Collins, L. (2003). Suxamethonium and donepezil: a cause of prolonged paralysis. *Anesthesiology* 98 (2): 574–575. https://doi.org/10.1097/00000542-200302000-00040.

59 Liu, M.M., Reidy, A.B., Saatee, S., and Collard, C.D. (2017). Perioperative steroid management: approaches based on current evidence. *Anesthesiology* 127 (1): 166–172. https://doi.org/10.1097/ALN.0000000000001659.

60 Chilkoti, G.T., Singh, A., Mohta, M., and Saxena, A.K. (2019). Perioperative "stress dose" of corticosteroid: pharmacological and clinical perspective. *J. Anaesthesiol. Clin. Pharmacol.* 35 (2): 147–152. https://doi.org/10.4103/joacp.JOACP_242_17.

61 Rowe, D.J. and Baker, A.C. (2009). Perioperative risks and benefits of herbal supplements in aesthetic surgery. *Aesthet. Surg. J.* 29 (2): 150–157. https://doi.org/10.1016/j.asj.2009.01.002.

62 Abebe, W. (2019). Review of herbal medications with the potential to cause bleeding: dental implications, and risk prediction and prevention avenues. *EPMA J.* 10 (1): 51–64. https://doi.org/10.1007/s13167-018-0158-2.

Section 5
The Perioperative Pharmacology

5.1 Inhalational Pharmacokinetics and Pharmacodynamics

Mechanism of Action

- Primarily augments $GABA_A$ receptors with various other protein and ion channel interactions
  - Except nitrous oxide which is primarily an NMDA-receptor antagonist

Minimum Alveolar Concentration (MAC)

- MAC is additive
- MAC is inversely proportional to potency (Figure 5.1)
- MAC is directly proportional to oil:gas coefficient (Figure 5.1)
- MAC can vary depending on a variety of factors (Figure 5.2)

	MAC (%)	Oil: Gas Coefficient	Potency
Nitrous Oxide	105	1.4	Least
Desflurane	6.6	29	
Sevoflurane	2.0	80	
Enflurane	1.7	98	
Isoflurane	1.2	98	
Halothane	0.75	224	Most

Figure 5.1 *Source:* Adapted from Peck and Harris [1].

Minimum Alveolar Concentration (Definitions)

- MAC
  - The concentration of volatile agent at one atmosphere which prevents movement in 50% of patients exposed to a surgical stimulus (Figure 5.1)
  - MAC ~1.0
- MAC Amnesia
  - The concentration of volatile agent at one atmosphere which prevents recall in 50% of patients
  - MAC ~0.2
- MAC Awake
  - The concentration of volatile agent at one atmosphere which prevents a wakeful response in 50% of patients
  - MAC ~0.3
- MAC_{90}
  - The concentration of volatile agent at one atmosphere which prevents movement in 90% of patients
  - MAC ~1.5

- MAC BAR
  - Prevents any adrenergic/autonomic response to surgical stimulus
  - MAC ~1.8

Factors Affecting MAC (Figure 5.2)

- MAC is the highest ~6 months of age and decreases by 6% per decade with a plateau/slight increase during puberty [3]

Factors Affecting Inhalational Onset

- Alveolar concentration of anesthetic gas (FA)
- Inspired concentration of inhaled anesthetic (FI)
- Solubility (Figure 5.3)
  - ↓ Blood:gas coefficient → ↓ Solubility → ↓ Uptake → ↑ FA/FI → ↑ Onset
  - ↑ Blood:gas coefficient → ↑ Solubility → ↑ Uptake → ↓ FA/FI → ↓ Onset

Anesthesia for Dental and Oral Maxillofacial Surgery, First Edition. Spencer D. Wade, Caroline M. Sawicki, Megann K. Smiley, Michael A. Cuddy, Steven Vukas, and Paul J. Schwartz.
© 2024 John Wiley & Sons, Inc. Published 2024 by John Wiley & Sons, Inc.

Increased MAC	No Change in MAC	Decreased MAC
		Advanced Age
		Hypothermia
Young Age		Hyponatremia
Hyperthermia		Hypercarbia
Hypernatremia	Sex	Anemia
Melanin Receptor Mutation	Hypothyroidism	Pregnancy
	Hyperthyroidism	Sedatives
Acute Stimulant Usage	Obesity	Opioids
Chronic Alcohol Usage		Chronic Stimulant Usage
		Neurodegeneration

Figure 5.2 *Source:* Adapted from Aranake et al. [2].

	Blood:Gas Coefficient	Solubility
Desflurane	0.45	Least
Nitrous Oxide	0.47	
Sevoflurane	0.70	
Isoflurane	1.40	
Enflurane	1.80	
Halothane	2.40	Most

Figure 5.3 *Source:* Adapted from Ekberg et al. [4].

- Cardiac Output
  - ↑ CO → ↑ Alveolar blood flow → ↓ FA/FI → ↓ Onset
  - ↓ CO → ↓ Alveolar blood flow → ↑ FA/FI → ↑ Onset
  - Changes in CO will have a lesser effect on more insoluble agents
  - Pulmonary shunt will have a greater effect on more insoluble agents
- Alveolar Gas and Venous Gas Concentrations Differential
  - ↑ Partial pressure difference → ↑ Uptake → ↓ FA/FI → ↓ Onset
  - ↓ Partial pressure difference → ↓ Uptake → ↑ FA/FI → ↑ Onset
- Ventilation
  - ↑ Ventilation → ↑ FA/FI → ↑ Onset
  - ↓ Ventilation → ↓ FA/FI → ↓ Onset
  - Changes in ventilation will have a lesser effect on more insoluble agents
- Second Gas Effect (Figure 5.4)
  - For this book's purposes, occurs with N_2O administration

- N_2O is taken up rapidly which "concentrates" the less soluble inhalational agent leading to a more rapid rise in FA during first few breaths
- Clinical relevance debated

Distribution

- Tissues with greater cardiac output will reach equilibrium the faster (Figure 5.5)
- Similar pharmacokinetics to intravenous infusions
- Vessel-Rich Group
  - ~10% Body mass
  - ~75% Cardiac output
  - Brain
  - Heart
  - Liver
  - Kidneys
- Muscle Group
  - ~50% Body mass
  - ~20% Cardiac output
  - Muscle
  - Skin
- Fat Group
  - ~20% Body mass
  - ~5% Cardiac output
  - Fat
- Vessel-Poor Group
  - ~20% Body mass
  - Negligible cardiac output
  - Cartilage
  - Bone
  - Teeth
  - Hair

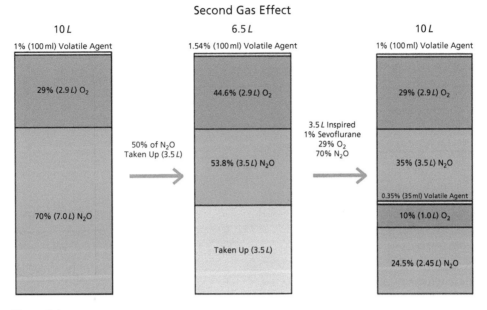

Figure 5.4

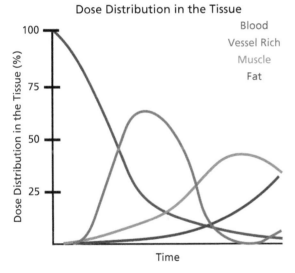

Figure 5.5

Metabolism

- Minimal for newer agents

Agent	Approximate liver metabolism (%)
Nitrous oxide	*0.002*
Desflurane	*0.02*
Isoflurane	*0.2*
Sevoflurane	*2*
Halothane	*20*

Elimination

- Primarily eliminated by exhalation

5.2 Inhalational Agents

Nitrous Oxide

- Clinical Considerations
  - Nonpungent
  - Low blood: gas coefficient allows for titration
- Cerebral
  - $\uparrow$ $CMRO_2$
  - $\uparrow$ CBF
- Cardiovascular
  - Minimal
  - Higher concentrations (>60%) [2]
    - $\uparrow$ HR
    - $\uparrow$ SV
    - $\uparrow$ MAP
  - May attenuate hemodynamic depressant effects of halogenated volatile agents
- Pulmonary
  - Least effect of the volatile agents
  - $\downarrow$ TV
  - $\uparrow$ RR
  - No change in minute ventilation unlike other volatile agents
- Renal
  - Minimal
- Hepatic
  - Minimal
- Neuromuscular
  - Not a triggering agent for malignant hyperthermia
- Contraindications
  - Pneumothorax
  - Small bowel obstruction
  - Otitis media
  - Air embolism
  - First trimester of pregnancy
  - Intraocular surgery with gas bubbles
    - No current guidelines on how long after the eye injection nitrous oxide administration should wait [5]

- B$_{12}$ deficiency and methyl tetrahydrofolate reductase deficiency
    - Debatable, but consider avoiding in this population [6]
- Board Facts
  - Prolonged N_2O can cause vitamin B_{12} deficiency and peripheral sensory and motor dysfunction, especially in chronic nitrous oxide abusers [7]
  - May increase risk of PONV especially at high concentrations [8]
  - Diffuses into endotracheal tube cuff over procedure and can lead to tracheal morbidity [9]
    - Consider inflating cuff with saline instead of air
  - Critical temperature is 36.5 °C
    - Temperature at which gas cannot be liquefied by pressure alone
  - *For N_2O e cylinder volume readings, see page 16*
  - Nitrous oxide stays in the atmosphere for 114 years [9]

Isoflurane

- Clinical Considerations
  - Pungent
  - Poor for inhalation induction
- Cerebral
  - $\uparrow$ CBF
  - $\downarrow$ $CMRO_2$
- Cardiovascular [10–12]
  - $\downarrow$ MAP
  - CO maintained up to 1 MAC before decreasing
  - $\downarrow$ SVR
- Pulmonary
  - Relaxes bronchial smooth muscle
  - $\downarrow$ TV
  - $\uparrow$ RR
  - $\downarrow$ MV

- Renal [13]
  - ↓ GFR
- Hepatic [14]
  - ↓ HBF
- Neuromuscular
  - Malignant hyperthermia trigger
  - Potentiates nondepolarizing NMBs
- Contraindications
  - Malignant hyperthermia susceptibility
  - Mask induction
- Board Facts
  - Coronary steal phenomenon
    - Debunked [15]

Desflurane

- Clinical Considerations
  - Pungent
  - Poor for inhalation induction
  - Lowest blood:gas solubility coefficient for inhaled anesthetics and nitrous oxide
- Cerebral
  - ↑ CBF
  - ↓ CMRO$_2$
- Cardiovascular [10–12]
  - ↓ MAP
  - CO maintained up to 1 MAC before decreasing
  - ↓ SVR
- Pulmonary
  - Bronchial smooth muscle irritant
  - ↓ TV
  - ↑ RR
  - ↓ MV
- Renal [16]
  - ↓ GFR
- Hepatic [17]
  - ↓ HBF
- Neuromuscular
  - Malignant hyperthermia trigger
  - Potentiates nondepolarizing NMBs
- Contraindications
  - Malignant hyperthermia susceptibility
  - Mask induction

- Reactive airway disease [18]
- Board Facts
  - Desflurane reacts with desiccated NaOH and KOH to form carbon monoxide particularly in desiccated CO$_2$ absorbers [19]
  - Associated with increased risk of laryngospasm [20]
  - Desflurane stays in the atmosphere for 9–21 years [21]

Sevoflurane

- Clinical Considerations
  - Nonpungent
  - Relatively low blood:gas coefficient
  - Ideal agent for smooth, rapid inhalation induction
- Cerebral Effects
  - ↑ CBF
  - ↓ CMRO$_2$
- Cardiovascular [10–12, 22]
  - ↓ MAP
  - CO maintained up to 1 MAC before decreasing
  - ↓ SVR
  - Least effect on cardiac output compared to the other halogenated volatile agents
- Pulmonary
  - Relaxes bronchial smooth muscle
  - ↓ TV
  - ↑ RR
  - ↓ MV
- Renal [16]
  - ↓ GFR
- Hepatic [14]
  - ↓ HBF
- Neuromuscular
  - Malignant hyperthermia triggering agent
  - Potentiates nondepolarizing NMB
- Contraindications
  - Malignant hyperthermia susceptibility
- Board Facts
  - Sevoflurane reacts with NaOH and KOH to form compound A
    - Likely little relevance under typically clinical conditions

5.3   Intravenous Pharmacokinetics and Pharmacodynamics

- Effective Dose$_{50}$ (ED50) (Figure 5.6)
  - The median drug dose which is effective in 50% of the population
  - Similar to MAC for inhalational agents
- Toxic Dose$_{50}$ (TD50) (Figure 5.6)
  - The median drug dose which has a toxic side effect in 50% of the population
- Lethal Dose$_{50}$ (LD50) (Figure 5.6)
  - The median drug dose which is lethal in 50% of the population

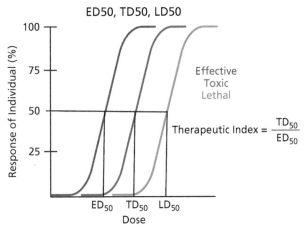

The higher therapeutic index, the greater
the medication's safety window

Figure 5.6

Factors Affecting Onset

- Drug Solubility
  - ↓ Blood solubility → ↑ Blood saturation rate → ↑ Tissue uptake → ↑ Onset
- Drug Concentration
  - ↑ Concentration → ↑ Onset
- Tissue pH
  - Drugs ionization dependent on pH of surrounding tissues

- ↑ Nonionized drug → ↑ Onset
  - o Nonionized drugs more readily cross cell membranes and the BBB to exert their effects
- Henderson–Hasselbalch equation determines nonionized/ionized drug ratio (Figure 5.7)
- Plasma Protein Binding
  - ↑ Drug binding → ↓ Free drug in blood → ↓ Tissue uptake → ↑ Onset
  - Bound drugs cannot permeate tissues and exert their effects
  - Predominantly **α**–1 acid glycoprotein (basic drugs) and albumin (acidic drugs)
- Site of Absorption (Figure 5.8)

Henderson–Hasselbalch Equation

$$pH = pKa + log\frac{[Conjugate\ Base]}{[Weak\ Acid]}$$

pKa = Acid Dissociation Constant

Figure 5.7

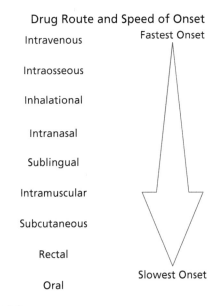

Figure 5.8

Distribution

- Tissues receiving greater cardiac output reach equilibrium the fastest
- Similar pattern of distribution as with intravenous agents (Figure 5.5)

Hepatic Metabolism

- Many intravenous drugs are metabolized by the liver
  - Accomplished by a variety of enzymes
    o Phase I: Cytochrome P_{450} family
      - P_{450} can be induced and inhibited by a variety of substrates and medications (Figure 5.9)
    o Phase II: Conjugation reactions (Glucuronidation)

P_{450} Inhibitors	P_{450} Inducers
Clarithromycin	
Erythromycin	
Antiretrovirals	Carbamazepine
Antidepressants	Phenobarbital
Diltiazem	Phenytoin
Verapamil	Rifampin
Metronidazole	Griseofulvin
Grapefriut Juice	Tobacco
Intraconazole	
Fluconazole	
Cimetidine	
St John's Wort	

Figure 5.9 *Source:* Adapted from Zhou [23]; Lynch and Price [24].

Hepatic Clearance

- Hepatic Clearance
  - Volume of blood cleared of a drug per unit of time
  - Hepatic clearance is either flow limited or capacity limited which is dictated by the extraction ratio of that drug (Figure 5.10)

Flow-Limited Drugs High Extraction Ratio	Capacity-Limited Drugs Low Extraction Ratio
Propofol	Diazepam
Fentanyl	Valproic acid
Ketamine	Carbamazepine
Morphine	Phenytoin
Meperidine	Ethanol
Lidocaine	Digitoxin
Propranolol	Acetaminophen
Verapamil	Warfarin
Nitroglycerin	Theophylline

Figure 5.10 *Source:* Adapted from Gershman and Steeper [25]; Mather [26].

   o Extraction ratio is the ratio of drug that gets cleared per pass through the liver
     - High extraction ratio > 0.7
     - Low extraction ratio < 0.3
  - Newer agents tend to be flow limited
  - More predictable to use flow-limited agents with intrinsic hepatic disease

Renal Clearance (Figure 5.11)

Dependent on Renal Clearance
Vecuronium
Pancuronium
Neostigmine
Sugammadex
Morphine
Hydromorphone
Meperidine
Diazepam
NSAIDs

Figure 5.11 *Source:* Adapted from Staals et al. [27].

5.4 Intravenous Induction Agents

- All benzodiazepines and intravenous induction agents are GABA$_A$ receptor allosteric modulators augmenting GABA function (Figure 5.12)
  - Except ketamine

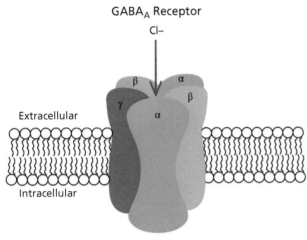

GABA$_A$ Receptor

Cl–

Extracellular

Intracellular

Ligand-gated (GABA) ion channel which Influxes chloride

Figure 5.12

Propofol

- Clinical Indications
  - General anesthesia induction
    - 2–4 mg/kg IV
  - Intravenous infusion
  - Antiemetic
  - Antiepileptic
- Cerebral
  - ↓ CBF
  - ↓ CMRO$_2$
  - Antiemetic
  - Antiepileptic
- Cardiovascular
  - ↓ CO
  - ↓ MAP

  - ↓ SVR
  - ↓ Baroreceptor reflex
- Pulmonary
  - ↓ TV
  - ↓ RR
- Renal
  - Minimal
- Hepatic
  - Primary site of metabolism
- Contraindications
  - Poor cardiac reserve
    - Especially with induction dosage
  - Not contraindicated with egg, soy, or peanut allergies [28]
- Board Facts
  - Pain on injection
    - Can be attenuated with lidocaine [29]
  - Lipid vehicle supports bacterial growth
  - Fospropofol
    - H$_2$O soluble prodrug
    - Decreased burning sensation on injection
  - Propofol infusion syndrome
    - Rare syndrome that typically occurs in prolonged propofol sedation (>48 hours), but can occur under clinical circumstances
      - Dyslipidemia
      - Metabolic acidosis
      - Right bundle branch block
      - Death
  - Extrahepatic metabolism [30]
    - Kidneys
    - Small intestines

Ketamine

- Mechanism of Action
  - NMDA-receptor antagonist
- Clinical Indications
  - General anesthesia induction
    - 1–2 mg/kg IV

- Pre-procedural sedation for uncooperative patient
  - Peds: 2–4 mg/kg IM
- Analgesia
  - Adult: 10–20 mg bolus IV titrated
  - Peds: 0.2 mg/kg IV
  - Infusion: 1–4 mcg/kg/min
- Cerebral
  - ↑ $CMRO_2$
  - ↑ CBF
  - Myoclonic activity
  - Delirium
  - Analgesia
- Cardiovascular
  - Direct myocardial depression
    - Masked by indirectly releasing catecholamines in healthy patients
  - ↑ CO
  - ↑ MAP
- Pulmonary
  - Bronchodilator
  - ↑ Secretions
- Renal
  - Minimal
- Hepatic
  - Primary site for metabolism
- Contraindications
  - Untreated psychosis
  - Porphyria
  - Uncontrolled hypertension
  - Unstable cardiac disease
  - Dysrhythmias
  - CHF
  - Advanced CAD
- Board Facts
  - Benzodiazepines may attenuate myoclonic activity and hallucinations
  - ↑ Secretions can be attenuated with anticholinergics
  - Ideal in asthmatics for bronchodilation effects
  - Ketamine is now considered safe to use in epileptic patients [31, 32]
  - Nor-ketamine is an active metabolite with 20% potency

Etomidate

- Clinical Indications
  - General anesthesia induction
    - 0.2–0.3 mg/kg IV

- Cerebral
  - ↓ $CMRO_2$
  - ↓ CBF
- Cardiovascular
  - Least effect on cardiac output and MAP compared to other IV induction agents
- Pulmonary
  - ↓ TV
  - ↓ RR
- Renal
  - Minimal
- Hepatic
  - Primary site of metabolism
- Contraindications
  - No real contraindications, but adrenal suppression has been noticed even after one bolus injection [33]
- Board Facts
  - ↓ Cortisol synthesis by 11β–hydroxylase in long-term infusions
  - Partially metabolized hepatic and by plasma esterases
  - ↑ Myoclonic activity

Methohexital

- Clinical Indications
  - General anesthesia induction
    - 1–1.5 mg/kg IV
- Cerebral
  - ↓ CBF
  - ↓ $CMRO_2$
  - ↓ Seizure threshold at lower doses
- Cardiovascular
  - ↓ CO
  - ↓ MAP
- Pulmonary
  - ↓ TV
  - ↓ RR
- Renal
  - Minimal
- Hepatic
  - Primary site of metabolism
- Contraindications
  - Seizure history
  - Acute intermittent porphyria/variegate porphyria
- Board Facts
  - Less commonly used today due to the favorable side effect profile of propofol
  - Can cause hiccups (singultus) on induction

5.5 Benzodiazepines

- All benzodiazepines are GABA$_A$ receptor allosteric modulators augmenting GABA function
  - *GABA receptor see Figure 5.12*
- Active Metabolites
  - Chlordiazepoxide
  - Clorazepate
  - Diazepam
  - Flurazepam
  - Midazolam
  - Triazolam
- No Active Metabolites
  - Alprazolam
  - Bromazepam
  - Clonazepam
  - Eszopiclone
  - Lorazepam
  - Oxazepam
  - Remimazolam
  - Temazepam
  - Zaleplon
  - Zolpidem

- Cardiovascular
  - Minimal
- Pulmonary
  - Minimal, in slowly titrated smaller doses
  - Historically, used as induction agent in high doses
- Renal
  - Minimal
- Hepatic
  - Primary site of metabolism
  - Enterohepatic circulation may cause "resedation" effects after hepatic clearance (Figure 5.13)
- Contraindications
  - Acute angle glaucoma
  - Hepatic dysfunction
- Board Facts
  - Diazepam requires propylene glycol solvent
    - Propylene glycol can cause venous thrombophlebitis and irritation on injection
  - Desmethyldiazepam is an active metabolite

Diazepam

- Clinical Indications
  - Pre-procedural sedation
    - Adult: 2.5–5 mg IV
    - Adult: 5–10 mg PO
  - Moderate sedation
    - Adult: 2.5–10 mg IV
  - Antiepileptic
- Cerebral
  - ↓ CBF
  - ↓ CMRO$_2$
  - Sedation
  - Anterograde amnesia
  - Antiepileptic
  - Muscle relaxant

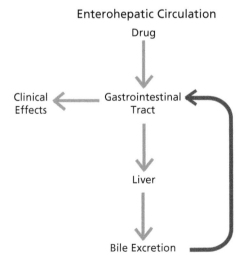

Figure 5.13

– Midazolam is more generally used due to more rapid amnesia, less active metabolites, and no pain on injection

Midazolam

- Clinical Indications
  - Pre-procedural sedation
    - Adult: 2–5 mg IV
    - Peds: 0.05–0.1 mg/kg IV
    - Peds: 0.5–1.0 mg/kg PO (Max 20 mg)
    - Peds: 0.2–0.3 mg/kg IN (Max 10 mg)
    - Peds: 0.2 mg/kg IM
  - Moderate sedation
    - Adult: 2–5 mg IV; titrate
    - Peds: 0.03–0.05 mg/kg IV (max 2 mg/dose) titrate
  - Antiepileptic
- Cerebral
  - ↓ CBF
  - ↓ $CMRO_2$
  - Sedation
  - Anterograde amnesia
  - Antiepileptic
  - Muscle relaxant
- Cardiovascular
  - Minimal
- Pulmonary
  - Minimal
- Renal
  - Minimal
- Hepatic
  - Primary site of metabolism
- Contraindications
  - Acute angle glaucoma
  - Hepatic dysfunction
- Board Facts
  - Midazolam has an active metabolite (α–hydroxymidazolam) which may build up in ESRD at a high dose or infusion

Remimazolam

- Clinical Indications
  - Pre-procedural sedation
    - 0.1–0.2 mg/kg IV
  - Anesthesia adjunct

  - 0.4–2.0 mg/kg/h IV
  - Antiepileptic
- Cerebral
  - ↓ CBF
  - ↓ $CMRO_2$
  - Sedation
  - Anterograde amnesia
  - Antiepileptic
  - Muscle relaxant
- Cardiovascular
  - Minimal
- Pulmonary
  - Minimal
- Renal
  - Minimal
- Hepatic
  - Minimal
- Contraindications
  - Acute angle glaucoma
- Board Facts
  - Approved by the FDA in 2020
  - Metabolized by esterases which allows for rapid offset independent of hepatic or renal function
  - Context sensitive half-time is ~5 minutes regardless of duration of infusion

Flumazenil

- Mechanism of Action
  - Benzodiazepine receptor antagonist on the GABA complex
- Clinical Indications
  - Mild benzodiazepine overdose
    - Airway still maintained
    - Adults: 0.1 mg IV every 2–5 minutes
    - Peds: 0.01 mg/kg (Max 0.1 mg) IV every 2–5 minutes
  - Severe benzodiazepine overdose
    - Apnea or severe hypopnea
    - Adults: 0.5 mg IV every 2–5 minutes
    - Peds: 0.05 mg/kg IV (Max 0.5 mg) every 2–5 minutes
- Contraindications
  - Epilepsy controlled by benzodiazepines
- Board Facts
  - Ensure prolonged post-procedure recovery to monitor for resedation
    - Especially with longer acting benzodiazepines
  - Flumazenil clinical half-life is about 30 minutes

5.6 Opioids

Opioid Receptor

- G-coupled protein receptor
- All opioids bind to the opioid receptor
- Receptor Subtypes
  - μ Receptor
    - o Analgesia
    - o Euphoria/addiction
    - o Nausea
    - o Respiratory depression
    - o Constipation
  - δ Receptor
    - o Analgesia
  - K Receptor
    - o Dysphoria
    - o Miosis

Equianalgesic

	Parenteral (mg)	Oral (mg)
Morphine	*10*	*30*
Hydromorphone	*1.5*	*7.5*
Fentanyl	*0.1*	*N/A*
Codeine	*100*	*200*
Alfentanil	*1*	*N/A*
Sufentanil	*0.01*	*N/A*

Morphine

- Clinical Indications
  - Analgesia
    - o Adult: 2.5–5 mg IV
    - o Peds: 0.05–0.2 mg/kg IV
  - Myocardial ischemia

- Cerebral
  - ↓ CBF
  - ↓ CMRO$_2$
  - Nausea
- Cardiovascular
  - Minimal
- Pulmonary
  - ↓ RR
  - ↓ TV
- Renal
  - Minimal
- Hepatic
  - Primary site of metabolism
- Contraindications
  - Asthma [34]
    - o Controversial
  - ↓ Renal activity
- Board Facts
  - ↑ Risk of PONV
  - Pruritus, more common with neuraxial opioids, can be treated with propofol, diphenhydramine, hydroxyzine, nalbuphine, or naloxone [35]
  - Active metabolites can accumulate in decreased renal function
    - o Morphine-6-glucuronide has analgesic activity [36]
    - o Morphine-3-glucuronide has neuroexcitatory effects [37]

Fentanyl

- Clinical Indications
  - Analgesia
    - o Adult: 25–100 mcg IV
    - o Peds: 0.5–1.0 mcg/kg IV
  - Myocardial ischemia
- Cerebral
  - ↓ CBF
  - ↓ CMRO$_2$
  - Nausea

- Cardiovascular
  - ↓ HR
    - Vagal effects
    - Central effects
  - ↓ MAP in the setting of hypovolemia
- Pulmonary
  - ↓ RR
  - ↓ TV
- Renal
  - Minimal
- Hepatic
  - Primary site of metabolism
- Contraindications
  - No "real" contraindications
- Board Facts
  - ↑ Risk of PONV
    - Less likely with fentanyl than morphine
  - Constipation is rare in an acute setting
  - Can cause chest wall rigidity especially at high doses
    - *Chest wall rigidity emergency covered on page 265*

Hydromorphone

- Clinical Indications
  - Analgesia
    - Adult: 0.2–1.0 mg IV
    - Peds: 0.10–0.15 mg/kg IV
- Cerebral
  - ↓ CBF
  - ↓ $CMRO_2$
  - Nausea
- Cardiovascular
  - Minimal
- Pulmonary
  - ↓ RR
  - ↓ TV
- Renal
  - Minimal
- Hepatic
  - Primary site of metabolism
- Contraindications
  - ↓ Renal activity
- Board Facts
  - Increased risk of PONV
  - Active metabolite can accumulate in decreased renal function
    - Hydromorphone-3-glucuronide and may lead to neuroexcitatory effects [38]

Remifentanil

- Clinical Indications
  - Analgesia adjunct
    - 0.04–0.2 mcg/kg/min IV
- Cerebral
  - Minimal decrease in CBF and $CMRO_2$ unless at high dosage [39]
  - Nausea not as pronounced as with other opioids [40]
- Cardiovascular
  - Minimal
  - Bolus
    - ↓ HR
      - Vagal effects
      - Central effects
- Pulmonary
  - ↓ RR
  - ↓ TV
- Renal
  - Minimal
- Hepatic
  - Minimal
- Contraindications
  - No "real" contraindications
- Board Facts
  - ↑ Risk of PONV
  - Metabolized by plasma and tissue esterases which allows for rapid offset not dictated by hepatic or renal function
  - Context sensitive half-time is ~5 minutes regardless of duration
  - Can cause chest wall rigidity even at low doses
    - *Chest wall rigidity emergency covered on page 265*

Naloxone

- Clinical Indications
  - Mild opioid overdose reversal
    - Airway maintained
    - Adults: 40 mcg IV every 2–5 minutes
    - Peds: 1–4 mcg/kg IV every 2–5 minutes
  - Severe opioid overdose reversal
    - Apnea or severe hypopnea
    - Adults: 400 mcg IV every 5 minutes
    - Peds: 10–20 mcg/kg IV every 5 minutes
- Contraindications
  - None

- Board Facts
  - Ensure prolonged post-procedure recovery to monitor for returning opioid affects
    o Especially with longer acting opioids
  - Naloxone half-life is about 60 minutes
  - Administration of naloxone can trigger acute pain especially if given after invasive procedure
    o Severe sudden HTN may result resulting in acute CHF

Other Opioids

- Methylnaltrexone
  - Opioid receptor antagonist that does not readily cross the BBB
  - Ideal for constipation treatment in chronic opioid users

- Hydrocodone
  - Metabolized to hydromorphone in the liver by P_{450} 2D6
- Codeine
  - Metabolized to morphine in the liver by enzyme P_{450} 2D6
    o Variable genetic metabolic rates (slow metabolizers, fast metabolizers) produce variable levels of morphine metabolite
  - Current black box warning and should be avoided as there are other medications with better safety profiles
- Meperidine
  - Meperidine toxicity with MAOIs can lead to serotonin syndrome [41]
  - Multiple black box warnings
  - Useful in treatment of postoperative shivering [42]
  - Current black box warning and should be avoided as there are other medications with better safety profiles

5.7 Non-opioid IV Analgesics

Ketamine

Already mentioned

Acetaminophen

- Mechanism of Action
  - Multifactorial
- Clinical Indications
  - Mild-moderate pain
    - Adult: 1000 mg PO/IV every 6 hours
      - Max daily dose: 3000–4000 mg
    - Peds: 15 mg/kg (Max 1000 mg) PO/IV every 6 hours
      - Max daily dose 2–12 years old: 75 mg/kg/d not to exceed 3750 mg
- Cerebral
  - Minimal
- Cardiovascular
  - Minimal
- Pulmonary
  - Minimal
- Renal
  - Minimal
- Hepatic
  - Primary site of metabolism
- Contraindications
  - Hepatic dysfunction
  - Alcoholics
- Board Facts
  - Acute liver failure with overdose (single or multiple dosing) is treated by n-acetylcysteine
  - Consider lower dosing or alternative treatment in those with alcohol abuse or hepatic dysfunction

Ketorolac

- *PO NSAIDS covered on page 88*
- Mechanism of Action
  - Nonselective COX inhibitor
- Clinical Indications
  - Mild-moderate pain
    - Adult: 15–30 mg IV
    - Peds: 0.5–1.0 mg/kg IV (Max 30 mg)
- Cerebral
  - Minimal
- Cardiovascular
  - Minimal
- Pulmonary
  - Minimal
- Renal
  - ↓ GFR
- Hepatic
  - Primary site of metabolism
- Contraindications
  - Allergy to NSAIDs
  - ↓ Kidney function
  - Platelet dysfunction
  - Bleeding disorders
  - Anticoagulation therapy
  - Ulcerative gastrointestinal disease
    - Peptic ulcers
    - Crohn's disease
    - Ulcerative colitis
  - Asthma
    - Controversial [43]
- Board Facts
  - ↑ Risk of postoperative bleeding
    - Debatable [44]
  - Ketorolac 30 mg = >10 mg morphine with less side effects [45, 46]

Dexmedetomidine

- Mechanism of Action
  - α_2 adrenergic receptor agonist
- Clinical Indications
  - Pre-procedural sedation
    - 1–2 mcg/kg IM
    - 1–3 mcg/kg IN

- Anesthesia adjunct
  ○ 0.1–0.3 mcg/kg IV
    • Important to infuse over 10 minutes to avoid bradycardia
  ○ 0.2–0.6 mcg/kg/h IV
- Postoperative delirium
- Cerebral
  - ↓ CBF
  - ↓ CMRO$_2$ [47]
- Cardiovascular
  - Bradycardia, especially after bolus dosing [48]
- Pulmonary
  - Minimal [49]
- Renal
  - Minimal
- Hepatic
  - Primary site of metabolism
- Contraindications
  - Myocardial dysfunction
- Board Facts
  - 1620 : 1 specificity for α_2 to α_1 [50]
  - Analgesic and anti-inflammatory properties [51]

5.8 Neuromuscular Monitoring

- Short-term paralysis is useful for intubation
- Longer procedural paralysis may be useful for controlled ventilation, lowering anesthesia dosage, and surgical relaxation
- It is always important to discuss with the surgeon neuromuscular blockade (paralysis) beyond the need for facilitation of endotracheal intubation as the surgical team may want to perform peripheral nerve testing

Clinical Evaluation

- Should not be used alone, but in conjunction with nerve monitoring
  - Sustained head lift longer than five seconds
  - Good grip strength
  - Adequate tidal volumes
  - An effective cough to clear secretions
  - A negative inspiratory force of -25 cm H_2O

Peripheral Nerve Stimulator

- Assists in qualitative assessment of neuromuscular blockade recovery
- Twitch
  - A single burst to a muscle group

- Tetanus
  - A sustained burst to a muscle group
- Train of Four
  - Four consecutive twitches
  - The most common method for evaluating neuromuscular blockade reversal (Figure 5.14)
- Fade
  - The presence of a decreased twitch response in the fourth twitch compared to the first twitch during train of four stimulation
- Post-Tetanic Twitch
  - Twitch stimulation immediately after tetanus stimulation
  - Exaggerates true neuromuscular recovery due to the recent stimulation of the muscle

Train of Four

- 0 Twitches indicates over >95% suppression
- 1 Twitch indicates 90–95% suppression
- 2 Twitches indicate 80–90% suppression
- 3 Twitches indicate 70–80% suppression
- 4 Twitches indicate 60–70% suppression
- The ratio of fade of the fourth twitch to the first twitch is the gold standard
  - Ideal to have at least 0.9 [52]

Twitch Response

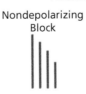
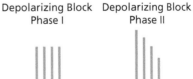

Normal Response   Nondepolarizing Block   Depolarizing Block Phase I   Depolarizing Block Phase II

Figure 5.14

Nerves

- Facial Nerve
  - Orbicularis oculi m.
    - Closes the eyelid
  - Facial nerve is a good indicator of pharyngeal neuro-muscular blockade
    - May be intrusive during head and neck procedures
- Tibial Nerve
  - Abductor hallucis m.
    - Hallux (big toe) dorsiflexion
  - Ideal for head and neck procedures with difficult access [53]
- Ulnar Nerve
  - Adductor pollicis m.
    - Adduction of the thumb
- Most to Least Resistant to Neuromuscular Blockade
  - Diaphragm m. = Laryngeal mm. > Orbicularis oculi m. (Facial n.) > Abductor hallucis m. (Tibial n.) > Adductor pollicis m. (Ulnar n.) [54]

Quantitative Neuromuscular Monitoring [60]

- Novel quantitative modalities to evaluate neuromuscular blockade
- Mechanomyography
  - Measures the force generated by a stimulated muscle
- Accelerometry
  - Measure the acceleration of a stimulated muscle
- Electromyography
  - Measures the sum of action potentials of a muscle following stimulation
- Phonomyography
  - Measures the low-frequency sounds emitted by a stimulated muscle

Factors Affecting Neuromuscular Blockade
(Figure 5.15)

Prolonged Block	Resistant to Block
Hypothermia	
Aminoglycosides	Hyperthermia
Tetracyclines	Phenytoin
Volatile Anesthetics	Carbamazepine
Local Anesthetics	Stroke
Magnesium	Myasthenia Gravis*
Lithium	Immobilization
Neuromuscular Weakness	Thermal Injury
Cholinesterase Inhibitors**	
Pseudocholinesterase Deficiency**	

*Patients with myasthenia gravis may display resistance to succinylcholine due to decreased receptors for the medication to act on. However, for patients who are on cholinesterase inhibitors could possibly see a prolonged block
**Will only affect succinylcholine, not nondepolarizing NMB

Figure 5.15 *Source:* Adapted from Lee et al. [55]; Motamed and Donati [56]; Blichfeldt-Lauridsen and Hansen [57]; Spacek et al. [58]; Ammundsen et al. [59].

5.9 Neuromuscular Blocking Agents

- Antagonize postsynaptic type 1 nicotinic acetylcholine receptors

Succinylcholine

- Clinical Indications
  - Rapid sequence intubation
    - 1.5–2.0 mg/kg IV
  - Intubation
    - 1.0–1.5 mg/kg IV (Figure 5.16)
  - Laryngospasm
    - 4 mg/kg IM
    - 0.1–2.0 mg/kg IV
      - Depending on degree of hypoxia, age, and comorbidities
- Cerebral
  - Minimal
- Cardiac
  - ↑ Risk of severe bradycardia in pediatrics, especially with second dose
- Pulmonary
  - ↓ RR
  - ↓ TV
  - Respiratory arrest
- Renal
  - Minimal

- Hepatic
  - Minimal
- Contraindications
  - Chronic trauma
    - Stroke
    - Burns
    - Spinal cord injuries
    - Debatable on how long the injury must be present to have hyperkalemic effects
  - Hyperkalemia
  - Parkinson's disease [61]
  - Muscular dystrophy
  - Malignant hyperthermia risk
  - Pseudocholinesterase deficiency
  - Emergency use only in pediatrics, with special precautions to males younger than age eight years of age, due to possibly undiagnosed muscular dystrophy and subsequent hyperkalemia
- Board Facts
  - Ok to use for open eye injuries [62]
  - Ok to use with cerebral palsy [63]
  - Dose on total body weight [64]
  - Muscle pain secondary to fasciculations
  - Metabolized by pseudocholinesterase
  - Pseudocholinesterase deficiency
    - Can do a clinical test which is measured by dibucaine and this measures the % amount that dibucaine can inhibit pseudocholinesterase
      - >80% inhibition
        - Normal
        - ~5-minute block
      - 20–80% inhibition
        - Heterozygous
        - ~20-minute block
      - <20% inhibition
        - Homozygous
        - ~3-hour block [65]
  - Acetylcholinesterase inhibitors can theoretically increase the duration of action by inhibiting pseudocholinesterase
    - Clinical relevance is debatable

Dose, Intubating, Duration of NMBs

	Intubating Dose (mg/kg)	Onset (Seconds)	Duration (Minutes)
Succinylcholine	1.0–1.5	60	10
Pancuronium*	0.1	200	60
Cisatracurium	0.1	150	45
Rocuronium	0.6–1.2	90	35
Vecuronium	0.1	120	35

* Not discussed this text

Figure 5.16

- o Donepezil
- o Rivastigmine
- o Galantamine
- o Tacrine
- o Edrophonium
- o Neostigmine
- – Consider using atropine in pediatrics to avoid succinylcholine-induced bradycardia
  - o Debatable [66]
- – FDA warning for patients who undergo cardiac arrest after administration and anesthetic overdose and inadequate ventilation are not causative, it is likely due to hyperkalemia and should be treated as such

Rocuronium

- Clinical Indications
  - – Rapid sequence intubation
    - o 1–1.2 mg/kg IV
  - – Intubation
    - o 0.6 mg/kg IV (Figure 5.16)
  - – Paralysis maintenance
    - o Adult: 10–20 mg IV
    - o Peds: 0.1–0.2 mg/kg IV
- Cerebral
  - – Minimal
- Cardiovascular
  - – Minimal
  - – Potential ↑ HR from weak vagolytic activity [67]
- Pulmonary
  - – ↓ RR
  - – ↓ TV
  - – Respiratory arrest
- Renal
  - – ~30% eliminated unchanged by the kidneys [68]
- Hepatic
  - – ~70% eliminated by the liver in bile [68]
- Contraindications
  - – Advanced renal disease
  - – Advanced hepatic disease
- Board Facts
  - – Priming dose may minimize fasciculations with succinylcholine, but will not prevent postoperative myalgia [69]

Vecuronium

- Clinical Indications
  - – Intubation
    - o 0.1 mg/kg IV (Figure 5.16)

- – Paralysis maintenance
  - o Adult: 1–2 mg IV
  - o Peds: 0.01–0.02 mcg/kg IV
- Cerebral
  - – Minimal
- Cardiovascular
  - – Minimal
- Respiratory
  - – ↓ RR
  - – ↓ TV
  - – Respiratory arrest
- Renal
  - – ~35% eliminated unchanged in the urine
- Hepatic
  - – ~50% eliminated by the liver in bile
- Contraindications
  - – Advanced renal disease
  - – Advanced hepatic disease
- Board Facts
  - – Metabolite 3-desacetyl vecuronium can cause sustained paralysis in renal failure

Cisatracurium

- Clinical Indications
  - – Intubation
    - o 0.1 mg/kg IV (Figure 5.16)
  - – Paralysis maintenance
    - o Adult: 1–2 mg IV
    - o Peds: 0.01–0.02 mcg/kg IV
- Cerebral [70]
  - – ↓ CBF
- Cardiovascular [70]
  - – ↓ CO
  - – ↓ MAP
  - – ↑ HR
- Pulmonary
  - – ↓ RR
  - – ↓ TV
  - – Respiratory arrest
- Renal
  - – Minimal
- Hepatic
  - – Minimal
- Contraindications
  - None
- Board Facts
  - – Less histamine release than atracurium
  - – Metabolized by nonspecific esterases and Hoffman degradation
  - – Laudanosine metabolite increases risk of seizures
    - o Produces less laudanosine than atracurium

5.10   Neuromuscular Reversal Agents

Sugammadex

- Mechanism of Action
  - Binds and antagonizes rocuronium and vecuronium
- Clinical Indications
  - Reversal of neuromuscular blockade
    - ○ Depends on the degree of blockade
    - ○ 2–4 mg/kg IV
  - Rapid reversal of neuromuscular blockade
    - ○ 16 mg/kg IV
- Cerebral
  - Minimal
- Cardiovascular
  - Case reports of bradycardia and PEA after administration
- Pulmonary
  - Possible acute bronchospasm from anaphylactoid reaction
- Renal
  - Eliminated unchanged by the kidneys
- Hepatic
  - Minimal
- Contraindications
  - Renal disease [27]
- Board Facts
  - Fastest neuromuscular blockade reversal agent [71]
  - Antimuscarinic coadministration is not necessary
  - ↓ Birth control efficacy [72]
  - After sugammadex administration, larger dose of rocuronium/vecuronium, cisatracurium or succinyl-choline will be required for re-paralysis
  - ↓ Incidence of PONV compared to neostigmine [73]

Neostigmine

- Neostigmine
- Pyridostigmine
- Edrophonium
- Physostigmine
- Mechanism of Action
  - Inhibits acetylcholinesterase

- Clinical Indications
  - Reversal of neuromuscular blockade
    - ○ Neostigmine
      - 0.02–0.08 mg/kg IV (Max dose 5 mg)
    - ○ Pyridostigmine
      - 0.1–0.25 mg/kg IV (Max dose 20 mg)
    - ○ Edrophonium
      - 0.5 mg/kg IV
    - ○ Physostigmine
      - 0.03–0.07 mg/kg IV [74]
- Cerebral
  - Physostigmine
    - ○ Only acetylcholinesterase inhibitor that can cross the blood–brain barrier
    - ○ Useful for the treatment of central anticholinergic syndrome
- Cardiovascular
  - Bradycardia
- Pulmonary
  - Bronchoconstriction
- Renal
  - Neostigmine
    - ○ ~50% eliminated by renal excretion
- Hepatic
  - Primary site of metabolism
- Contraindications
  - Advanced renal disease
  - Profound neuromuscular blockade
- Board Facts
  - Acetylcholinesterase inhibitors must be administered with anticholinergics (antimuscarinics) to avoid bradycardia and other parasympathetic effects
  - Onset fast to slow
    - ○ Edrophonium > Neostigmine > Pyridostigmine
  - Anticholinesterase inhibitors cross the placenta and can lead to fetal bradycardia
    - ○ Prevent with atropine coadministration
  - As physostigmine can cross the BBB, it can be useful in treating central anticholinergic effects

Atropine

- Mechanism of Action
  - Muscarinic receptor antagonist
- Clinical Indications
  - *ACLS indications covered on page 146*
  - Coadministration with neuromuscular reversal
    - 2.0–12 mcg/kg IV (Max 1 mg)
- Cerebral
  - May present as excitation or sedation in high doses
- Cardiovascular
  - ↑ CO
  - ↑ HR
  - Low-dose atropine may cause bradycardia [75]
- Pulmonary
  - Bronchodilator
  - ↓ Secretions and thicken them
- Renal
  - Minimal
- Hepatic
  - Primary site of metabolism
- Contraindications
  - Significant cardiac disease
  - Acute angle glaucoma
  - Cardiac transplantation due to denervation
    - Paradoxical bradycardia can occur [76]
- Board Facts
  - Atropine coadministration with neostigmine can prevent fetal bradycardia as both cross the placenta

Glycopyrrolate

- Mechanism of Action
  - Muscarinic receptor antagonist
- Clinical Indications
  - Coadministration with neuromuscular reversal
    - 2.0–12 mcg/kg IV (Max 1 mg)
- Cerebral
  - Minimal
- Cardiovascular
  - ↑ CO
  - ↑ HR
- Pulmonary
  - Bronchodilator
  - Thicker, decreased secretions
- Renal
  - Minimal
- Hepatic
  - Primary site of metabolism
- Contraindications
  - Significant cardiac disease
  - Acute angle glaucoma
  - Cardiac transplantation due to denervation
    - Paradoxical bradycardia can occur [76]
- Board Facts
  - Does not cross BBB or placenta

5.11   Hypertensive Agents

Phenylephrine

- Mechanism of Action
  - α_1 adrenergic receptor agonist (Figure 5.17)
- Clinical Indications
  - Mild-moderate hypotension
    - Adult: 100–200 mcg IV
    - Peds: 1–5 mcg/kg IV
    - Infusion: 0.05–0.7 mcg/kg/min IV
- Cerebral
  - ↓ CBF
- Cardiovascular
  - ↑ MAP
  - Baroreflex-induced bradycardia
  - ↓ CO
- Pulmonary
  - ↑ PAP [78, 79]
- Renal
  - ↓ RBF
- Hepatic
  - Partial metabolism
- Contraindications
  - Hypotension in the setting of bradycardia as can further worsen bradycardia
- Board Facts
  - Metabolized primarily by monoamine oxidase
  - Extravasation can lead to tissue necrosis

Norepinephrine

- Mechanism of Action
  - Primarily α_1, modest β_1, and β_2 adrenergic receptor agonist (Figure 5.17)
- Clinical Indications
  - Moderate-severe hypotension
    - Adult: 5–15 mcg IV
    - Peds: 0.05–0.2 mcg/kg IV
    - Infusion: 0.1–0.5 mcg/kg/min IV
- Cerebral
  - Minimal [80]
- Cardiovascular
  - ↑ MAP
  - Minimal HR change
  - ↑ CO
- Pulmonary
  - ↑ PAP [78]
- Renal
  - Minimal [81]
- Hepatic
  - Minimal [82]
- Contraindications
  - No "real" contraindications
- Board Facts
  - Does not cause baroreflex-induced bradycardia due to subsequent mild β_1 stimulation
  - Eliminated by reuptake and metabolized by monoamine oxidase and COMT

Epinephrine

- Mechanism of Action
  - α_1, β_1, and β_2 adrenergic receptor agonist (Figure 5.17)
- Clinical Indications
  - Moderate-severe hypotension
    - Adult: 10–100 mcg IV
    - Peds: 0.1–1 mcg/kg IV
    - Infusion: 0.1–0.5 mcg/kg/min IV

Receptor Agonism

	α_1	β_1	β_2	VR*
Phenylephrine	++++	–	–	–
Norepinephrine	+++	++	+	–
Epinephrine	++	++	++	–
Ephedrine	++	++	++	–
Vasopressin	–	–	–	++++

*Vasopressin receptor

Figure 5.17   *Source:* Adapted from McPherson et al. [77].

- Moderate-severe allergic reaction
  - 1 mcg/kg IV; increase and repeat as needed
  - Adult: 300 mcg IM (Figure 5.18)
  - Peds: 150 mcg IM (Figure 5.18)
- Bradycardia
  - Second-line pharmacologic treatment behind atropine in ACLS Bradycardia Algorithm
  - Adult: 10–20 mcg IV
  - Peds: 0.1–1 mcg/kg IV
- Bronchospasm
  - 0.1–1 mcg/kg IV
- Cardiac arrest
  - Adult: 1 mg IV q3–5 minutes
  - Peds: 10 mcg/kg IV q3–5 minutes (Max 1 mg)
- Cerebral
  - Variable effect on CBF [83, 84]
- Cardiovascular
  - ↑ MAP
  - ↑ HR
  - ↑ CO
- Pulmonary
  - Bronchodilation
- Renal
  - ↓ RBF
- Hepatic
  - Minimal
- Contraindications
  - Myocardial infarction with a pulse
  - Coadministration with nonselective beta blockers can cause hypertensive crisis
  - Coadministration with alpha-1 antagonists, phenothiazines, butyrophenones can cause hypotension (epinephrine reversal)
- Board Facts
  - More useful in treating bradycardia in transplanted hearts/denervated hearts than anticholinergics as β_1 is still intact on the myocardium [85]
  - Can be given endotracheally

Autoinjector Dosing

Pediatrics 150 mcg Autoinjector 10–30 kg (25–66 lbs)
Adults 300 mcg Autoinjector >20 kg (>66 lbs)

Figure 5.18

- Eliminated by reuptake and metabolized by monoamine oxidase and COMT
- In the event an adult epi pen is only what is available, they can safely be used in kids

Ephedrine

- Mechanism of Action (Figure 5.17)
  - α_1, β_1, and β_2 adrenergic receptor agonist
  - Indirect release of norepinephrine from postsynaptic neurons with some direct action
- Clinical Indications
  - Mild-moderate hypotension
    - Adult: 5–20 mg IV
    - Peds: 0.1–0.2 mcg/kg IV
- Cerebral
  - ↑ CBF [86]
- Cardiovascular
  - ↑ MAP
  - ↑ HR
  - ↑ CO
- Pulmonary
  - Bronchodilation
  - ↑ PAP [79]
- Renal
  - Minimal
- Hepatic
  - Minimal
- Contraindications
  - Coadministration with monoamine oxidase inhibitors
  - Pulmonary hypertension
- Board Facts
  - Tachyphylaxis can occur after multiple uses
  - Metabolized by monoamine oxidase and COMT
  - Antiemetic properties when given IM [87]

Vasopressin

- Mechanism of Action
  - Vasopressin receptor agonist (Figure 5.17)
    - Directly contracts vascular smooth muscle
    - ↑ Water reabsorption in the kidneys
- Clinical Indications
  - Refractory/severe hypotension
    - Adults: 1–4 units IV
    - Infusion 0.01–0.04 units/min IV
- Cerebral
  - ↓ CBF

- Cardiovascular
  - ↑ MAP
  - Baroreflex-induced bradycardia
- Pulmonary
  - Minimal [88]
- Renal
  - ↓ RBF [89]
- Hepatic
  - Primary site of metabolism
  - ↓ HBF [89]

- Contraindications
  - No "real" contraindications
- Board Facts
  - Generally used in cases of refractory hypotension where previous attempts to treat were not successful
  - Could lead to dilutional hyponatremia

5.12   Antihypertensive Agents

- Many of the following agents can also play a role in hypotensive anesthesia

Clevidipine

- Mechanism of Action
  - Dihydropyridine calcium channel antagonist (Figure 5.19)
- Clinical Indications
  - Hypertension
    - Infusion: 1–2 mg/h
- Cerebral
  - Minimal [90]

- Cardiovascular
  - ↓ MAP
  - Minimal effect on CO
- Pulmonary
  - ↓ PVR [91]
- Renal
  - Minimal
- Hepatic
  - Minimal
- Contraindications
  - No "real" contraindications
- Board Facts
  - Metabolized by plasma and tissue esterases
  - Ideal to use in patients with renal or hepatic dysfunction

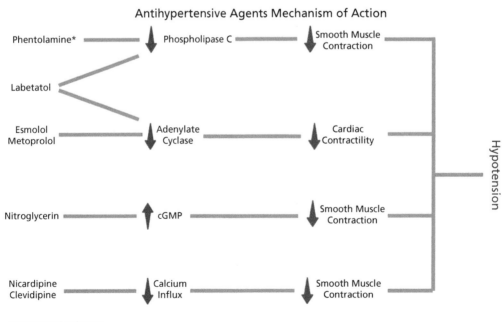

Figure 5.19

Esmolol

- Mechanism of Action
  - β_1 receptor antagonist (Figure 5.19)
- Clinical Indications
  - Tachycardia with a pulse
    - Adult: 10–50 mg IV
  - Brief sympathetic hemodynamic control
    - Adult: 10–50 mg IV
- Cerebral
  - Minimal
- Cardiovascular
  - ↓ CO
  - ↓ HR
- Pulmonary
  - Minimal
- Renal
  - Minimal
- Hepatic
  - Minimal
- Contraindications
  - Long-term hemodynamic control
  - Bradycardia
  - Cardiac conduction delays
  - WPW syndrome
- Board Facts
  - ↓ PONV
  - ↓ Postoperative pain [92]
  - Rapid metabolism by esterases in RBCs

Metoprolol

- Mechanism of Action
  - β_1 receptor antagonist (Figure 5.19)
- Clinical Indications
  - Stable atrial fibrillation
    - Adult: Metoprolol 2.5–5 mg IV (Max 15 mg)
  - Stable atrial flutter
    - Adult: Metoprolol 2.5–5 mg IV (Max 15 mg)
  - Stable AVNRT/AVRT
    - Adult: Metoprolol 2.5–5 mg IV (Max 15 mg)
- Cerebral
  - Minimal
- Cardiovascular
  - ↓ CO
  - ↓ HR
- Pulmonary
  - Minimal
- Renal
  - Minimal

- Hepatic
  - Primary site of metabolism
- Contraindications
  - Bradycardia
  - Cardiac conduction delays
  - WPW syndrome
- Board Facts
  - Beta blockade made mask hypoglycemia symptoms in diabetics

Labetalol

- Mechanism of Action
  - α_1, β_1, and β_2 adrenergic receptor antagonist (Figure 5.19)
- Clinical Indications
  - Hypertension
    - Adult: 5–20 mg IV
- Cerebral
  - Minimal [93]
- Cardiovascular
  - ↓ MAP
  - ↓ HR
  - ↓ CO
- Pulmonary
  - Bronchoconstriction [94, 95]
  - ↓ PVR
- Renal
  - Minimal
- Hepatic
  - Primary site of metabolism
- Contraindications
  - Bradycardia
  - Asthma [94]
- Board Facts
  - Ideal to use in the setting of hypertension with tachycardia due to the β_1 antagonism
  - β_2 antagonism may exacerbate asthma

Nicardipine

- Mechanism of Action
  - Dihydropyridine calcium channel antagonist (Figure 5.19)
- Clinical Indications
  - Hypertension
    - Adult: 100–500 mcg IV
    - Infusion: 1–5 mcg/kg/min
- Cerebral
  - ↑ CBF [96]

- Cardiovascular
  - ↓ MAP
  - Minimal effect on CO [97]
- Pulmonary
  - ↓ PVR [98]
- Renal
  - ↑ RBF [99]
- Hepatic
  - Primary site of metabolism
  - ↑ HBF [100]
- Contraindications
  - No "real" contraindications
- Board Facts
  - Inhibitor of P_{450} system [101]

Hydralazine

- Mechanism of action
  - Direct-acting vasodilator primarily on arterioles
  - Exact mechanism is not well established
- Clinical Indications
  - Hypertension
    o Adults: 5–20 mg IV
- Cerebral
  - ↑ CBF [102]
- Cardiovascular
  - ↓ MAP
  - Baroreflex-induced tachycardia
  - ↑ CO [103]
- Pulmonary
  - ↓ PVR [104]
- Renal
  - ↑ RBF [105]
- Hepatic
  - Primary site of metabolism

- Contraindications
  - Tachycardia
- Board Facts
  - Slow onset
  - Can cause drug-induced lupus [106]

Nitroglycerin

- Mechanism of Action
  - Inhibits vascular smooth muscle contraction (Figure 5.19)
- Clinical Indications
  - Myocardial ischemia
    o Adult: 0.3–0.6 mg SL
    o Adult: 25–50 mcg IV
    o Infusion: 1–40 mcg/min IV
  - Hypertension
    o Adult: 25–50 mcg IV
    o Infusion: 1–40 mcg/min IV
- Cerebral
  - ↑ CBF
- Cardiovascular [107]
  - ↓ MAP
  - Minimal effect on HR
  - ↓ CO
- Pulmonary
  - ↓ PVR [107]
- Renal
  - Minimal
- Hepatic
  - Primary site of metabolism
- Contraindications
  - Coadministration with phosphodiesterase inhibitors like sildenafil
  - Myocardial ischemia in the setting of hypotension
- Board Facts
  - Inhibits platelet aggregation

5.13 Antidysrhythmics

- *Esmolol and metoprolol discussed on page 143*
- See Figure 4.12 for antidysrhythmics classifications

Adenosine

- Mechanism of Action
  - Adenosine receptor agonist
- Clinical Indications
  - Stable AVNRT/AVRT
    - First dose
      - Adult: 6 mg IV
      - Peds: 0.1 mg/kg IV
    - Second dose
      - Adult: 12 mg IV
      - Peds: 0.2 mg/kg IV
- Cerebral
  - Minimal
- Cardiovascular
  - Transient conduction cessation at the SA and AV node
  - ↓ MAP
  - ↓ HR
  - ↓ CO
- Pulmonary
  - Bronchoconstriction
- Renal
  - Minimal
- Hepatic
  - Minimal
- Contraindications
  - Any rhythm that is not AVRT/AVNRT
  - WPW syndrome
  - Asthma
- Board Facts
  - Rapid injection following by a saline flush
  - Raise limb to facilitate adenosine movement into central circulation
  - If AVRT/AVNRT rhythm does not terminate after second dose of adenosine, consider monomorphic ventricular tachycardia

- Methylxanthines antagonize adenosine requiring an increased dose
- Carbamazepine and dipyridamole potentiate adenosine action and thus require a reduced dose [108]
- Transplanted hearts/denervated hearts require a reduced dose [109]

Amiodarone

- Mechanism of Action
  - Na^+, K^+, and Ca^{2+} channel antagonist (Figure 4.12)
- Clinical Indications
  - VF/pulseless VT
    - First dose
      - Adult: 300 mg IV
      - Peds: 5 mg/kg IV
    - Second dose
      - Adult: 150 mg IV
      - Peds 2.5 mg/kg IV
  - Stable wide QRS tachycardia with a pulse
    - Adult: 150 mg IV over 10 minutes
    - Peds: 5 mg/kg IV over 20–60 minutes
  - Atrial fibrillation
- Cerebral
  - Minimal
- Cardiovascular [110]
  - ↓ MAP
  - Minimal change in HR
  - ↑ CO
- Pulmonary
  - Pulmonary fibrosis (in chronic use)
- Renal
  - ↓ RBF [111]
  - Renal toxicity [112]
- Hepatic
  - Primary site of metabolism
  - Hepatic toxicity (primarily with chronic use) [113]
- Contraindications
  - Pregnancy

- – Renal pathology
- – Pulmonary pathology
- – Hepatic pathology
- – Thyroid pathology
- Board Facts
  - – Chronic use may cause blue–gray skin discoloration and toxic toxicity [114, 115]
    - o Amiodarone toxicity is mostly related to chronic oral, rarely occurs with acute administration

Atropine

- Mechanism of Action
  - – Muscarinic receptor antagonist
- Clinical Indications
  - – Bradycardia with a pulse
    - o Adult: 0.5 mg IV (Max 3 mg)
    - o Peds: 0.02 mg/kg IV (Max 1 mg)
    - o Peds: 0.02 mg/kg IM
  - – Coadministration with neuromuscular reversal
    - o *Neuromuscular reversal covered on page 138*
- Cerebral
  - – May present as excitation or sedation in high doses
- Cardiovascular
  - – ↑ CO
  - – ↑ HR
  - – Low-dose atropine may cause bradycardia [75]
- Pulmonary
  - – Bronchodilator
  - – ↓ Secretions and thicken them
- Renal
  - – Minimal
- Hepatic
  - – Primary site of metabolism
- Contraindications
  - – Acute angle glaucoma
  - – Cardiac transplantation due to denervation
    - o Paradoxical bradycardia can occur [76]
- Board Facts
  - – Crosses placenta and BBB

Diltiazem

- Mechanism of Action
  - – Non-dihydropyridine calcium channel antagonist (Figure 4.12)
- Clinical Indications
  - – Stable atrial flutter
    - o 5–10 mg IV; Titrate, Max 50 mg
      - 0.25 mg/kg initial; 0.35 mg/kg next

- – Stable atrial fibrillation
  - o 5–10 mg IV; Titrate, Max 50 mg
    - 0.25 mg/kg initial; 0.35 mg/kg next
- – Stable AVNRT/AVRT
  - o 5–10 mg IV; Titrate, Max 50 mg
    - 0.25 mg/kg initial; 0.35 mg/kg next
- Cerebral
  - – ↑ CBF
- Cardiovascular
  - – ↑ CO
  - – ↓ HR
  - – ↓ MAP
- Pulmonary
  - – Minimal
- Renal
  - – Minimal
- Hepatic
  - – Primary site of metabolism
- Contraindications
  - – WPW syndrome
  - – Bradycardia
  - – Cardiac conduction delays
- Board Facts
  - – Gingival overgrowth is generally caused by chronic administration [116]
  - – Diltiazem can increase blood digoxin levels [117]

Verapamil

- Mechanism of Action
  - – Non-dihydropyridine calcium channel antagonist (Figure 4.12)
- Clinical Indications
  - – Stable atrial flutter
    - o 2.5–5 mg IV; Titrate to max 20 mg
  - – Stable AVNRT/AVRT
    - o 2.5–5 mg IV; Titrate to max 20 mg
- Cerebral
  - – ↑ CBF
- Cardiovascular [118]
  - – ↓ CO
  - – ↓ HR
  - – ↓ MAP
- Pulmonary
  - – Minimal
- Renal
  - – Minimal
- Hepatic
  - – ↑ HBF [119]
- Contraindications
  - – WPW syndrome

- Bradycardia
- Cardiac conduction delays
- Board Facts

        – Gingival overgrowth is generally caused by chronic administration [120]
        – Inhibitor of P_{450} system [121]

References

1 Peck, T.E. and Harris, B. (2021). *Pharmacology for Anaesthesia and Intensive Care*, 5e. Cambridge University Press.

2 Aranake, A., Mashour, G.A., and Avidan, M.S. (2013). Minimum alveolar concentration: ongoing relevance and clinical utility. *Anaesthesia* 68 (5): 512–522. https://doi.org/10.1111/anae.12168.

3 Cameron, C.B., Robinson, S., and Gregory, G.A. (1984). The minimum anesthetic concentration of isoflurane in children. *Anesth. Analg.* 63 (4): 418–420.

4 Ekberg, E., Nilsson, I.M., Michelotti, A. et al. (2023). Diagnostic criteria for temporomandibular disorders – INfORM recommendations: comprehensive and short-form adaptations for adolescents. *J. Oral Rehabil.* https://doi.org/10.1111/joor.13488.

5 Fu, A.D., McDonald, H.R., Eliott, D. et al. (2002). Complications of general anesthesia using nitrous oxide in eyes with preexisting gas bubbles. *Retina* 22 (5): 569–574. https://doi.org/10.1097/00006982-200210000-00006.

6 Nagele, P., Brown, F., Francis, A. et al. (2013). Influence of nitrous oxide anesthesia, B-vitamins, and MTHFR gene polymorphisms on perioperative cardiac events: the vitamins in nitrous oxide (VINO) randomized trial. *Anesthesiology* 119 (1): 19–28. https://doi.org/10.1097/ALN.0b013e31829761e3.

7 Hathout, L. and El-Saden, S. (2011). Nitrous oxide-induced B_{12} deficiency myelopathy: perspectives on the clinical biochemistry of vitamin B_{12}. *J. Neurol. Sci.* 301 (1–2): 1–8. https://doi.org/10.1016/j.jns.2010.10.033.

8 Divatia, J.V., Vaidya, J.S., Badwe, R.A., and Hawaldar, R.W. (1996). Omission of nitrous oxide during anesthesia reduces the incidence of postoperative nausea and vomiting. A meta-analysis. *Anesthesiology* 85 (5): 1055–1062. https://doi.org/10.1097/00000542-199611000-00014.

9 Combes, X., Schauvliege, F., Peyrouset, O. et al. (2001). Intracuff pressure and tracheal morbidity: influence of filling with saline during nitrous oxide anesthesia. *Anesthesiology* 95 (5): 1120–1124. https://doi.org/10.1097/00000542-200111000-00015.

10 Brioni, J.D., Varughese, S., Ahmed, R., and Bein, B. (2017). A clinical review of inhalation anesthesia with sevoflurane: from early research to emerging topics. *J. Anesth.* 31 (5): 764–778. https://doi.org/10.1007/s00540-017-2375-6.

11 Torri, G. (2010). Inhalation anesthetics: a review. *Minerva Anestesiol.* 76 (3): 215–228.

12 Tanaka, S., Tsuchida, H., Nakabayashi, K. et al. (1996). The effects of sevoflurane, isoflurane, halothane, and enflurane on hemodynamic responses during an inhaled induction of anesthesia via a mask in humans. *Anesth. Analg.* 82 (4): 821–826. https://doi.org/10.1097/00000539-199604000-00025.

13 Tateishi, T., Asoh, M., Nakura, H. et al. (1999). Carbamazepine induces multiple cytochrome P450 subfamilies in rats. *Chem. Biol. Interact.* 117 (3): 257–268. https://doi.org/10.1016/s0009-2797(98)00110-0.

14 Frink, E.J., Morgan, S.E., Coetzee, A. et al. (1992). The effects of sevoflurane, halothane, enflurane, and isoflurane on hepatic blood flow and oxygenation in chronically instrumented greyhound dogs. *Anesthesiology* 76 (1): 85–90. https://doi.org/10.1097/00000542-199201000-00013.

15 Agnew, N.M., Pennefather, S.H., and Russell, G.N. (2002). Isoflurane and coronary heart disease. *Anaesthesia* 57 (4): 338–347. https://doi.org/10.1046/j.1365-2044.2002.02469.x.

16 Burchardi, H. and Kaczmarczyk, G. (1994). The effect of anaesthesia on renal function. *Eur. J. Anaesthesiol.* 11 (3): 163–168.

17 Merin, R.G., Bernard, J.M., Doursout, M.F. et al. (1991). Comparison of the effects of isoflurane and desflurane on cardiovascular dynamics and regional blood flow in the chronically instrumented dog. *Anesthesiology* 74 (3): 568–574. https://doi.org/10.1097/00000542-199103000-00027.

18 von Ungern-Sternberg, B.S., Saudan, S., Petak, F. et al. (2008). Desflurane but not sevoflurane impairs airway and respiratory tissue mechanics in children with susceptible airways. *Anesthesiology* 108 (2): 216–224. https://doi.org/10.1097/01.anes.0000299430.90352.d5.

19 Keijzer, C., Perez, R.S., and de Lange, J.J. (2005). Carbon monoxide production from desflurane and six types of carbon dioxide absorbents in a patient model. *Acta Anaesthesiol. Scand.* 49 (6): 815–818. https://doi.org/10.1111/j.1399-6576.2005.00690.x.

20 de Oliveira, G.S., Girao, W., Fitzgerald, P.C., and McCarthy, R.J. (2013). The effect of sevoflurane versus desflurane on the incidence of upper respiratory morbidity in patients undergoing general anesthesia with a Laryngeal Mask Airway: a meta-analysis of randomized controlled trials. *J. Clin. Anesth.* 25 (6): 452–458. https://doi.org/10.1016/j.jclinane.2013.03.012.

21 Varughese, S. and Ahmed, R. (2021). Environmental and occupational considerations of anesthesia: a narrative review and update. *Anesth. Analg.* 133 (4): 826–835. https://doi.org/10.1213/ANE.0000000000005504.

22 Li, F. and Yuan, Y. (2015). Meta-analysis of the cardioprotective effect of sevoflurane versus propofol during cardiac surgery. *BMC Anesthesiol.* 15: 128. https://doi.org/10.1186/s12871-015-0107-8.

23 Zhou, S.F. (2008). Drugs behave as substrates, inhibitors and inducers of human cytochrome P450 3A4. *Curr. Drug Metab.* 9 (4): 310–322. https://doi.org/10.2174/138920008784220664.

24 Lynch, T. and Price, A. (2007). The effect of cytochrome P450 metabolism on drug response, interactions, and adverse effects. *Am. Fam. Physician* 76 (3): 391–396.

25 Gershman, H. and Steeper, J. (1991). Rate of clearance of ethanol from the blood of intoxicated patients in the emergency department. *J. Emerg. Med.* 9 (5): 307–311. https://doi.org/10.1016/0736-4679(91)90371-l.

26 Mather, L.E. (1983). Clinical pharmacokinetics of fentanyl and its newer derivatives. *Clin. Pharmacokinet.* 8 (5): 422–446. https://doi.org/10.2165/00003088-198308050-00004.

27 Staals, L.M., Snoeck, M.M., Driessen, J.J. et al. (2010). Reduced clearance of rocuronium and sugammadex in patients with severe to end-stage renal failure: a pharmacokinetic study. *Br. J. Anaesth.* 104 (1): 31–39. https://doi.org/10.1093/bja/aep340.

28 Asserhøj, L.L., Mosbech, H., Krøigaard, M., and Garvey, L.H. (2016). No evidence for contraindications to the use of propofol in adults allergic to egg, soy or peanut†. *Br. J. Anaesth.* 116 (1): 77–82. https://doi.org/10.1093/bja/aev360.

29 King, S.Y., Davis, F.M., Wells, J.E. et al. (1992). Lidocaine for the prevention of pain due to injection of propofol. *Anesth. Analg.* 74 (2): 246–249. https://doi.org/10.1213/00000539-199202000-00013.

30 Raoof, A.A., van Obbergh, L.J., de Ville de Goyet, J., and Verbeeck, R.K. (1996). Extrahepatic glucuronidation of propofol in man: possible contribution of gut wall and kidney. *Eur. J. Clin. Pharmacol.* 50 (1–2): 91–96. https://doi.org/10.1007/s002280050074.

31 Corssen, G., Little, S.C., and Tavakoli, M. (1974). Ketamine and epilepsy. *Anesth. Analg.* 53 (2): 319–335.

32 Kurdi, M.S., Sushma, K.S., Ranjana, R., and Kiran, P.B. (2017). Ketamine: a convulsant? *Anesth. Essays Res.* 11 (1): 272–273. https://doi.org/10.4103/0259-1162.200241.

33 Komatsu, R., You, J., Mascha, E.J. et al. (2013). Anesthetic induction with etomidate, rather than propofol, is associated with increased 30-day mortality and cardiovascular morbidity after noncardiac surgery. *Anesth. Analg.* 117 (6): 1329–1337. https://doi.org/10.1213/ANE.0b013e318299a516.

34 Mitchell, H.S. and Dejong, J.D. (1954). The effect of morphine on bronchial muscle. *J. Allergy* 25 (4): 302–305. https://doi.org/10.1016/0021-8707(54)90130-6.

35 George, R.B., Allen, T.K., and Habib, A.S. (2009). Serotonin receptor antagonists for the prevention and treatment of pruritus, nausea, and vomiting in women undergoing cesarean delivery with intrathecal morphine: a systematic review and meta-analysis. *Anesth. Analg.* 109 (1): 174–182. https://doi.org/10.1213/ane.0b013e3181a45a6b.

36 Abdallah, C. (2014). Considerations in perioperative assessment of valproic acid coagulopathy. *J. Anaesthesiol. Clin. Pharmacol.* 30 (1): 7–9. https://doi.org/10.4103/0970-9185.125685.

37 Smith, M.T. (2000). Neuroexcitatory effects of morphine and hydromorphone: evidence implicating the 3-glucuronide metabolites. *Clin. Exp. Pharmacol. Physiol.* 27 (7): 524–528. https://doi.org/10.1046/j.1440-1681.2000.03290.x.

38 Wright, A.W., Mather, L.E., and Smith, M.T. (2001). Hydromorphone-3-glucuronide: a more potent neuro-excitant than its structural analogue, morphine-3-glucuronide. *Life Sci.* 69 (4): 409–420. https://doi.org/10.1016/s0024-3205(01)01133-x.

39 Paris, A., Scholz, J., von Knobelsdorff, G. et al. (1998). The effect of remifentanil on cerebral blood flow velocity. *Anesth. Analg.* 87 (3): 569–573. https://doi.org/10.1097/00000539-199809000-00013.

40 Rama-Maceiras, P., Ferreira, T.A., Molíns, N. et al. (2005). Less postoperative nausea and vomiting after propofol + remifentanil versus propofol + fentanyl anaesthesia during plastic surgery. *Acta Anaesthesiol. Scand.* 49 (3): 305–311. https://doi.org/10.1111/j.1399-6576.2005.00650.x.

41 Rogers, K.J. and Thornton, J.A. (1969). The interaction between monoamine oxidase inhibitors and narcotic analgesics in mice. *Br. J. Pharmacol.* 36 (3): 470–480. https://doi.org/10.1111/j.1476-5381.1969.tb08003.x.

42 Kurz, A., Ikeda, T., Sessler, D.I. et al. (1997). Meperidine decreases the shivering threshold twice as much as the vasoconstriction threshold. *Anesthesiology* 86 (5): 1046–1054. https://doi.org/10.1097/00000542-199705000-00007.

43 Haddow, G.R., Riley, E., Isaacs, R., and McSharry, R. (1993). Ketorolac, nasal polyposis, and bronchial asthma: a cause for concern. *Anesth. Analg.* 76 (2): 420–422.

44 Gobble, R.M., Hoang, H.L.T., Kachniarz, B., and Orgill, D.P. (2014). Ketorolac does not increase perioperative bleeding: a meta-analysis of randomized controlled trials. *Plast. Reconstr. Surg.* 133 (3): 741–755. https://doi.org/10.1097/01.prs.0000438459.60474.b5.

45 Watcha, M.F., Jones, M.B., Lagueruela, R.G. et al. (1992). Comparison of ketorolac and morphine as adjuvants during pediatric surgery. *Anesthesiology* 76 (3): 368–372. https://doi.org/10.1097/00000542-199203000-00008.

46 Jelinek, G.A. (2000). Ketorolac versus morphine for severe pain. Ketorolac is more effective, cheaper, and has fewer side effects. *BMJ* 321 (7271): 1236–1237. https://doi.org/10.1136/bmj.321.7271.1236.

47 Drummond, J.C., Dao, A.V., Roth, D.M. et al. (2008). Effect of dexmedetomidine on cerebral blood flow velocity, cerebral metabolic rate, and carbon dioxide response in normal humans. *Anesthesiology* 108 (2): 225–232. https://doi.org/10.1097/01.anes.0000299576.00302.4c.

48 Gong, M., Man, Y., and Fu, Q. (2017). Incidence of bradycardia in pediatric patients receiving dexmedetomidine anesthesia: a meta-analysis. *Int. J. Clin. Pharm.* 39 (1): 139–147. https://doi.org/10.1007/s11096-016-0411-5.

49 Hsu, Y.W., Cortinez, L.I., Robertson, K.M. et al. (2004). Dexmedetomidine pharmacodynamics: part I: crossover comparison of the respiratory effects of dexmedetomidine and remifentanil in healthy volunteers. *Anesthesiology* 101 (5): 1066–1076. https://doi.org/10.1097/00000542-200411000-00005.

50 Gertler, R., Brown, H.C., Mitchell, D.H., and Silvius, E.N. (2001). Dexmedetomidine: a novel sedative-analgesic agent. *Proc. (Bayl. Univ. Med. Cent.)* 14 (1): 13–21. https://doi.org/10.1080/08998280.2001.11927725.

51 Li, S., Yang, Y., Yu, C. et al. (2015). Dexmedetomidine analgesia effects in patients undergoing dental implant surgery and its impact on postoperative inflammatory and oxidative stress. *Oxidative Med. Cell. Longev.* 2015: 186736. https://doi.org/10.1155/2015/186736.

52 Lien, C.A. and Kopman, A.F. (2014). Current recommendations for monitoring depth of neuromuscular blockade. *Curr. Opin. Anaesthesiol.* 27 (6): 616–622. https://doi.org/10.1097/ACO.0000000000000132.

53 Fuchs-Buder, T., Schreiber, J.U., and Meistelman, C. (2009). Monitoring neuromuscular block: an update. *Anaesthesia* 64 (Suppl 1): 82–89. https://doi.org/10.1111/j.1365-2044.2008.05874.x.

54 Hemmerling, T.M., Schmidt, J., Hanusa, C. et al. (2000). Simultaneous determination of neuromuscular block at the larynx, diaphragm, adductor pollicis, orbicularis oculi and corrugator supercilii muscles. *Br. J. Anaesth.* 85 (6): 856–860. https://doi.org/10.1093/bja/85.6.856.

55 Lee, J.H., Lee, S.I., Chung, C.J. et al. (2013). The synergistic effect of gentamicin and clindamycin on rocuronium-induced neuromuscular blockade. *Korean J. Anesthesiol.* 64 (2): 143–151. https://doi.org/10.4097/kjae.2013.64.2.143.

56 Motamed, C. and Donati, F. (2002). Sevoflurane and isoflurane, but not propofol, decrease mivacurium requirements over time. *Can. J. Anaesth.* 49 (9): 907–912. https://doi.org/10.1007/BF03016872.

57 Blichfeldt-Lauridsen, L. and Hansen, B.D. (2012). Anesthesia and myasthenia gravis. *Acta Anaesthesiol. Scand.* 56 (1): 17–22. https://doi.org/10.1111/j.1399-6576.2011.02558.x.

58 Spacek, A., Neiger, F.X., Krenn, C.G. et al. (1999). Rocuronium-induced neuromuscular block is affected by chronic carbamazepine therapy. *Anesthesiology* 90 (1): 109–112. https://doi.org/10.1097/00000542-199901000-00016.

59 Ammundsen, H.B., Sørensen, M.K., and Gätke, M.R. (2015). Succinylcholine resistance. *Br. J. Anaesth.* 115 (6): 818–821. https://doi.org/10.1093/bja/aev228.

60 Murphy, G.S. (2018). Neuromuscular monitoring in the perioperative period. *Anesth. Analg.* 126 (2): 464–468. https://doi.org/10.1213/ANE.0000000000002387.

61 Gravlee, G.P. (1980). Succinylcholine-induced hyperkalemia in a patient with Parkinson's disease. *Anesth. Analg.* 59 (6): 444–446.

62 Chidiac, E.J. and Raiskin, A.O. (2006). Succinylcholine and the open eye. *Ophthalmol. Clin. N. Am.* 19 (2): 279–285. https://doi.org/10.1016/j.ohc.2006.02.015.

63 Theroux, M.C., Brandom, B.W., Zagnoev, M. et al. (1994). Dose response of succinylcholine at the adductor pollicis of children with cerebral palsy during propofol and nitrous oxide anesthesia. *Anesth. Analg.* 79 (4): 761–765. https://doi.org/10.1213/00000539-199410000-00024.

64 Lemmens, H.J. and Brodsky, J.B. (2006). The dose of succinylcholine in morbid obesity. *Anesth. Analg.* 102 (2): 438–442. https://doi.org/10.1213/01.ane.0000194876.00551.0e.

65 Viby-Mogensen, J. (1981). Succinylcholine neuromuscular blockade in subjects homozygous for atypical plasma cholinesterase. *Anesthesiology* 55 (4): 429–434. https://doi.org/10.1097/00000542-198110000-00015.

66 McAuliffe, G., Bissonnette, B., and Boutin, C. (1995). Should the routine use of atropine before succinylcholine in children be reconsidered? *Can. J. Anaesth.* 42 (8): 724–729. https://doi.org/10.1007/BF03012672.

67 Mirakhur, R.K. (1994). Safety aspects of non-depolarizing neuromuscular blocking agents with special reference to rocuronium bromide. *Eur. J. Anaesthesiol. Suppl.* 9: 133–140.

68 Proost, J.H., Eriksson, L.I., Mirakhur, R.K. et al. (2000). Urinary, biliary and faecal excretion of rocuronium in humans. *Br. J. Anaesth.* 85 (5): 717–723. https://doi.org/10.1093/bja/85.5.717.

69 Joshi, G.P., Hailey, A., Cross, S. et al. (1999). Effects of pretreatment with cisatracurium, rocuronium, and d-tubocurarine on succinylcholine-induced fasciculations and myalgia: a comparison with placebo. *J. Clin. Anesth.* 11 (8): 641–645. https://doi.org/10.1016/s0952-8180(99)00109-9.

70 Schramm, W.M., Papousek, A., Michalek-Sauberer, A. et al. (1998). The cerebral and cardiovascular effects of cisatracurium and atracurium in neurosurgical patients. *Anesth. Analg.* 86 (1): 123–127. https://doi.org/10.1097/00000539-199801000-00025.

71 Flockton, E.A., Mastronardi, P., Hunter, J.M. et al. (2008). Reversal of rocuronium-induced neuromuscular block with sugammadex is faster than reversal of cisatracurium-induced block with neostigmine. *Br. J. Anaesth.* 100 (5): 622–630. https://doi.org/10.1093/bja/aen037.

72 Webber, A.M. and Kreso, M. (2018). Informed consent for sugammadex and oral contraceptives: through the looking glass. *Anesth. Analg.* 127 (3): e52. https://doi.org/10.1213/ANE.0000000000003608.

73 Yağan, Ö., Taş, N., Mutlu, T., and Hancı, V. (2017). Comparison of the effects of sugammadex and neostigmine on postoperative nausea and vomiting. *Braz. J. Anesthesiol.* 67 (2): 147–152. https://doi.org/10.1016/j.bjane.2015.08.003.

74 Salmenperä, M. and Nilsson, E. (1981). Comparison of physostigmine and neostigmine for antagonism of neuromuscular block. *Acta Anaesthesiol. Scand.* 25 (5): 387–390. https://doi.org/10.1111/j.1399-6576.1981.tb01671.x.

75 Carron, M. and Veronese, S. (2015). Atropine sulfate for treatment of bradycardia in a patient with morbid obesity: what may happen when you least expect it. *BMJ Case Rep.* 2015: https://doi.org/10.1136/bcr-2014-207596.

76 Bernheim, A., Fatio, R., Kiowski, W. et al. (2004). Atropine often results in complete atrioventricular block or sinus arrest after cardiac transplantation: an unpredictable and dose-independent phenomenon. *Transplantation* 77 (8): 1181–1185. https://doi.org/10.1097/01.tp.0000122416.70287.d9.

77 McPherson, G.A., Molenaar, P., and Malta, E. (1985). The affinity and efficacy of naturally occurring catecholamines at beta-adrenoceptor subtypes. *J. Pharm. Pharmacol.* 37 (7): 499–501. https://doi.org/10.1111/j.2042-7158.1985.tb03051.x.

78 Kwak, Y.L., Lee, C.S., Park, Y.H., and Hong, Y.W. (2002). The effect of phenylephrine and norepinephrine in patients with chronic pulmonary hypertension*. *Anaesthesia* 57 (1): 9–14. https://doi.org/10.1046/j.1365-2044.2002.02324.x.

79 Tanaka, M. and Dohi, S. (1994). Effects of phenylephrine and ephedrine on pulmonary arterial pressure in patients with cervical or lumbar epidural anesthesia, or enflurane anesthesia. *J. Anesth.* 8 (2): 125–131. https://doi.org/10.1007/BF02514698.

80 Myburgh, J.A., Upton, R.N., Grant, C., and Martinez, A. (1998). A comparison of the effects of norepinephrine, epinephrine, and dopamine on cerebral blood flow and oxygen utilisation. *Acta Neurochir. Suppl.* 71: 19–21. https://doi.org/10.1007/978-3-7091-6475-4_6.

81 Albanèse, J., Leone, M., Garnier, F. et al. (2004). Renal effects of norepinephrine in septic and nonseptic patients. *Chest* 126 (2): 534–539. https://doi.org/10.1378/chest.126.2.534.

82 Zhang, H., Smail, N., Cabral, A. et al. (1997). Effects of norepinephrine on regional blood flow and oxygen extraction capabilities during endotoxic shock. *Am. J. Respir. Crit. Care Med.* 155 (6): 1965–1971. https://doi.org/10.1164/ajrccm.155.6.9196103.

83 Ristagno, G., Tang, W., Huang, L. et al. (2009). Epinephrine reduces cerebral perfusion during cardiopulmonary resuscitation. *Crit. Care Med.* 37 (4): 1408–1415. https://doi.org/10.1097/CCM.0b013e31819cedc9.

84 Berkowitz, I.D., Gervais, H., Schleien, C.L. et al. (1991). Epinephrine dosage effects on cerebral and myocardial blood flow in an infant swine model of cardiopulmonary resuscitation. *Anesthesiology* 75 (6): 1041–1050. https://doi.org/10.1097/00000542-199112000-00017.

85 Leenen, F.H., Davies, R.A., and Fourney, A. (1998). Catecholamines and heart function in heart transplant patients: effects of β_1– versus nonselective beta-blockade. *Clin. Pharmacol. Ther.* 64 (5): 522–535. https://doi.org/10.1016/S0009-9236(98)90135-7.

86 Koch, K.U., Mikkelsen, I.K., Aanerud, J. et al. (2020). Ephedrine versus phenylephrine effect on cerebral blood flow and oxygen consumption in anesthetized brain tumor patients: a randomized clinical trial. *Anesthesiology* 133 (2): 304–317. https://doi.org/10.1097/ALN.0000000000003377.

87 Rothenberg, D.M., Parnass, S.M., Litwack, K. et al. (1991). Efficacy of ephedrine in the prevention of postoperative nausea and vomiting. *Anesth. Analg.* 72 (1): 58–61. https://doi.org/10.1213/00000539-199101000-00010.

88 Siehr, S.L., Feinstein, J.A., Yang, W. et al. (2016). Hemodynamic effects of phenylephrine, vasopressin, and epinephrine in children with pulmonary hypertension: a pilot study. *Pediatr. Crit. Care Med.* 17 (5): 428–437. https://doi.org/10.1097/PCC.0000000000000716.

89 Krejci, V., Hiltebrand, L.B., Jakob, S.M. et al. (2007). Vasopressin in septic shock: effects on pancreatic, renal, and hepatic blood flow. *Crit. Care* 11 (6): R129. https://doi.org/10.1186/cc6197.

90 Vadasz, E., Moss, J., Chang, N. et al. (2023). Effect of clevidipine on intracranial pressure in pediatric neurosurgical patients: a single-center retrospective review. *J. Neurosurg. Pediatr.* 31 (3): 252–257. https://doi.org/10.3171/2022.11.PEDS22255.

91 Bailey, J.M., Lu, W., Levy, J.H. et al. (2002). Clevidipine in adult cardiac surgical patients: a dose-finding study. *Anesthesiology* 96 (5): 1086–1094. https://doi.org/10.1097/00000542-200205000-00010.

92 Watts, R., Thiruvenkatarajan, V., Calvert, M. et al. (2017). The effect of perioperative esmolol on early postoperative pain: a systematic review and meta-analysis. *J. Anaesthesiol. Clin. Pharmacol.* 33 (1): 28–39. https://doi.org/10.4103/0970-9185.202182.

93 Olsen, K.S., Svendsen, L.B., Larsen, F.S., and Paulson, O.B. (1995). Effect of labetalol on cerebral blood flow,

oxygen metabolism and autoregulation in healthy humans. *Br. J. Anaesth.* 75 (1): 51–54. https://doi.org/10.1093/bja/75.1.51.

94 Larsson, K. (1982). Influence of labetalol, propranolol and practolol in patients with asthma. *Eur. J. Respir. Dis.* 63 (3): 221–230.

95 Jackson, S.H. and Beevers, D.G. (1983). Comparison of the effects of single doses of atenolol and labetalol on airways obstruction in patients with hypertension and asthma. *Br. J. Clin. Pharmacol.* 15 (5): 553–556. https://doi.org/10.1111/j.1365-2125.1983.tb02089.x.

96 Abe, K., Iwanaga, H., and Inada, E. (1994). Effect of nicardipine and diltiazem on internal carotid artery blood flow velocity and local cerebral blood flow during cerebral aneurysm surgery for subarachnoid hemorrhage. *J. Clin. Anesth.* 6 (2): 99–105. https://doi.org/10.1016/0952-8180(94)90004-3.

97 Cheung, A.T., Guvakov, D.V., Weiss, S.J. et al. (1999). Nicardipine intravenous bolus dosing for acutely decreasing arterial blood pressure during general anesthesia for cardiac operations: pharmacokinetics, pharmacodynamics, and associated effects on left ventricular function. *Anesth. Analg.* 89 (5): 1116–1123.

98 Uren, N.G., Ludman, P.F., Crake, T., and Oakley, C.M. (1992). Response of the pulmonary circulation to acetylcholine, calcitonin gene-related peptide, substance P and oral nicardipine in patients with primary pulmonary hypertension. *J. Am. Coll. Cardiol.* 19 (4): 835–841. https://doi.org/10.1016/0735-1097(92)90528-u.

99 van Schaik, B.A., van Nistelrooy, A.E., and Geyskes, G.G. (1984). Antihypertensive and renal effects of nicardipine. *Br. J. Clin. Pharmacol.* 18 (1): 57–63. https://doi.org/10.1111/j.1365-2125.1984.tb05022.x.

100 García-Pagán, J.C., Feu, F., Luca, A. et al. (1994). Nicardipine increases hepatic blood flow and the hepatic clearance of indocyanine green in patients with cirrhosis. *J. Hepatol.* 20 (6): 792–796. https://doi.org/10.1016/s0168-8278(05)80151-5.

101 Katoh, M., Nakajima, M., Shimada, N. et al. (2000). Inhibition of human cytochrome P450 enzymes by 1,4-dihydropyridine calcium antagonists: prediction of in vivo drug-drug interactions. *Eur. J. Clin. Pharmacol.* 55 (11–12): 843–852. https://doi.org/10.1007/s002280050706.

102 Overgaard, J. and Skinhoj, E. (1975). A paradoxical cerebral hemodynamic effect of hydralazine. *Stroke* 6 (4): 402–410. https://doi.org/10.1161/01.str.6.4.402.

103 Leier, C.B., Magorien, R.D., Desch, C.E. et al. (1981). Hydralazine and isosorbide dinitrate: comparative central and regional hemodynamic effects when administered alone or in combination. *Circulation* 63 (1): 102–109. https://doi.org/10.1161/01.cir.63.1.102.

104 Lupi-Herrera, E., Sandoval, J., Seoane, M., and Bialostozky, D. (1982). The role of hydralazine therapy for pulmonary arterial hypertension of unknown cause. *Circulation* 65 (4): 645–650. https://doi.org/10.1161/01.cir.65.4.645.

105 Cogan, J.J., Humphreys, M.H., Carlson, C.J., and Rapaport, E. (1980). Renal effects of nitroprusside and hydralazine in patients with congestive heart failure. *Circulation* 61 (2): 316–323. https://doi.org/10.1161/01.cir.61.2.316.

106 He, Y. and Sawalha, A.H. (2018). Drug-induced lupus erythematosus: an update on drugs and mechanisms. *Curr. Opin. Rheumatol.* 30 (5): 490–497. https://doi.org/10.1097/BOR.0000000000000522.

107 Williams, D.O., Amsterdam, E.A., and Mason, D.T. (1975). Hemodynamic effects of nitroglycerin in acute myocardial infarction. *Circulation* 51 (3): 421–427. https://doi.org/10.1161/01.cir.51.3.421.

108 Watt, A.H., Bernard, M.S., Webster, J. et al. (1986). Intravenous adenosine in the treatment of supraventricular tachycardia: a dose-ranging study and interaction with dipyridamole. *Br. J. Clin. Pharmacol.* 21 (2): 227–230. https://doi.org/10.1111/j.1365-2125.1986.tb05180.x.

109 Flyer, J.N., Zuckerman, W.A., Richmond, M.E. et al. (2017). Prospective study of adenosine on atrioventricular nodal conduction in pediatric and young adult patients after heart transplantation. *Circulation* 135 (25): 2485–2493. https://doi.org/10.1161/CIRCULATIONAHA.117.028087.

110 Côté, P., Bourassa, M.G., Delaye, J. et al. (1979). Effects of amiodarone on cardiac and coronary hemodynamics and on myocardial metabolism in patients with coronary artery disease. *Circulation* 59 (6): 1165–1172. https://doi.org/10.1161/01.cir.59.6.1165.

111 Pollack, A.Z., Mumford, S.L., Mendola, P. et al. (2015). Kidney biomarkers associated with blood lead, mercury, and cadmium in premenopausal women: a prospective cohort study. *J. Toxicol. Environ. Health A* 78 (2): 119–131. https://doi.org/10.1080/15287394.2014.944680.

112 Morales, A.I., Barata, J.D., Bruges, M. et al. (2003). Acute renal toxic effect of amiodarone in rats. *Pharmacol. Toxicol.* 92 (1): 39–42. https://doi.org/10.1034/j.1600-0773.2003.920107.x.

113 Babatin, M., Lee, S.S., and Pollak, P.T. (2008). Amiodarone hepatotoxicity. *Curr. Vasc. Pharmacol.* 6 (3): 228–236. https://doi.org/10.2174/157016108784912019.

114 Enseleit, F., Wyss, C.A., Duru, F. et al. (2006). Images in cardiovascular medicine. The blue man: amiodarone-induced skin discoloration. *Circulation* 113 (5): e63. https://doi.org/10.1161/CIRCULATIONAHA.105.554303.

115 Martino, E., Bartalena, L., Bogazzi, F., and Braverman, L.E. (2001). The effects of amiodarone on the thyroid.

Endocr. Rev. 22 (2): 240–254. https://doi.org/10.1210/edrv.22.2.0427.

116 Livada, R. and Shiloah, J. (2014). Calcium channel blocker-induced gingival enlargement. *J. Hum. Hypertens.* 28 (1): 10–14. https://doi.org/10.1038/jhh.2013.47.

117 Rameis, H., Magometschnigg, D., and Ganzinger, U. (1984). The diltiazem-digoxin interaction. *Clin. Pharmacol. Ther.* 36 (2): 183–189. https://doi.org/10.1038/clpt.1984.160.

118 Busse, D., Templin, S., Mikus, G. et al. (2006). Cardiovascular effects of (R)- and (S)-verapamil and racemic verapamil in humans: a placebo-controlled study. *Eur. J. Clin. Pharmacol.* 62 (8): 613–619. https://doi.org/10.1007/s00228-006-0154-7.

119 Meredith, P.A., Elliott, H.L., Pasanisi, F. et al. (1985). Verapamil pharmacokinetics and apparent hepatic and renal blood flow. *Br. J. Clin. Pharmacol.* 20 (2): 101–106. https://doi.org/10.1111/j.1365-2125.1985.tb05038.x.

120 Miller, C.S. and Damm, D.D. (1992). Incidence of verapamil-induced gingival hyperplasia in a dental population. *J. Periodontol.* 63 (5): 453–456. https://doi.org/10.1902/jop.1992.63.5.453.

121 Wang, Y.H., Jones, D.R., and Hall, S.D. (2004). Prediction of cytochrome P450 3A inhibition by verapamil enantiomers and their metabolites. *Drug Metab. Dispos.* 32 (2): 259–266. https://doi.org/10.1124/dmd.32.2.259.

Section 6
Adult Disease and Syndromes

Obstructive Sleep Apnea is mentioned in Section X
Pediatric Disease and Syndromes are mentioned in section VII

6.1 Neurologic Disease

Epilepsy

- Etiology/Risk Factors
  - Genetic
  - Structural
    - Trauma
    - Ischemia
    - Hemorrhage
  - Metabolic
    - Febrile
      - 3–5% of children will have a febrile seizure before age 5
      - 30% of those will have additional febrile seizures
      - ↑ Risk of developing epilepsy
  - Infection
  - Immature brain (Neonates and infants) more prone to seizures
- Pathophysiology
  - Abnormal, excessive, or synchronous discharge of neurons
    - Intermittent and usually self-limiting
    - Provoked
      - Identifiable systemic illness or brain insult
    - Unprovoked (Figure 6.1)
      - Unknown etiology
      - Preexisting brain lesion or progressive nervous system disorder
    - Status epilepticus
      - Prolonged or recurrent without return of consciousness
- Treatment
  - Avoid seizure triggers
  - Antiepileptics
  - Vagal nerve stimulator
  - Focal resection
- Primary Concerns
  - Perioperative seizure
  - The presence of developmental delay may make cooperation difficult
  - Medication interactions
    - Anesthetics
    - Oral contraception

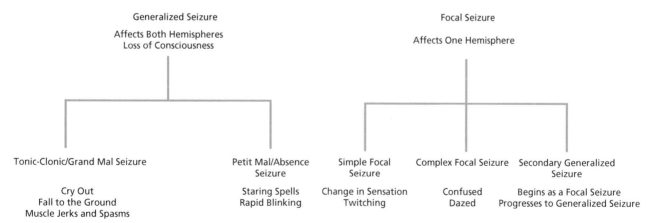

CDC Seizure Categorization

Generalized Seizure
Affects Both Hemispheres
Loss of Consciousness

Focal Seizure
Affects One Hemisphere

Tonic-Clonic/Grand Mal Seizure
Cry Out
Fall to the Ground
Muscle Jerks and Spasms

Petit Mal/Absence Seizure
Staring Spells
Rapid Blinking

Simple Focal Seizure
Change in Sensation
Twitching

Complex Focal Seizure
Confused
Dazed

Secondary Generalized Seizure
Begins as a Focal Seizure
Progresses to Generalized Seizure

Figure 6.1

Anesthesia for Dental and Oral Maxillofacial Surgery, First Edition. Spencer D. Wade, Caroline M. Sawicki, Megann K. Smiley, Michael A. Cuddy, Steven Vukas, and Paul J. Schwartz.
© 2024 John Wiley & Sons, Inc. Published 2024 by John Wiley & Sons, Inc.

- o Liver function
- o Coagulopathy
- o Electrolyte abnormalities
- Evaluation
  - Consider neurologist consultation
  - CBC
  - LFT
  - BMP
  - Careful history
    - o Type of seizure (Figure 6.1)
    - o Typical presentation
    - o Last seizure
    - o How often they occur
    - o How long they last
    - o Identifiable triggers
    - o Recognizable "aura"
    - o Self-resolving vs. need for intervention
    - o Hospitalizations
- Anesthesia Management
  - Consider premedication for uncooperative patient
  - Continue antiepileptics perioperatively
  - Avoid seizure triggers
  - Most anesthetics have antiseizure activity
  - Consider avoiding cisatracurium as its metabolite, laudanosine, is a proconvulsant
  - Ketamine is now considered safe to use in epileptic patients [1]
  - *Seizure management covered on page 268*

Neurofibromatosis Type 1

- Etiology/Risk Factors
  - Autosomal dominant
- Pathophysiology (Figure 6.2)
  - Café-au-lait macules
  - Diffuse, benign, cutaneous neurofibromas which can interfere with physiologic functions and cause cosmetic problems

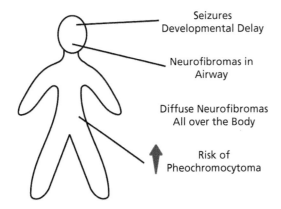

Seizures
Developmental Delay

Neurofibromas in Airway

Diffuse Neurofibromas All over the Body

Risk of Pheochromocytoma

Figure 6.2

- ↑ Incidence of CHD
- ↑ Incidence of essential HTN
- Treatment
  - Antiepileptics
  - Removal of tumors interfering with function and/or esthetics
- Primary Concerns
  - The presence of developmental delay may make cooperation difficult
  - Chronic pain
  - Neurofibromas
    - o Airway obstruction and difficult intubation
    - o Compress spinal nerves
  - Presence of pheochromocytoma
  - ↑ risk of seizures
- Evaluation
  - Often cared for by multidisciplinary team
  - Consider neurologist consultation
  - Consider endocrinologist consultation
  - Neurofibromas in airway
    - o Past airway/endoscopy notes
    - o Stridor
    - o Direct visualization in the mouth
    - o Consider oral intubation
  - Note any sensory/motor deficits
  - Evaluate for signs and symptoms of pheochromocytoma
    - o Hypertension
    - o Hypermetabolism
    - o Hyperglycemia
    - o Headache
    - o Hyperhidrosis
- Anesthesia Management
  - Consider premedication for uncooperative patients
  - Be prepared for unknown upper airway obstruction from laryngeal neurofibromas [2]
  - Neuromuscular blocking agents are considered OK
    - o No prolongation of neuromuscular blocking agents [3, 4]
  - No specific contraindications to induction or maintenance agents

Alzheimer's Disease

- Etiology/Risk Factors
  - Idiopathic/multifactorial
  - Genetic
    - o Down syndrome
      - Additional copy of amyloid precursor protein gene due to trisomy of chromosome 21
  - Older age
  - Cardiovascular disease

- Pathophysiology
  - Most common cause of dementia
  - Progressive loss of memory and cognition
  - Formation of beta amyloid neuritic plaques and neurofibrillary tangles
- Treatment
  - Symptom amelioration, no cure
  - Memory care
  - Memantine
    - NMDA receptor antagonist
  - Cholinesterase inhibitors
    - Donepezil
    - Tacrine
    - Rivastigmine
    - Galantamine
- Primary Concerns
  - Inability to give informed consent
  - The presence of cognitive decline may make cooperation difficult
  - Medication interactions may affect depolarizing neuromuscular blockade *(see page 106)*
- Evaluation
  - Evaluate baseline cognition
- Anesthesia Management
  - Consider premedication for uncooperative patients
  - Continue Alzheimer's medications
  - Avoid centrally acting anticholinergics like promethazine, atropine, and diphenhydramine
  - Consider shorter acting anesthetics with more conservative titration
  - ↑ Duration of succinylcholine may occur in this population if they currently taking a cholinesterase inhibitor, but it is unlikely to be clinically relevant

Parkinson's Disease

- Etiology/Risk Factors [5]
  - Idiopathic
  - ↑ Age
  - Male
  - Traumatic brain injury
  - Genetic
- Pathophysiology
  - Progressive neurodegenerative loss of dopaminergic neurons of the basal ganglia, especially substantia nigra
    - Dopamine depletion disrupts connections to thalamus and motor cortex
  - Resting tremor (Figure 6.3)
  - Rigidity
  - Bradykinesia
  - Postural instability

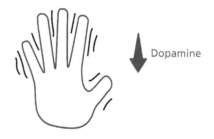

Figure 6.3

- Mask-like facial expression
- Shuffling small-stepped gait
- Treatment

Amantadine	↑ Dopamine release
Carbidopa/levodopa	Decarboxylase inhibitor
Entacapone Tolcapone	COMT inhibitor
Rasagiline Selegiline Safinamide	MAO-B Inhibitor
Pramipexole Ropinirole	Dopamine receptor agonist

- Deep brain stimulator
- Primary Concerns
  - The presence of severe cognitive decline may make cooperation difficult
  - Global muscle weakness
  - ↑ Risk of aspiration [6]
    - Pharyngeal muscle weakness
    - ↓ Respiratory muscle function [7]
    - ↓ Gastric emptying [8]
  - Autonomic dysregulation
    - Orthostatic hypotension
    - Tachycardia
- Evaluation
  - Consider neurologist consultation
  - Evaluate baseline cognition
  - Evaluate degree of tremor
  - Evaluate autonomic dysfunction
    - Heart rate variability with deep breathing and moving from supine to standing position
  - History
    - Episodes of aspiration or chronic pulmonary infections from silent aspiration
    - Difficulty handling secretions or swallowing food
  - Assess extremity strength
- Anesthesia Management
  - Consider premedication for uncooperative patient
  - Continue Parkinson's medications

- Consider rapid sequence induction to minimize aspiration risk
- Dyskinesias may be treated with dexmedetomidine and propofol [9, 10]
- Phenylephrine is an excellent treatment for hypotension [11]
- Avoid anti-dopaminergic medications
  - Haloperidol
  - Droperidol
  - Metoclopramide

Huntington's Disease

- Etiology/Risk Factors
  - Autosomal dominant
  - Trinucleotide repeat expansion in the HTT gene on chromosome 4p (Figure 6.4)

CAGCAGCAGCAG
├───────┤

Figure 6.4

- Pathophysiology
  - Progressive neuronal degenerative disease which can lead to coordination, muscle, and cognitive dysfunction
    - Chorea
      - Involuntary, irregular, jerky movements
    - Dementia
- Treatment
  - Symptomatic and supportive, no known cure
    - Haloperidol [11]
    - Olanzapine [12]
    - Aripiprazole [13]
    - Tetrabenazine [14]
    - Deep brain stimulator
- Primary Concerns
  - The presence of severe cognitive delay may make cooperation difficult
  - Progression of cardiac amyloidosis [15]
  - Global muscle weakness
  - ↑ Risk of aspiration
    - Pharyngeal muscle weakness
    - ↓ Respiratory muscle function [16]
    - ↓ Gastric emptying [17]
- Evaluation
  - Often cared for by multidisciplinary team
  - Consider neurologist consultation
  - Consider cardiologist consultation

- Evaluate baseline cognition
- History
  - Episodes of aspiration or chronic pulmonary infections from silent aspiration
  - Difficulty swallowing or handling secretions
- Assess extremity strength
- Anesthesia Management
  - Continue Huntington's medications
    - Withdrawal can precipitate neuroleptic malignant syndrome (*Covered in emergencies/urgencies see page 275*)
  - Consider rapid sequence induction to reduce risk of aspiration
  - Consider short-acting medications if possible
  - ↑ Sensitivity to benzodiazepines [18]
  - ↑ Duration of succinylcholine due to atypical pseudocholinesterase
    - Clinical relevance is debatable [19]

Previous Stroke

- *Active stroke management covered on page 272*
- Etiology/Risk Factors
  - Diabetes
  - HTN
  - Atrial fibrillation
  - Smoking
  - Lifestyle/diet
  - Older age
  - Anticoagulants
  - Trauma
- Pathophysiology
  - Cerebral hypoxia
    - Ischemia due to thrombosis, embolism, systemic hypoperfusion, and/or hemorrhage (Figure 6.5)

Types of Strokes

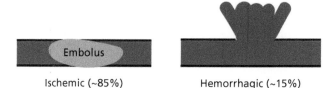

Ischemic (~85%)   Hemorrhagic (~15%)

Figure 6.5

- Treatment
  - Physical therapy
  - Antiplatelet therapy (ischemic stroke)
    - Aspirin

- o Aspirin plus extended-release dipyridamole
- o Clopidogrel
  - – Anticoagulants (ischemic stroke)
- o Rivaroxaban
- Primary Concerns
  - – The presence of cognitive deficit may make cooperation difficult
  - – Anticoagulants/antiplatelet therapy
  - – ↑ Risk of aspiration depending on long-term symptoms
  - – Muscle weakness
- Evaluation
  - – Consider neurologist consultation
  - – Consider PT/PTT/INR
  - – Evaluate baseline cognition
  - – History
    - o When the stroke occurred
    - o Type of stroke
    - o Residual long-term effects
      - Has there been any improvement?
    - o Past episodes of aspiration or chronic pulmonary infections from silent aspiration
    - o Difficulty swallowing or handling secretions
  - – Assess extremity strength
- Anesthesia Management [20]
  - – Delay elective surgery at least three months after stroke [21]
  - – Consider risk/benefit of continuing anticoagulant/antiplatelets
  - – Avoid succinylcholine in the setting of significant motor deficits
  - – Consider short-acting agents as recovery may be prolonged in these patients

6.2 Cardiac Disease

Stable Angina Pectoris

- *MI/unstable angina covered in emergencies/urgencies*
- Etiology/Risk Factors
  - Lifestyle/diet
  - Genetic
  - Smoking
  - Hyperlipidemia
- Pathophysiology
  - Imbalance of coronary O_2 blood supply and demand resulting in chest pain from myocardial ischemia
    - Determinants of supply
      - Oxygen-carrying capacity of blood
      - Degree of oxygen unloading from hemoglobin
      - Coronary artery blood flow (Figure 6.6)
    - Determinants of demand
      - Heart rate
      - Afterload
      - Myocardial wall tension
      - Contractility
  - Stable angina should be relieved with rest and, if needed, nitroglycerin
- Treatment
  - Lifestyle/diet modifications
  - Antiplatelets
    - Aspirin
    - Clopidogrel
  - Nitrates, long acting
  - Nitroglycerin
  - β-blockers
  - Calcium channel blockers
  - Revascularization
    - CABG
    - PCI stent
- Primary Concerns
  - ↑ Risk of MI
  - Current antiplatelet medications
  - Previous PCI
- Evaluation
  - Consider cardiologist consult
  - Consider preoperative ECG
    - May be normal when patient is asymptomatic
  - Consider echocardiogram
  - *Establish DASI/METs on pages 67–68*
  - History
    - Provoking factors
    - Alleviating factors
    - Duration of pain discomfort
    - Last time patient had symptoms
    - Previous interventions
- Anesthesia Management
  - Avoid tachycardia/high normal HR
  - Avoid significant hypertension or hypotension
  - Attempt to keep epinephrine usage to under 40 μg [22]. Carefully observe patient response

Normal Coronary Blood Flow

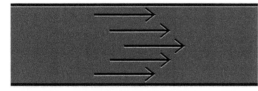

Stable Angina

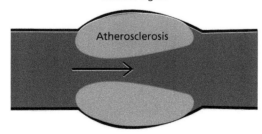

Atherosclerosis

Figure 6.6

Congestive Heart Failure

- Etiology/Risk Factors
  - Lifestyle/diet
  - Smoking
  - Genetics
  - Diabetes
  - Cardiac ischemia
  - Cardiomyopathies
  - Valvular abnormalities
  - Arrhythmias
  - Chronic systemic HTN
  - Pulmonary HTN
- Pathophysiology (Figures 6.7 & 6.8)
  - Clinical signs and symptoms due to fluid accumulation
  - All heart failure
    - Fatigue
    - Weakness

Types of Congestive Heart Failure

Heart Failure with Reduced Ejection Fraction
LVEF < 40%
(Previously Called Systolic Heart Failure)

Heart Failure with Preserved Ejection Fraction
LVEF > 50%
(Previously Called Diastolic Heart Failure)

Figure 6.7

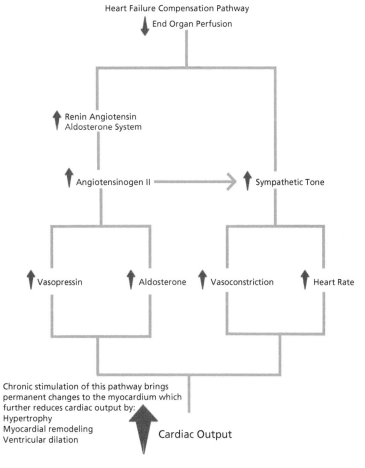

Figure 6.8

- Left-sided heart failure
  - o Dyspnea
  - o Orthopnea
  - o Rales heard on lung auscultation
- Right-sided heart failure
  - o Peripheral edema
  - o Abdominal distension and discomfort
  - o Jugular venous distension
- Treatment
  - Lifestyle/diet modifications
  - Treat underlying cause (e.g. valve replacement)
  - ACEi
  - ARB
  - β-blockers
  - Diuretics
  - Statins
  - Left Ventricular Assist Device (LVAD)
  - Heart transplant
- Primary Concerns
  - Poor cardiac reserve that may not tolerate anesthesia
  - Volume status
  - Acute pulmonary edema
- Evaluation
  - Consider cardiology consult
  - Consider preoperative ECG
  - Consider echocardiogram
  - *Establish DASI/METs on pages 67–68*
  - Type of CHF

	New York heart association functional classification of congestive heart failure
Class I	*No symptoms and no limitation in ordinary physical activity such as shortness of breath when walking or climbing stairs*
Class II	*Mild symptoms* *Mild shortness of breath and/or angina* *Slight limitation during ordinary activity*
Class III	*Marked limitation in activity due to symptoms, even during less-than-ordinary activity* *Walking short distances* *Comfortable only at rest*
Class IV	*Severe limitations. Experiences symptoms even while at rest. Mostly bedbound patients*

- Evaluate for signs of volume overload
  - o Peripheral edema
  - o Dyspnea
  - o Jugular venous distension
- Anesthesia Management
  - Continue statins
  - Continue β-blockers
  - Consider holding diuretics, ACEi, and ARBs
  - Careful titration of anesthetics as they can decrease cardiac contractility and CO
  - Avoid excessive fluid administration
  - *For LVAD management see page 177*

6.3 Valvular Disease

Optimal Hemodynamic Goals

	HR	MAP
Aortic stenosis	Low	Normal/high
Mitral valve stenosis	Low	Normal/high
Mitral valve regurgitation	High	Low
Aortic regurgitation	High	Low

Mitral Valve Stenosis

- Etiology/Risk Factors
  - Most common cause is rheumatic heart disease
- Pathophysiology
  - Non-compliant mitral valve requiring excess pressure from the left atrium to open leading to left atrial hypertrophy which can lead to:
    - ↑ Risk of atrial fibrillation
    - ↑ Risk of thrombosis
    - Hoarseness secondary to impingement on the left recurrent laryngeal nerve
  - ↓ CO
  - Pulmonary HTN
  - Pulmonary edema
  - Dyspnea
  - Murmur is low-pitched diastolic rumble heard best at apex
- Treatment
  - Regular follow-up and monitoring
  - Diuretics
  - β-blockers
  - Calcium channel blockers
  - Anticoagulants
  - Valve replacement
- Primary Concerns
  - Anesthetics further decreasing CO
  - Maintaining diastolic kick

- Volume status
- Current anticoagulation status
- *For management of pulmonary HTN see page 180*
- Evaluation
  - Consider cardiology consult
  - Consider preoperative ECG
  - Consider echocardiogram
  - Consider PT/PTT/INR
  - *Establish DASI/METs on pages 67–68*
  - Evaluate for pulmonary edema
- Anesthesia Management
  - Discuss anticoagulation management with surgeon
  - Continue β-blockers and CCBs
  - Careful titration of anesthetics as they can decrease cardiac contractility and CO
  - Optimize atrial kick of diastole
    - Relatively low heart rate
    - Maintain normal sinus rhythm
  - Avoid tachycardia
    - Ketamine
    - Catecholamines (stress)
    - Anticholinergics
  - Avoid excessive fluids
  - Avoid Trendelenburg position

Mitral Valve Regurgitation

- Etiology/Risk Factors
  - Genetic
  - Congenital malformation
  - Rheumatic fever
  - Papillary muscle dysfunction
  - Previous MI
- Pathophysiology
  - Incompetent mitral valve allowing for regurgitation of blood into left atria during systole
  - Left ventricle dilates to compensate for increased volume which eventually decreases contraction and CO

– Common early symptoms:
  o Exertional dyspnea
  o Fatigue
– Holosystolic murmur heard best at apex but highly variable
• Treatment [23]
– Serial monitoring
  o Often asymptomatic until left ventricle dysfunction, pulmonary HTN, or atrial fibrillation develop
– ACEi
– ARBs
– Nitrates [24]
– Valve replacement
• Primary Concerns
– Anesthetics further decreasing CO
• Evaluation
– Consider cardiology consult
– Consider preoperative ECG
– Consider echocardiogram
– *Establish DASI/METs on pages 67–68*
• Anesthesia Management
– ↓ Regurgitant time
  o Heart rate relatively high
  o MAP relatively low
– Careful titration of anesthetics as they can decrease cardiac contractility and CO
– Avoid increases in systemic vascular resistance (SVR)
– Maintain euvolemia

Aortic Stenosis

• Etiology/Risk Factors
– Natural calcification from aging
– Bicuspid aortic valve
– Rheumatic fever
• Pathophysiology
– Stenotic valve causing left ventricular hypertrophy due to increased left ventricular pressure
– Symptoms uncommon until stenosis is severe leading to the classic triad:
  o Angina
  o Dyspnea on exertion
  o Syncope
– Systolic murmur heard best at right intercostal space
• Treatment
– β-blockers
– Valve replacement
• Primary Concerns
– Anesthetic agents decreasing CO
– Maintaining an elevated MAP
– Preventing tachycardia

• Evaluation
– Consider cardiology consult
– Consider preoperative ECG
– Consider echocardiogram
– Evaluate severity of lesion [25]

Severity	Aortic jet velocity (m/s)	Mean gradient (mmHg)	Aortic valve area (cm [2])
Normal	<2.5	—	3–4
Mild	2.5–2.9	<25	1.5–2
Moderate	3–4	25–40	1–1.5
Severe	>4	>40	<1

– *Establish DASI/METs on pages 67–68*
• Anesthesia Management
– Continue β-blockers
– Careful titration of anesthetics as they can decrease cardiac contractility and CO
– ↑ Systole duration to overcome stenotic valve
  o Avoiding tachycardia
– Avoid decrease in SVR as this reduces coronary blood flow
– Consider
  o Etomidate
  o Opioids
– Avoid
  o Ketamine
  o Catecholamines (Stress)
  o Anticholinergics
– Treat hypotension with α_1 adrenergic agonists like phenylephrine
  o No tachycardia and possibly rebound bradycardia
  o ↑ SVR
– Cardiopulmonary resuscitation may be ineffective across stenotic valve
  o CPR should still be attempted

Aortic Regurgitation

• Etiology/Risk Factors
– Advanced age
– Bicuspid valve
– Marfan syndrome
– Aortic root dilation
– Rheumatic heart disease
• Pathophysiology
– Inadequate closure of aortic valve leaflets allowing for regurgitation of blood into left ventricle during diastole

- Increase in left ventricle end-diastolic volume
- Compensatory eccentric hypertrophy of left ventricle
- May remain asymptomatic until adaptive changes result in systolic dysfunction
  - Common early symptoms of decompensation:
  - Exertional dyspnea
  - Angina
  - Fatigue
  - Peripheral edema
  - Early diastolic murmur
- Treatment [26]
  - ACEi
  - ARBs
  - CCBs
  - Valve replacement
  - Serial monitoring of symptoms
- Primary Concerns
  - Anesthetics further decreasing CO
  - Periods of hypertension causing increased regurgitation

- Evaluation
  - Consider cardiology consult
  - Consider preoperative ECG
  - Consider echocardiogram
  - *Establish DASI/METs on pages 67–68*
- Anesthesia Management
  - ↓ Regurgitant volume
    - Heart rate high normal
    - MAP low normal
  - Careful titration of anesthetics as they can decrease cardiac contractility and CO
  - Avoid increases in SVR
    - Avoid phenylephrine
  - Consider an adrenergic agent for hypotension
  - Consider nitrates or hydralazine if needed to treat hypertension
    - Avoid β-blockers
  - Maintain euvolemia
    - Over-hydration may worsen regurgitation

6.4 Bradydysrhythmias

- *Unstable bradycardia covered on page 251*

Sinus Bradycardia

- Etiology/Risk Factors
  - Genetic
  - Athletic conditioning
  - Degenerative changes
  - Advanced age
  - Medications [26]
    ○ β-blockers
    ○ Non-dihydropyridine calcium channel blockers
    ○ Amiodarone
    ○ Digoxin
    ○ Opioids
    ○ Sedatives
  - Electrolyte imbalance
- Pathophysiology
  - Heart rate less than 60 beats/min (Figure 6.9)

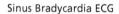

Sinus Bradycardia ECG

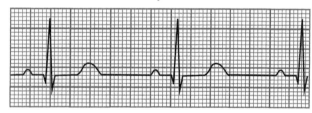

Rhythm: (Regular)
Rate (Bradycardic)
P-wave before every QRS complex (Yes)
P-wave similar size and shape (Yes)
QRS after every P-wave (Yes)
QRS (Narrow)
PR Interval (Normal)
QT Interval (Normal)

Figure 6.9

- ↓ Heart rate can lead to systemic signs of poor CO such as:
  ○ Syncope
  ○ Lightheadedness
  ○ Angina
- Treatment
  - Generally none, unless symptomatic
  - Pacemaker
- Primary Concerns
  - Anesthetic medications further decreasing CO
- Evaluation
  - Consider cardiology consult
  - Consider preoperative ECG
  - Consider BMP
  - *Establish DASI/METs on pages 67–68*
  - *Perioperative pacemaker management covered on pages 176–177*
- Anesthesia Management
  - Avoid rapid inhalation induction as cardiac depression could enhance bradycardia
  - Slow titration of bradycardia-inducing medications
    ○ Fentanyl and derivatives
    ○ Dexmedetomidine

Sick Sinus Syndrome (Sinus Node Dysfunction)

- Etiology/Risk Factors
  - Degenerative changes
- Pathophysiology
  - Irregular SA node propagation which can lead to patterns of bradycardic and/or tachycardic rhythms (Figure 6.10)
    ○ Inappropriate heart rate response to physiologic state
  - Symptoms typically intermittent with gradual progression
    ○ Fatigue
    ○ Lightheadedness

Sick Sinus Syndrome ECG

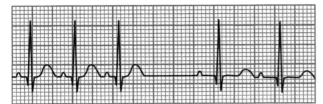

Rhythm: Irregular
Rate (Bradycardic/Tachycardic)
P-wave before every QRS complex (Yes)
P-wave similar size and shape (Yes)
QRS after every P-wave (Yes)
QRS (Narrow)
PR Interval (Normal)
QT Interval (Normal)

Figure 6.10

- ○ Palpitations
- ○ Syncope
- ○ Dyspnea on exertion
- ○ Chest pain

- Treatment
  - Generally, none unless symptomatic
  - Pacemaker
- Primary Concerns
  - Maintaining adequate HR to avoid decreased CO and organ hypoperfusion
- Evaluation
  - Consider cardiology consult
  - Consider preoperative ECG
  - Consider echocardiogram
  - Consider BMP
  - *Establish DASI/METs on pages 67–68*
  - *Perioperative pacemaker management covered on pages 176–177*
- Anesthesia Management [27]
  - Careful titration of anesthetics as they can decrease HR, cardiac contractility, and CO
  - Slow titration of bradycardia-inducing medications
    - ○ Fentanyl and derivatives
    - ○ Dexmedetomidine
  - Bradycardia may be refractory to atropine
    - ○ Consider ephedrine or epinephrine

6.5   Tachydysrhythmias

- *Tachycardia with a pulse covered on page 252*

Sinus Tachycardia

- Etiology/Risk Factors
  - Catecholamines
    - o Stress
    - o Pain
    - o Medications
      - Norepinephrine reuptake blockers
      - Recreational drugs
  - Hypovolemia
  - Endocrine abnormalities
  - Metabolic derangements
  - Anemia
  - Hypoxia
- Pathophysiology
  - Heart rate greater than 100 beats/min (Figure 6.11)
    - o Can precipitate angina by increasing myocardial oxygen demand

Sinus Tachycardia ECG

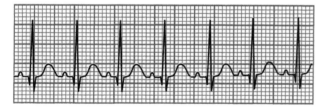

Rhythm (Regular)
Rate (Tachycardia)
P-wave before every QRS complex (Yes)
P-wave similar size and shape (Yes)
QRS after every P-wave (Yes)
QRS (Narrow)
PR Interval (Normal)
QT Interval (Normal)

Figure 6.11

- Treatment
  - Generally no long-term treatment unless symptomatic
  - Stress management exercises
  - Treat underlying cause
  - β-blockers
- Primary Concerns
  - ↑ CO and stress on the heart
  - The underlying cause contributing to the tachycardia
- Evaluation
  - Consider cardiology consult
  - Consider preoperative ECG
  - Consider BMP
  - Establish underlying source of preoperative tachycardia
- Anesthesia Management
  - Anxiety
    - o Behavioral
    - o Sedative-hypnotics
  - Pain
    - o Analgesics
    - o Local anesthetics
  - Hypovolemia
    - o Fluids
  - If ischemia develops, consider β-blockers if MAP is adequate
    - o *MI treatment covered on page 254*

Atrial Fibrillation

- Etiology/Risk Factors
  - Atrial enlargement
  - Hypertension
  - Coronary artery disease
  - Rheumatic heart disease
  - Valvular stenosis or regurgitation
  - Heart failure
  - Previous atrial flutter
  - Ischemic changes

- Electrolyte imbalances
- Hyperthyroidism
- Chronic alcohol use
- Obstructive sleep apnea
- Obesity
- Diabetes
- Genetics
- Pathophysiology
  - The atria fibrillate with some impulses propagated by the AV node (Figure 6.12)
    - HR may be in normal range or have rapid ventricular response (RVR)

Atrial Fibrillation ECG

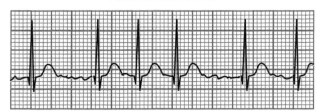

Rhythm (Irregular)
Rate (Tachycardia)
P-wave before every QRS complex (N/A)
P-wave similar size and shape (N/A)
QRS after every P-wave (N/A)
QRS (Narrow)
PR Interval (N/A)
QT Interval (Normal)

Figure 6.12

- Episodic (intermittent)
  - Terminates spontaneously or with intervention within seven days
- Persistent
  - Fails to self-terminate within seven days
  - Often requires intervention
- Long-standing
  - Persists more than 12 months
- Permanent
  - Rhythm control strategies are no longer being pursued
- Clinical symptoms usually associated with RVR
  - Palpitations
  - Tachycardia
  - Fatigue
  - Weakness
  - Lightheadedness
  - Polyuria
  - Dyspnea on exertion or rest
  - Angina
    - Syncope
    - Symptoms of stroke or heart failure
  - Irregularly irregular pulse may be noted during symptomatic episodes
- Treatment
  - Diet/exercise
  - Ablation
  - Anticoagulation
  - β-blockers
  - Non-dihydropyridine calcium channel blockers
  - Digoxin
- Primary Concerns
  - Anesthetic agents worsening CO
  - Anticoagulation status
  - Rapid ventricular response
- Evaluation
  - Consider cardiologist consult
  - Consider PT/PTT/INR
  - History
    - Date of diagnosis
    - Precipitating factors
    - Frequency and duration of episodes
    - Typical symptoms
  - *DASI/METs on pages 67–68*
- Anesthesia Management
  - Make sure patient is adequately rate controlled
  - Continue β-blockers
  - Continue CCB used for rate control
  - Decision to continue or discontinue anticoagulation based on surgical bleeding risk and type of anticoagulation
  - Careful titration of anesthetics as they can decrease cardiac contractility and CO
  - ↑ Risk of hypotension under sedation due to lack of atrial kick

Multifocal Atrial Tachycardia

- Etiology/Risk Factors
  - Highly associated with COPD [28, 29]
  - Methylxanthine toxicity [30]
  - Electrolyte abnormality [28]
- Pathophysiology
  - Heart rate greater than 100 beats/min
  - Irregular rhythm with multiple ectopic atrial pacemakers generating multiple P-wave morphologies on ECG (Figure 6.13)
  - Right atrial distension secondary to COPD-related pulmonary HTN
- Treatment
  - Treat underlying cause
  - β-blockers [31]

Multifocal Atrial Tachycardia ECG

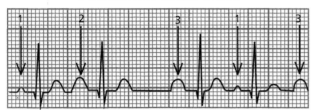

Rhythm (Irregular)

Rate (Tachycardia)

P-wave before every QRS complex (Yes)

P-wave similar size and shape (No)

QRS after every P-wave (Yes)

QRS (Narrow)

PR Interval (Variable)

QT Interval (Normal)

Figure 6.13

- Primary Concerns
  - Anesthetic agents worsening CO
- Evaluation
  - Consider cardiologist consultation
  - Consider preoperative ECG
  - Consider BMP
  - *DASI/METs on pages 67–68*
- Anesthesia Management
  - Make sure the patient is adequately rate controlled
  - Continue β-blockers
  - Careful titration of anesthetics as they can decrease cardiac contractility and CO

6.6 Cardiac Conduction Defects

Long QT Syndrome

- Etiology/Risk Factors
  - Congenital
  - Acquired
    - Patients may have underlying pathology
    - Drug induced is the most common cause of acquired long QT syndrome [32, 33]
      - Antibiotics
        - Macrolides
        - Fluoroquinolones
        - Antifungals
      - Antidysrhythmics
      - Antidepressants
      - Antihistamines [34]
      - Methadone [35, 36]
    - Electrolyte disturbance
      - Eating disorders
    - Coronary artery disease
    - Bradydysrhythmias
    - Advanced age
- Pathophysiology
  - Typical mechanism is interaction with potassium channels on myocardium

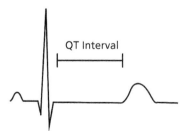

Prolonged QT Interval

≥ 460 ms Birth to Adolescence
≥ 470 ms in Men
≥ 480 ms in Women

QT Interval

Figure 6.14

- Prolonged QT interval (Figure 6.14)
- Athletes may be initially diagnosed based on pre-sports participation screening
- Treatment
  - Treat underlying cause
  - Discontinue precipitating medication
  - β-blockers
  - Implantable cardioverter-defibrillator (ICD)
- Primary Concerns
  - Anesthetic medications and adjuncts increasing QT interval
    - ↑ Risk of torsades de pointes
- Evaluation
  - Consider cardiology consultation
  - History
    - Episodes of syncope
    - Family history of sudden cardiac death
- Anesthesia Management [37]
  - Consider delay of elective procedure if underlying cause is treatable
  - Magnesium readily available
  - Continue β-blocker
  - Avoid significant increases in HR
    - Prolongs the QT interval
  - Considered safe:
    - Propofol
    - Midazolam
    - Fentanyl [38]
    - Sevoflurane [39]
    - Isoflurane [40]
    - Phenylephrine [41]
    - Vecuronium
  - Consider avoiding as elongates QT interval
    - Ondansetron [42]
    - Pancuronium [43]
    - Anticholinergics [44]
    - Cholinesterase inhibitors [45]
      - Can use in conjunction with anticholinergics
    - Haloperidol [46]

- o Droperidol
- o Antihistamines [34]
- o Albuterol [47]
- o Ephedrine
- o Epinephrine [41]
- o Norepinephrine
- o Macrolide antibiotics
- *ICD management covered on page 175.*

Wolff–Parkinson–White Syndrome

- Etiology/Risk Factors
  - Genetic
- Pathophysiology
  - Accessory conduction pathway which connects atria to ventricles, bypassing AV node (Figure 6.15)
    - o Bundle of Kent

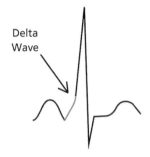

Wolff–Parkinson–White Syndrome

Delta Wave

Rhythm (Regular)
Rate (Normal)
P-wave before every QRS complex (Yes)
P-wave similar size and shape (Yes)
QRS after every P-wave (Yes)
QRS (Narrow and δ wave)
PR Interval (Shortened)
QT Interval (Normal)

Figure 6.15

- Wolff–Parkinson–White pattern
  - o Preexcitation (delta wave) on ECG without symptomatic arrhythmias
- Wolff–Parkinson–White syndrome
  - o Both preexcitation (delta wave) on ECG and symptomatic arrhythmias
- Treatment [48]
  - Ablation
  - Medical management possible for patients who prefer not to undergo ablation [49]

- Primary Concerns
  - SVT
  - Atrial fibrillation
  - Atrial flutter
- Evaluation
  - Consider cardiologist consult
  - Consider preoperative ECG
- Anesthesia Management [48, 50]
  - Delay elective case until after ablation
  - Electrical cardioversion equipment readily available
  - Avoid:
    - o Sympathetic stimulation
    - o Ketamine
    - o Anticholinergics
    - o Adrenergic agonists
    - o Avoid calcium channel blockers and β-blockers which interfere with normal AV conduction
  - Consider
    - o Propofol
    - o Benzodiazepines
    - o Rocuronium
    - o Vecuronium
    - o Inhalational agents
      - Well tolerated as they do not slow conduction through AV node
  - For patients who experience perioperative SVT, adenosine, CCBs, and β-blockers are considered first-line therapy. However, for those with WPW and SVT, these therapies may worsen the patients' condition
    - o Procainamide is a more efficacious agent in those with SVT and WPW

First-Degree AV Block

- Etiology/Risk Factors
  - Slow resting heart rate
    - o Including athletic conditioning
  - Medications that slow nodal conduction
  - Cardiac disease
  - Degenerative changes
- Pathophysiology
  - Delayed or slowed AV conduction resulting in a PR interval longer than 200 ms at rest (Figure 6.16)
  - No interruption in atrial to ventricular conduction
- Treatment
  - Generally none, if asymptomatic
- Primary Concerns
  - ↑ Vagal tone may result in severe, symptomatic bradycardia
- Evaluation
  - Consider cardiology consult
  - History

First-Degree Heart Block ECG

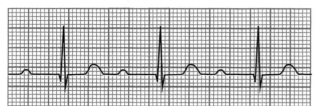

Rhythm (Regular)
Rate (Normal)
P-wave before every QRS complex (Yes)
P-wave similar size and shape (Yes)
QRS after every P-wave (Yes)
QRS (Narrow)
PR Interval (Prolonged)
QT Interval (Normal)

Figure 6.16

- o Heart disease
- o Recent cardiac procedures
- o Medications
- Anesthesia Management
  - Avoid increases in vagal tone [51]
  - Vagolytic and chronotropic agents immediately available

Second-Degree AV Block: Mobitz Type I

- Etiology/Risk Factors
  - Degenerative changes
  - Myocardial ischemia/infarction
  - Cardiomyopathy
  - Hyperkalemia
  - Medications
  - High vagal tone
- Pathophysiology
  - Progressive PR interval prolongation until a beat is entirely blocked/dropped (Figure 6.17)
  - Rarely produces symptoms
- Treatment
  - Generally, none indicated
- Primary Concerns
  - Vagal stimulation or AV nodal blocking agents could precipitate symptomatic bradycardia
- Evaluation
  - Consider cardiologist consult
  - History
    - o History of heart disease
    - o Recent cardiac procedures
    - o Medications
- Anesthesia Management
  - Avoid increase in vagal tone
  - Vagolytic and chronotropic agents readily available

Mobitz Type I ECG

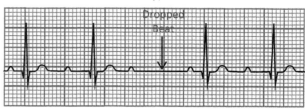

Rhythm (Regular)
Rate (Normal/Bradycardic)
P-wave befoe every QRS complex (Yes)
P-wave similar size and shape (Yes)
QRS after every P-wave (No)
QRS (Narrow)
PR Interval (Variable)
QT Interval (Normal)

Figure 6.17

Second-Degree AV Block: Mobitz Type II

- Etiology/Risk Factors
  - Conduction system disease below level of AV node
  - Degenerative changes
  - Myocardial ischemia/infarction
  - Cardiomyopathy
  - Hyperkalemia
  - Medications
  - High vagal tone
- Pathophysiology
  - Consistent, unchanging PR interval with P-waves that fail to conduct to the ventricles (Figure 6.18)
  - Variable degree of symptoms
    - o Fatigue
    - o Dyspnea
    - o Chest pain

Mobitz Type II ECG

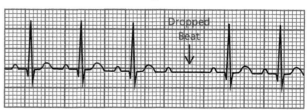

Rhythm (Regular)
Rate (Normal/Bradycardic)
P-wave before every QRS complex (Yes)
P-wave similar size and shape (Yes)
QRS after every P-wave (No)
QRS (Narrow)
PR Interval (Variable)
QT Interval (Normal)

Figure 6.18

o Presyncope
o Sudden cardiac arrest
- Treatment
  - Pacemaker
- Primary Concerns
  - ↑ Risk of deterioration to complete heart block
  - Vagal stimuli could precipitate symptomatic bradycardia
- Evaluation
  - Consider cardiologist consult
  - Perioperative pacemaker management covered on pages 176–177
  - History
    o History of heart disease
    o Recent cardiac procedures
    o Medications
- Anesthesia Management
  - Consider treatment in hospital
  - Postpone elective surgery until after pacer placement
  - Avoid increase in vagal tone
  - Bradycardia may be unresponsive to atropine
    o Consider epinephrine or ephedrine for first-line treatment of symptomatic bradycardia

Third-Degree AV Block

- Etiology/Risk Factors
  - MI
  - Idiopathic fibrosis
  - Myocarditis (e.g. Lyme disease)
  - Medications
  - Overdose
  - High vagal tone
- Pathophysiology
  - No conduction of impulses from atria to ventricles (Figure 6.19)

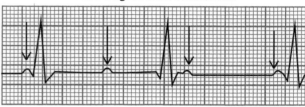

Third-Degree Heart Block ECG

Rhythm (Regular)
Rate (Usually brady)
P-wave before every QRS complex (No)
P-wave similar size and shape (Yes)
QRS after every P-wave (No)
QRS (Usually wide)
PR Interval (N/A)
QT Interval (Normal)

Figure 6.19

- Treatment
  - Pacemaker
- Primary Concerns
  - Significantly reduced CO
- Evaluation
  - Consider cardiologist consult
  - *Perioperative pacemaker management covered on pages 176–177*
- Anesthesia Management
  - Consider treatment in hospital
  - Postpone elective surgery until after pacemaker placement
  - Avoid increase in vagal tone
  - Bradycardia will be refractory to antimuscarinics as they act at the AV node
    o Consider epinephrine or ephedrine for first-line treatment of symptomatic bradycardia

6.7 Cardiac Equipment and Transplants [51]

- *For stent management, see page 69*

Implantable Cardioverter-Defibrillator (Figure 6.20) (ICD)

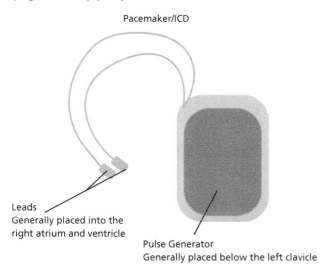

Pacemaker/ICD

Leads
Generally placed into the
right atrium and ventricle

Pulse Generator
Generally placed below the left clavicle

Figure 6.20

- Indications
  - Prevention of sudden cardiac death due to VT/VF
- Primary Concerns
  - Electromagnetic interference
    - Device could misinterpret as tachyarrhythmia and deliver shock
    - Electrosurgery units
      - Monopolar more likely to interfere than bipolar
      - Coagulation setting more likely to interfere than cutting setting
    - Peripheral nerve stimulators
    - Dental equipment generally considered safe [52]
- Evaluation
  - Pulse generator will most likely be in a left prepectoral, subcutaneous position
    - Placed on right side for left-handed patients

- History
  - Cardiac history
  - Cardiac procedures
  - Interrogation by cardiac care team within three to six months of procedure to reveal:
    - Manufacturer
    - Model number
    - Function
    - Magnet response of device (Figure 6.21)
    - Battery life
    - Significant events
    - Treatments delivered
    - Underlying rhythm

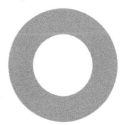

Magnets and ICDs/PPMs

Magnet effect is variable for ICDs and
PPMs but generally disables the device
Magnet can be unreliable as it can move
Always consult the device manufacturer
Best to disable through interrogation, if required

Figure 6.21

- Anesthesia Management
  - Consider treating in hospital setting
  - Cardiology consultation
  - Obtain recent baseline ECG
  - In coordination with cardiac care team, devices may be disabled or reprogrammed to suspend anti-tachyarrhythmia mode
  - Attach defibrillator pads before induction as there is a reason the patient has an ICD

- In the event of an arrhythmia, if a magnet has been placed, remove magnet to allow for reactivation of anti-tachyarrhythmia function of ICD
- Limit epinephrine in local anesthetic to 40 μg
- External defibrillator with transcutaneous pacing capability readily available
- Reactivate or reprogram prior to discharge

Permanent Pacemaker (PPM)

Most modern devices are a pacemaker and ICD
- If an ICD has pacing capability, magnet will suspend anti-tachyarrhythmia therapy but will not affect pacing mode
- Pacemakers have a specific code to understand their functionality (Figure 6.22)
- Indications
- Treat various symptomatic bradydysrhythmias
- Older pacemakers did not sense, only fired
  ○ VOO
- Newer pacemakers sense and pace
  ○ DDO
  ○ Allows a natural underlying rhythm if possible
- Primary Concerns
- Electromagnetic interference
  ○ Inhibition of pacing due to device misinterpretation as native electrical activity
  ○ Electrosurgery units
    • Monopolar more likely to interfere than bipolar
    • Coagulation setting more likely to interfere than cutting setting
  ○ Peripheral nerve stimulators
  ○ Dental equipment generally considered safe [52]

- Evaluation
- Pulse generator will most likely be in a left prepectoral, subcutaneous position
  ○ Placed on right side for left-handed patients
- Baseline ECG
  ○ Location of the pacemaker spikes on ECG lets the provider know where the patient is currently being paced (Figure 6.23)

Pacing Modes

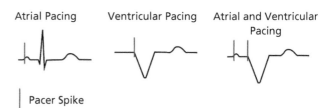

Atrial Pacing   Ventricular Pacing   Atrial and Ventricular Pacing

| Pacer Spike

Figure 6.23

- History
  ○ Cardiac history
  ○ Cardiac procedures
  ○ Interrogation by cardiac care team within three to six months of procedure to reveal:
    • Manufacturer
    • Model number
    • Function
    • Magnet response of device
    • Battery life
    • Underlying rhythm
    • Pacing dependency
- Anesthesia Management [53]
  - Consider treating in hospital setting

Pacemaker Code

Position I Chamber Paced	Position II Chamber Sensed	Position III Sensing Response	Position IV Rate Modulation	Position V Anti-Tachycardiac
(V) Ventricular	(V) Ventricular	(T) Triggered	(P) Programmable	(P) Pacing
(A) Atrial	(A) Atrial	(I) Inhibited	(M) Multiprogrammable	(S) Shock
(D) Dual	(D) Dual	(D) Trigger/Inhibit	(C) Communicating	(D) Pacing/Shock
(O) None	(S) Single	(O) None	(R) Rate Modulated	(O) None
	(O) None			

Figure 6.22

- Cardiology consultation
- In coordination with cardiac care team, device may be placed in asynchronous mode by reprogramming or magnet placement
- Disable rate modulation function, if present [54]
- In the event of a bradydysrhythmias, if a magnet has been placed, remove magnet to allow for reactivation of pacing function
- Defibrillator with transcutaneous pacing capability readily available
- Succinylcholine may inhibit pacing function due to fasciculations [55]
- Intravenous or inhalation agents acceptable, will not alter pacemaker [56]
- Reactivate or reprogram prior to discharge

Left Ventricular Assist Device (LVAD)

- Indications
  - Hemodynamic support in advanced heart failure (Figure 6.24)

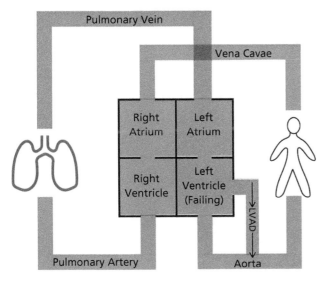

Figure 6.24

- Bridge to heart transplant or total artificial heart
- Current generations are non-pulsatile
  o Augments but does not replace heart function [57]
- Primary Concerns
  - Anticoagulation
  - High risk of stroke, infection, and GI bleeding
  - Exercise capacity limited as pump speed does not change
  - Acquired von Willebrand (vWF) syndrome secondary to intravascular shear forces

- Physiologic changes
  o Patients have no palpable pulse
  o Blood pressure difficult to measure by auscultation
  o Heart sounds are obscured by device hum
- Evaluation
  - Cardiac consultation
    o Recent echocardiogram results
    o Device interrogation
    o Patients require close follow-up and meticulous self-care
  - Obtain baseline ECG
  - Consider PT/PTT/INR
- Anesthesia Management [58, 59]
  - Consider treating in hospital setting
  - Antibiotic prophylaxis [60]
  - Anticoagulation
  - Avoid chest compressions
  - Can use an intra-arterial catheter or Doppler to monitor MAP
  - Pulse oximeter not useful with pulseless versions

Denervated Heart

- Indications
  - Cardiac transplantation as definitive therapy for end-stage heart failure
- Primary Concerns
  - No parasympathetic sensory innervation (Figure 6.25)
    o Neither carotid sinus massage nor Valsalva maneuver will have an effect
    o May re-innervate after three years

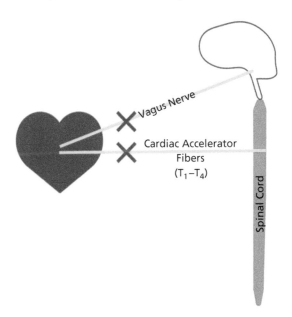

Figure 6.25

- Immunosuppression
- Adrenal axis suppression
- Evaluation
  - Cardiology consult
  - Consider preoperative ECG
  - Consider echocardiogram
  - ↑ Resting heart rate
    - 90–130 beats/min
  - Screen for pre-transplant comorbidities
    - Renal insufficiency
    - Liver dysfunction
    - HTN
  - Duration and dose of steroid regimen
- Anesthesia Management
  - Elective procedures deferred for 6–12 months after transplantation
  - Continue immunosuppressants

- Continue steroids
  - *Stress dose (page 108)*
- Avoid dehydration
- Carefully titrate agents with vasodilatory effects
- Inability to increase heart rate immediately after induction
  - No baroreceptor activity
  - Eventual response to circulating catecholamines as β receptors are still intact on donor heart
- Atropine, glycopyrrolate, neostigmine do not affect heart rate
- Epinephrine, dobutamine, isoproterenol will increase heart rate
- β-blockers and CCBs are assumed to work as well but meticulous care when using these
- Adenosine requires 1/5 the normal dose

6.8 Vascular Disease

Systemic Hypertension

Mean arterial blood pressure (MAP) = Cardiac output (CO) × Systemic vascular resistance (SVR) (Figure 6.26)

Systemic Blood Pressure Classification
(AHA)

	SBP (mmHg)		DBP (mmHg)
Normal	<120	and	<80
Elevated	120–129	and	<80
Stage I Hypertension	130–139	or	80–89
Stage II Hypertension	>140	or	>90
Hypertensive Urgency	>180	or	>120
Hypertensive Crisis*	>180	or	<120

*Also must include the presence of end organ damage

Figure 6.26

- Etiology/Risk Factors
  - Primary determinants of blood pressure
    o Sympathetic tone
    o Renin–angiotensin–aldosterone system
    o Plasma volume
  - Essential hypertension
    o Genetics
    o African American race
    o Diabetes
    o Lifestyle/diet
  - Secondary hypertension
    o Medications
    o Renal artery stenosis
    o Hyperthyroidism
    o Pheochromocytoma
    o Obstructive sleep apnea

- Pathophysiology
  - ↑ Shear forces on small microvascular beds
    o Ocular issues
    o Chronic kidney disease (CKD)
    o Cerebral infarctions
  - Increasing hypertrophy of cardiac myocytes
    o Left ventricular hypertrophy
    o Increased risk of CHF
- Treatment
  - Lifestyle/diet modifications
  - Thiazides
  - ACEi
  - ARBs
  - Nitrates
  - CCBs
  - β-blockers
- Primary Concerns
  - ↑ Autoregulation of MAP
  - Anesthetic medications excessively lowering MAP
  - Significant vascular event
    o MI
    o CVA
- Evaluation
  - Consider cardiology consult
  - Consider CMP
  - Measure baseline blood pressure
- Anesthesia Management [61]
  - Continue nitrates, calcium channel blockers, and β-blockers
  - Consider discontinuing thiazides, ACEi, and ARBs or could risk intraoperative hypotension [62]
  - Consider delaying elective cases if baseline systolic is above 180 mmHg or diastolic is above 110 mmHg [63]
  - Keep blood pressure close to baseline [64]
  - Treat acute intraoperative HTN and tachycardia instances with short-acting medications such as esmolol or propofol
  - For hypotension, treat appropriately with phenylephrine and ephedrine and escalate as needed
  - *For management of hypertensive urgency/emergency see page 253*

Pulmonary Hypertension [65]

- ↑ MAP within the pulmonary arterial system. Graded based on the systolic pulmonary arterial pressure

	Systolic pulmonary artery pressure (mmHg)
Normal	<35
Mild	35–50
Moderate	50–70
Severe	>70

- Etiology/Risk Factors
  - Left-sided heart dysfunction
  - Pulmonary disease
    - Emphysema
  - Obstructive sleep apnea
  - Obesity
  - Scleroderma
- Pathophysiology
  - Chronic disease characterized by vascular remodeling
  - ↑ Pulmonary artery pressure which can lead to:
    - Dyspnea
    - Fatigue
    - Right heart disease
      - Angina
      - Edema
  - Nonspecific symptoms and slow progression often lead to delay in diagnosis
- Treatment
  - Oxygen
  - Anticoagulants
  - Diuretics
  - PDEi
  - Prostacyclin analogs
  - Endothelin receptor antagonists
  - Surgery
- Primary Concerns
  - Right heart dysfunction
  - High risk of perioperative complications
    - MI
    - PE
    - Cardiogenic shock
- Evaluation
  - Cardiology and/or pulmonary consult
  - Consider preoperative ECG
  - Consider echocardiogram
  - Baseline pulmonary artery pressure
  - History
    - Symptoms
    - *DASi/METs on pages 67–68*
    - Comorbidities
- Anesthesia Management
  - Consider treatment in hospital setting

- Stress, pain, and surgery can exacerbate pulmonary arterial HTN
  - Consider preoperative sedation but titrate carefully to avoid hypoventilation [66]
- Continue anticoagulation
- Continue pulmonary medications
- Consider regional/local anesthesia technique
- Consider arterial line
- Avoid hypoxia and hypercarbia
- Careful fluid management
- Higher dose opioids and decreased volatile agent use to maintain CO [67]
  - Consider TIVA
- Avoid ketamine and nitrous oxide [68]
- Consider midazolam, propofol, and etomidate have minimal effect on PVR at appropriate doses [69]

Abdominal Aortic Aneurysm [70]

Aneurysm diameter (cm)	ACC/AHA guidelines
<3	No surveillance
3–3.9	Ultrasound every 2–3 years
4–5.4	Ultrasound every 6 months to a year
>5.4	Surgery

- Etiology/Risk Factors
  - Male gender
  - HTN
  - Atherosclerosis
  - Degenerative changes
  - Smoking
  - Marfan syndrome
  - Ehlers–Danlos syndrome
- Pathophysiology
  - Segmental, full-thickness dilation of aorta
    - Can lead to sudden life-threatening rupture
- Treatment
  - Lifestyle/diet modifications
  - Statins [71]
  - Antihypertensives
  - Surgery
- Primary Concerns
  - Sudden rupture
- Evaluation
  - Consider cardiology consult
  - Consider echocardiogram
  - Consider MRI
  - Current size
- Anesthesia Management
  - Consider delaying case depending on size and symptoms
  - Important to maintain MAP close to baseline

6.9 Pulmonary Disease

Asthma (Adult Patients)

- Etiology/Risk Factors [72]
  - Tobacco
  - Smoking
  - Air pollutants
  - Genetics
  - Stress
  - Obesity
- Pathophysiology
  - Acute inflammation and narrowing of conducting airways characterized by reversible airway obstruction
    - Hypoxia
    - Hypercarbia
  - ↓ Forced expiratory flow
- Treatment
  - β_2 receptor agonists
  - Corticosteroids
  - Cromolyn
  - Leukotriene receptor antagonists, e.g. Montelukast, Zileuton
  - Anticholinergics
  - Antihistamines
- Primary Concerns
  - Perioperative adverse respiratory event especially in uncontrolled asthma increases anesthesia risk [73]
  - Intraoperative bronchospasm and/or laryngospasm
- Evaluation
  - Consider pulmonologist consult in moderate–severe cases
  - PFTs rarely required
  - Assess for level of control
    - Medication use
    - Triggers
    - Frequency of rescue inhaler use
    - Hospitalizations/ED visits
    - Use of oral steroids
  - Smoke exposure [74]
  - Recent URI

- Baseline pulse oximetry
- Symptoms
  - Wheezing
  - Dyspnea
  - Chest discomfort
- Anesthesia Management
  - Continue bronchodilators and corticosteroids
    - *Consider stress dose (page 108)*
  - Consider preoperative albuterol
  - Consider anticholinergic in patients who can tolerate tachycardia to dry secretions and decrease parasympathetic airway constriction
  - Volatile agents are bronchodilators
    - Avoid desflurane [75]
  - Carefully monitor $ETCO_2$ (Figure 6.27)

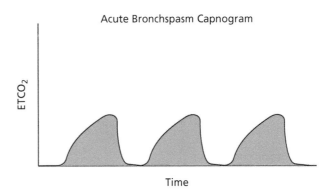

Acute Bronchspasm Capnogram

Figure 6.27

  - Consider IV lidocaine or LTA prior to intubation to reduce bronchoconstriction [76]
  - LMA may be less likely to trigger bronchospasm than an ETT [77]
  - Maintain deep level of anesthesia especially while manipulating airway
  - Ketamine has bronchodilator effects [78]
  - Propofol blunts airway reflexes [79]
  - Ketorolac may contribute to asthma exacerbations in aspirin-exacerbated respiratory disease [80]

- Caution with histamine-releasing compounds
  o Morphine
  o Meperidine
  o Codeine
  o Mivacurium
  o Cisatracurium
- Fentanyl, remifentanil, hydromorphone are preferred opioid choices due to lack of histamine release
- Choose selective β_1-blockers for HR and BP control if needed
- Consider deep extubation
- *For bronchospasm management see page 260*

Chronic Obstructive Pulmonary Disease

Global Initiative for Chronic Obstructive
Lung Disease (GOLD)
Stage Classification

	FEV$_1$/FVC	FEV$_1$ predicted (%)
I	<0.7	>80
II	<0.7	50–79
III	<0.7	30–49
IV	<0.7	>30

- Etiology/Risk Factors
  - Environmental
    o Smoking
    o Air pollutants
    o Occupational exposure
  - Chronic pulmonary infections
  - α_1 antitrypsin deficiency
- Pathophysiology
  - Chronic bronchitis – chronic airway inflammation with an accompanying partially reversible bronchoconstriction
  - Emphysema – destruction of lung parenchyma with disruption of gas exchange
    o V/Q mismatch
    o Hypoxemia
    o Hypercarbia
    o Hyperinflation secondary to air trapping
- Treatment
  - Goal is at least 88–92% SpO$_2$ or 55–60 PaO$_2$mmHg [81]
  - Smoking cessation
  - Oxygen
  - Corticosteroids
  - β_2 adrenergic agonists
  - Anticholinergics
  - Surgery

- Primary Concerns
  - High sensitivity to sedative agents
  - Intraoperative bronchospasm
  - Auto-PEEP (air trapping)
  - ↑ Risk of postoperative complications
    o Pneumonia
    o Inability to wean from ventilator
- Evaluation
  - Consider pulmonology consult
  - Recent PFTs
  - Baseline and current FEV$_1$
  - History
    o Smoke exposure [74]
    o Need for rescue inhalers
    o Recent URI
    o Last exacerbation
    o Last steroid use
    o Hospitalizations
  - Physical exam
    o Work of breathing
    o Baseline oxygen saturation
  - Symptoms
    o Wheezing
    o Dyspnea
    o Chest discomfort
- Anesthesia Management
  - Management similar to asthma
  - Continue inhaled bronchodilators and glucocorticoids
    o *Consider stress dose (page 108)*
  - Consider presedation but titrate carefully to avoid respiratory depression
  - Titrate supplemental oxygen to maintain SpO$_2$ 88–92% or close to preop baseline [82]
  - Consider using regional/local anesthesia technique [83, 84]
  - Consider TIVA, as propofol does not inhibit hypoxic pulmonary vasoconstriction [85]
  - Avoid endotracheal intubation if possible
  - *COPD exacerbation can present as Figure 6.27*
  - Consider IV lidocaine to reduce bronchoconstriction [76] for intubation
  - Deep level of anesthesia especially during airway manipulation
  - Avoid N$_2$O
  - Allow adequate time for exhalation to avoid auto-PEEP. To evaluate:
    o Look for rises in PEEP
    o EtCO$_2$ loses the "plateau"
    o Disconnect from ventilator to relieve excess PEEP
    o Reduce inspiratory to expiratory ratio
  - Avoid long-acting opioids due to prolonged respiratory depression

6.10 Neuromuscular Disease

Myasthenia Gravis

- Etiology/Risk Factors
  - Multifactorial
  - Genetic [86]
  - Thymoma [87]
  - Female gender
- Pathophysiology
  - Autoimmune antibodies target and destroy post-synaptic type 1 nicotinic receptors (Figure 6.28)
    o Fatigable weakness of skeletal muscles
- Treatment [88]
  - Cholinesterase inhibitors
    o Neostigmine
    o Pyridostigmine
    o Physostigmine
  - Thymectomy
  - Immunosuppressants
  - Steroids
  - IVIG
  - Plasmapheresis
- Primary Concerns
  - ↑ Risk of perioperative respiratory events from muscle weakness
    o ↑ Risk of upper airway obstruction due to decreased muscle tone [89]
  - ↑ Risk of aspiration
    o Swallowing difficulty
    o Pharyngeal weakness
- Evaluation
  - Consider neurology consult
  - May have recent PFTs
  - Evaluate baseline strength
  - History
    o Respiratory symptoms
    o Last crisis
    o Need for intubation during exacerbation

Myasthenia Gravis Neuromuscular Junction

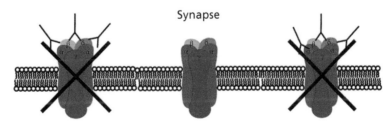

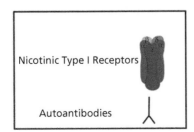

Figure 6.28

- Anesthesia Management
  - Consider hospital setting for patients with advanced disease
  - Delay elective surgery to stable phase of disease, if possible
  - Continue current glucocorticoids
    - *Consider stress dose (page 108)*
  - Continue anticholinesterase agents
  - Consider regional/local anesthetic technique
  - Best to avoid paralytics if possible [90]
    - ↑ ED95 of depolarizing NMB due to decreased number of receptors
    - ↓ ED95 of non-depolarizing NMB due to generalized muscle weakness
    - Anticholinesterase may prolong duration of depolarizing NMB
    - Consider sugammadex as anticholinesterase reversal could precipitate cholinergic crisis [91]
      - Confirm adequate reversal
    - Muscle relaxation can be achieved with potent inhalation agents alone in this population [92]
  - Short-acting anesthetic agents to avoid postoperative respiratory depression
  - Prolonged ventilatory support may be required

Spinal Cord Injury

- Etiology/Risk Factors
  - Trauma
- Pathophysiology
  - C_3–C_5
    - Loss diaphragmatic contraction
  - T_1–T_4
    - Loss of cardiac accelerator fibers
    - Bradycardia
  - T_1–L_2
    - Loss of vasoconstriction
    - Hypotension
  - T_6 and above
    - Autonomic dysreflexia (Figure 6.29)
  - T_{10} and above
    - Loss of chest wall musculature
    - ↓ FRC and tidal volumes in higher lesions
    - Hypothermia from lack of muscle mass
- Treatment
  - Spasmolytics
  - Support as needed
  - Physical therapy

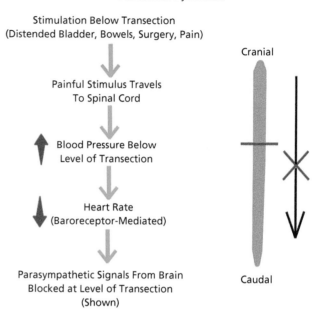

Figure 6.29

- Primary Concerns
  - Comfortable positioning of the patient
    - Contractures and muscle spasms common
  - Autonomic dysreflexia
    - Consider straight cath prior to surgery to avoid bladder distension
    - Treat with rapid, short-acting vasodilators
  - Chronic pain
    - May be treating with antiseizure, antidepressant, or analgesic medications
- Evaluation
  - Level of transection
  - Current sensory, motor deficits
  - Respiratory function
    - Aspiration
    - Pneumonia
- Anesthesia Management [93]
  - Titrate doses of anesthetic agents to avoid hypotension
  - Consider administration of fluid prior to induction to maintain CO
  - Consider vasopressors to combat systemic vasodilation
  - ↓ Vasoconstriction can lead to poor thermoregulation
  - Succinylcholine contraindicated as regions that have loss innervation will have a gross upregulation of postsynaptic nicotinic receptors
    - ↑ K^+ and myoglobinemia will lead to asystole and renal failure, respectively

6.11 Renal Disease

Chronic Kidney Disease (CKD)

- Etiology/Risk Factors [94]
  - Genetics
  - ↑ Age
  - Obesity
  - Smoking
  - Lifestyle/diet
  - Diabetes
  - HTN
- Pathophysiology
  - Progressive decline in kidney function
  - Symptoms appear when disease becomes advanced
    - o Volume overload
    - o Hyperkalemia
    - o Metabolic acidosis
    - o HTN
    - o Anemia
    - o Uremia
    - o CKD
- Treatment
  - Lifestyle/diet modifications
  - Dialysis
  - Kidney transplantation
- Primary Concerns
  - ↑ Cardiovascular risk
  - Coagulopathy secondary to uremia
  - Anesthetic medications and renal clearance
  - Metabolic derangement
    - o Especially hyperkalemia
- Evaluation
  - Consider nephrologist consult
  - Current GFR

Severity	Glomerular filtration rate (ml/min)
Stage 1	>90
Stage 2	60–89
Stage 3a	45–59
Stage 3b	30–44
Stage 4	15–29
Stage 5 (renal failure)	<15

  - Consider PT/PTT/INR
  - Consider CMP
  - Consider CBC
- Anesthesia Management
  - Avoid hypovolemia as to not worsen kidney function
  - Avoid aggressive intravenous fluids especially if GFR is low
  - Choice of IV fluid
    - o Consider balanced electrolyte solution unless patient has hyperkalemia
    - o Normal saline with caution to avoid hyperchloremic metabolic acidosis
  - ↑ Risk of perioperative bleeding, secondary to uremia and platelet dysfunction [95]
  - Avoid nephrotoxic medications:
    - o NSAIDs
    - o Aminoglycoside antibiotics
  - Avoid/decrease dose for medications or their metabolites which are dependent on renal clearance:
    - o Morphine
    - o Midazolam
    - o Hydromorphone

- o Meperidine
- o Vecuronium
- o Rocuronium
- o Neostigmine
- – Consider
  - o Volatile anesthetics
  - o Propofol
  - o Remimazolam
  - o Fentanyl
  - o Remifentanil
  - o Acetaminophen
  - o Cisatracurium

- o Succinylcholine
  - • Avoid in cases of hyperkalemia
- – For patients undergoing dialysis, it should be performed the day before the procedure to optimize volume and electrolytes [96]
- – Avoid IV access and BP cuff on arm used for dialysis vascular access
- – For patients with renal transplant, in addition to appropriate labs and specialists consultation, ensure patient continues immunosuppressant medications
  - o Otherwise, no special anesthesia considerations required when compared to a native kidney

6.12   Liver and Biliary Disease

Viral Hepatitis

- Etiology/Risk Factors

	Transmission	Acute/ chronic	Symptoms
Hepatitis A	Fecal-oral	Acute	Flu-like Self-limiting
Hepatitis B	Parenteral	Chronic	Can progress to cirrhosis
Hepatitis C	Parenteral	Chronic	Can progress to cirrhosis
Hepatitis D	Parental Co-Infection with Hepatitis B	Chronic	Can progress to cirrhosis
Hepatitis E	Fecal-oral	Acute	Flu-like Self-limiting ↑ Severity in pregnant women

- Pathophysiology
  - Inflammatory disease of liver parenchyma
  - Can be acute or chronic infection depending on virus
  - Hepatitis B, C, and D can lead to:
    o Cirrhosis
    o Hepatocellular carcinoma
    o Liver failure
- Treatment
  - Hepatitis A and E
    o Generally self-limiting
  - Hepatitis B, C, and D
    o Acute hepatitis becomes chronic after six months
    o Interferon and ribavirin
- Primary Concerns
  - ↓ Hepatic clearance/metabolism of anesthetics
- Evaluation
  - Consider hepatologist consult
  - Consider LFTs
  - Consider PT/PTT/INR
  - Consider CBC

- History
  o Etiology
  o Duration
  o Severity of hepatic dysfunction
- Anesthesia Management
  - Acute hepatitis episodes should delay elective treatment until resolved
  - Universal standards for PPE do not change for patients with diagnosed blood-borne transmissible diseases
    o Hepatitis B is the most communicable parenterally
  - ↑ Risk of bleeding perioperatively due to decreased clotting factors
  - Consider medications that are independent of hepatic metabolism/elimination
    o Remimazolam
    o Remifentanil
    o Cisatracurium
    o Succinylcholine
  - Judicious titration of medications requiring hepatic metabolism/elimination
    o Midazolam
    o Fentanyl
    o Dexmedetomidine
  - Succinylcholine duration may be prolonged due to decreased pseudocholinesterase [97]
  - Acetaminophen is considered ok if it is within the recommended therapeutic range [98]

Cirrhosis

- Etiology/Risk Factors (Figure 6.30)
  - Alcoholism
  - Viral
  - Nonalcoholic fatty liver disease
  - Acetaminophen overdose
  - Isoniazid
- Pathophysiology
  - Can be asymptomatic until decompensated cirrhosis (Figure 6.31)

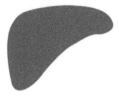

Healthy Liver

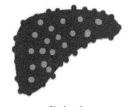

Cirrhosis

Figure 6.30

- Treatment
  - Salt restriction
  - Medications [99]
    - Spironolactone
    - Furosemide
    - Vaptans
    - β-blockers for esophageal varices
  - Esophageal banding
  - Paracentesis
  - Liver transplant
- Primary Concerns
  - ↑ Risk of cardiomyopathy [100]
  - Hyperdynamic circulation [101]
  - Coagulopathy
  - ↓ Plasma protein binding
  - ↓ Hepatic clearance/metabolism of anesthetic agents
- Evaluation
  - Consider hepatologist consult
  - LFTs
  - PT/PTT/INR
  - CBC
  - History
    - Etiology
    - Duration

- Severity of hepatic dysfunction
- Recent EGD
- Anesthesia Management
  - Only compensated cirrhosis discussed here
    - Patients with jaundice, ascites, hepatic encephalopathy, hepatorenal syndrome, or variceal hemorrhage should be considered for care in hospital
  - Similar management to viral hepatitis
  - Universal standards for PPE do not change for patients with diagnosed blood-borne transmissible diseases
  - ↑ Risk of bleeding perioperatively due to decreased clotting factors
  - Consider medications that are independent of hepatic metabolism/elimination
    - Remimazolam
    - Remifentanil
    - Esmolol
    - Cisatracurium
    - Succinylcholine
  - Judicious titration of medications requiring hepatic metabolism/elimination
    - Midazolam
    - Fentanyl
    - Dexmedetomidine
  - Succinylcholine duration may be prolonged due to decreased pseudocholinesterase [97]
  - Acetaminophen is considered ok if it is within the recommended therapeutic range [98]
  - For patients with liver transplant, in addition to appropriate labs and specialists consultation, ensure patient continue to take immunosuppressant medications
    - Otherwise, no special anesthesia considerations required when compared to a native liver

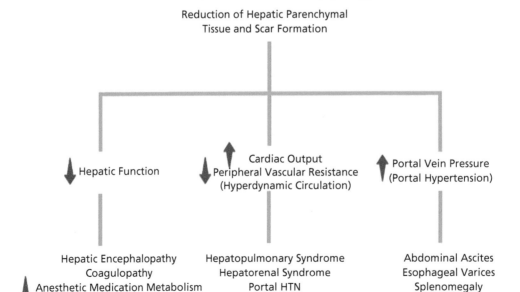

Decompensated Cirrhosis Pathophysiology

Reduction of Hepatic Parenchymal Tissue and Scar Formation

↓ Hepatic Function

↑ Cardiac Output
↓ Peripheral Vascular Resistance
(Hyperdynamic Circulation)

↑ Portal Vein Pressure
(Portal Hypertension)

Hepatic Encephalopathy
Coagulopathy
↓ Anesthetic Medication Metabolism

Hepatopulmonary Syndrome
Hepatorenal Syndrome
Portal HTN
Portopulmonary HTN

Abdominal Ascites
Esophageal Varices
Splenomegaly

Figure 6.31

6.13   Gastrointestinal Disease

Gastroesophageal Reflux Disease

- Etiology/Risk Factors
  - Hiatal hernia
  - Obesity
  - Diet
  - Pregnancy
- Pathophysiology
  - Reflux of gastric contents in esophagus (Figure 6.32)
    - Causes mucosal injury
    - Often occurs during sleep

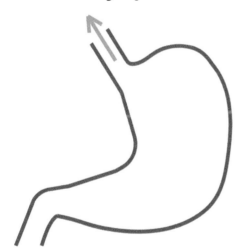

Figure 6.32

  - Chronic aspiration can lead to significant pulmonary pathology
    - Bronchial asthma
    - Chronic cough
    - Pharyngitis
    - Chronic bronchitis
    - Idiopathic pulmonary fibrosis
- Treatment
  - Dietary modifications
  - H_2 antagonists
  - PPIs
  - Surgery
- Primary Concerns
  - ↑ Risk of aspiration
  - Difficult airway
    - Eroded enamel
    - Inflamed pharyngeal/laryngeal structures [102]
  - ↑ Risk of pulmonary pathology
- Evaluation
  - History
    - Duration of symptoms
    - Triggers
    - When do symptoms occur
    - Current symptoms
- Anesthesia Management
  - Consider difficult airway [103]
  - Continue GERD medications day of surgery
  - Consider supplemental administration of an H_2 antagonists or proton pump inhibitors [104]
    - Premedication with nonparticulate antacids or antiemetics [105]
  - Consider elevated head position prior to induction
  - Consider intubation in uncontrolled patients
  - Consider rapid sequence induction [106]
  - Consider cricoid pressure [104, 107]
    - Debatable
  - Many anesthetics decrease lower esophageal sphincter tone
    - Anticholinergics
    - Benzodiazepines
    - Opioids
    - Volatile anesthetics
  - Succinylcholine is ok as it both increases lower esophageal sphincter pressure and gastric pressure during fasciculations, but they balance out [108]
  - Consider awake extubation

Inflammatory Bowel Disease: Ulcerative Colitis and Crohn's Disease

- Etiology/Risk Factors
  - Genetics
  - Diet
  - Autoimmune
- Pathophysiology
  - They are both inflammatory diseases of the gastrointestinal tract (Figure 6.33)

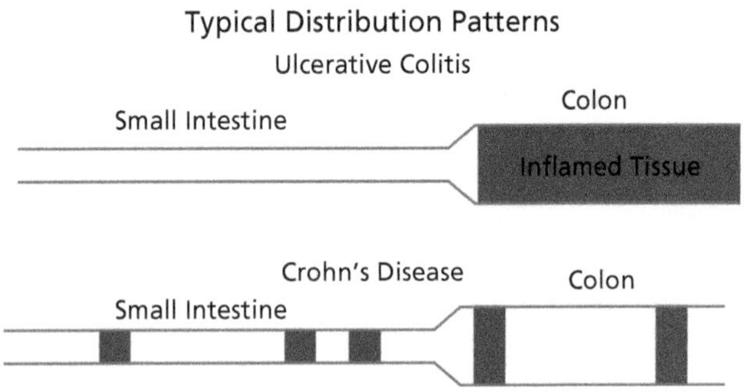

Typical Distribution Patterns

Figure 6.33

  - Ulcerative colitis
    o Affects colon and involves mucosal layer
  - Crohn's disease
    o Can involve any portion of the GI tract and is characterized by transmural inflammation

- Chronic inflammation leads to poor nutrient uptake resulting in:
  o Electrolyte abnormalities
  o Hypovolemia
  o Malnutrition
- Treatment
  - Opioids
  - Corticosteroids
  - Immunosuppressants
  - Surgery
- Primary Concerns
  - Adrenal axis suppression
  - Hypovolemia
  - Electrolyte imbalances
- Evaluation
  - History
    o Recent exacerbation of symptoms
    o Length, duration, and strength of most recent steroid course
  - Consider BMP
  - Consider CBC
- Anesthesia Management
  - Consider stress dose steroids
  - Consider pain management needs in the setting of chronic opioid use
  - Many patients will likely present with dehydration and electrolyte imbalances
  - IV ketorolac is ok, but avoid PO NSAIDs [109]

6.14 Endocrine Disease

Diabetes Mellitus (DM) Type II

- *DM Type I covered in pediatrics on page 232*
- Etiology/Risk Factors
  - Genetics
  - Lifestyle/diet
- Pathophysiology
  - Hyperglycemia
  - ↓ Insulin synthesis relative to increased tissue resistance (Figure 6.34)

Type I Diabetes 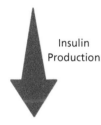   Insulin Production

Type II Diabetes 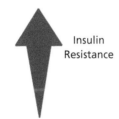   Insulin Resistance

Figure 6.34

  - Frequent comorbidities = metabolic syndrome
    o HTN
    o Dyslipidemia
    o Central obesity
  - Peripheral neuropathy
    o Distal
    o Symmetric
    o Often in stocking-glove distribution
  - Autonomic neuropathy
    o Hypotension
    o Orthostatic hypotension
    o Impaired vasoconstriction
    o Exercise intolerance
    o Resting tachycardia
    o Silent myocardial ischemia
    o Intraoperative cardiovascular instability

  - ↓ Immune function
  - Polyuria
  - ↑ Risk of coronary artery disease
  - ↑ Risk of cerebrovascular disease
  - Nephropathy
  - Retinopathy
- Treatment
  - Lifestyle/diet modifications
  - Hypoglycemic agents
    o Biguanides (metformin)
    o Sulfonylureas
    o Meglitinides
    o TZDs
    o GLP-1s
    o DPP-4s
    o α-Glucosidase inhibitors
    o SGLT2
    o Insulin
  - Bariatric surgery
- Primary Concerns
  - Perioperative glucose levels
  - Difficult airway
    o Glycosylation of cervical vertebrae and/or body habitus may limit neck extension
  - Atherosclerosis
    o ↑ Risk of coronary artery disease
    o ↑ Risk of CVA
    o Nephropathy
  - Autonomic neuropathy
    o Gastroparesis
    o ↑ Heart rate
- Evaluation
  - Consult endocrinologist
  - Blood glucose
  - HbA1c
    o Generally A1C ≤ 7% is target of glycemic control
  - History
    o Hypoglycemic episodes
      • Frequency

- Whether patient is aware
- At what blood glucose level
  - Medications
    o Exogenous insulin usage
  - Consider BMP
  - Evaluate for any sensory defects
  - Evaluate autonomic neuropathy
    o Check heart rate variability with deep breathing
    o Presence of postural hypotension
  - Evaluate for prayer sign
    o If present, increased risk of difficult airway due to decreased joint mobility [110]
- Anesthesia Management
  - *Oral medications to continue and discontinue covered on pages 99–102*
  - GLP-1 agonists markedly suppress gastric emptying and increase risk of aspiration
  - Preoperative blood glucose
    o Adjust if needed
  - No contraindications to certain anesthetic induction or maintenance agents
  - Relative contraindication to dexamethasone as may increase blood glucose postoperatively [111, 112]
  - Consider rapid sequence induction if intubating
  - Check blood glucose levels at least hourly
  - Ideal to maintain blood glucose between 140 and 180 mg/dl [113]
  - 1800 rule to calculate approximate blood glucose drop from rapid-acting insulin
    o Example: If they take 45 units of regular/fast acting a day, one unit should drop BG by ~40 mg/dl
      - 1800/45 = 40
  - 1 g dextrose raises BG by ~4 mg/dl
  - Stress of surgery will increase blood glucose
  - Check blood glucose prior to discharge

Hyperthyroidism

- Etiology/Risk Factors
  - Graves' disease (Figure 6.35)
  - Thyroid adenoma
  - Excessive exogenous levothyroxine
- Pathophysiology
  - ↑ T_3/T_4 which leads to the following:
    o ↓ TSH
      - Negative feedback
    o ↑ CO
    o ↑ Circulating blood volume
    o ↓ SVR
    o ↑ Anxiety
    o Sweating
    o Diarrhea

Graves' Disease

Systemic Autoimmune Disease Caused by Autoantibodies Binding to TSH Receptors

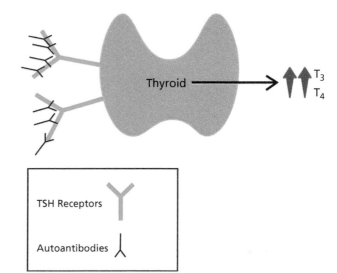

Figure 6.35

- Treatment
  - Methimazole
  - Propylthiouracil
  - β-blockers
  - Radioactive iodine therapy
  - Surgical removal of thyroid
- Primary Concerns
  - ↑ Risk of cardiovascular damage
    o Prone to sinus tachycardia and atrial fibrillation
    o May experience perioperative hemodynamic instability
    o Increased myocardial oxygen consumption
  - ↑ Sensitivity to catecholamines [114]
  - Respiratory muscle weakness
  - ↑ Risk of thyroid storm
- Evaluation
  - Consult endocrinologist
  - Consider TSH
  - Consider CMP
- Anesthesia Management
  - Establish euthyroid six to eight weeks prior to elective surgery
  - Hyperthyroidism does NOT increase MAC requirement
  - Consider difficult airway in patients with goiter obstruction
  - Avoid/reduce catecholaminergics due to increased sensitivity:
    o Ketamine

- Ephedrine
- Epinephrine
- No specific contraindications to volatile agents
- Monitor for thyroid storm
  - Under anesthesia, difficult to distinguish from MH
  - Hyperthermia
  - Cardiac dysfunction
    - Tachycardia
    - CHF
    - Hypotension
    - Dysrhythmias
  - No increased $EtCO_2$
    - Unlike MH
  - If diagnosis is unclear, okay to administer dantrolene
  - β-blockers and cooling measures available

Hypothyroidism

- Etiology/Risk Factors
  - Genetic
  - Iodine deficiency
  - Surgical removal
  - Hashimoto's thyroiditis
    - Autoimmune disease in which the thyroid gland is gradually destroyed
- Pathophysiology
  - ↓ T_3/T_4 which leads to the following (Figure 6.36):
  - ↑ TSH
    - Weight gain
    - Coarse facial features
    - Large tongue
    - Goiter
    - Left ventricular dysfunction [115]
    - Cold intolerance

- Bradycardia
- Hypotension
  - Peripheral edema
  - Significant reduction in exercise parameters [116]
  - Respiratory muscle weakness and reduced respiratory drive
  - ↑ Risk of coronary artery disease [117]
  - Myxedema coma
    - Rare severe form of hypothyroidism
- Treatment
  - Supplemental levothyroxine
- Primary Concerns
  - Cardiac dysfunction
  - Difficult airway
    - Enlarged tongue
    - Possible goiter
  - ↑ Sensitivity to anesthetic agents
  - ↑ Risk of hypothermia
- Evaluation
  - Consider endocrinologist consult
  - Consider TSH
  - Consider preoperative ECG
  - Consider CMP
- Anesthesia Management
  - Establish euthyroid six to eight weeks prior to elective surgery
    - ↓ Sensitivity [118]
  - They do NOT have decreased MAC requirement
  - ↑ Concern for a difficult airway, if goiter present
  - ↑ Sensitivity to opioids may lead to respiratory depression [119]
  - ↑ Risk for low blood pressure and CO on induction [120]
  - ↑ Hypothermia risk
  - ↓ Sensitivity to catecholamines [118]
    - ↑ Norepinephrine and epinephrine dosing
  - Patients may have delayed emergence

Cushing's Syndrome

- Etiology/Risk Factors
  - Long-term high-dose exogenous steroids
  - Cortisol secreting tumor
  - ACTH-secreting tumor
    - Pituitary adenoma
    - Pulmonary tumors [121]
- Pathophysiology
  - ↑ Circulating cortisol (Figure 6.37)
    - Inhibits secretion of CRH, ACTH, and vasopressin (ADH)
  - Physical changes:
    - Moon face

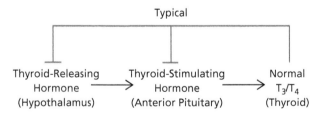

Typical

Thyroid-Releasing Hormone (Hypothalamus) → Thyroid-Stimulating Hormone (Anterior Pituitary) → Normal T_3/T_4 (Thyroid)

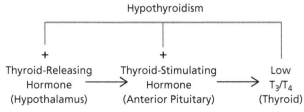

Hypothyroidism

+ Thyroid-Releasing Hormone (Hypothalamus) → + Thyroid-Stimulating Hormone (Anterior Pituitary) → Low T_3/T_4 (Thyroid)

Figure 6.36

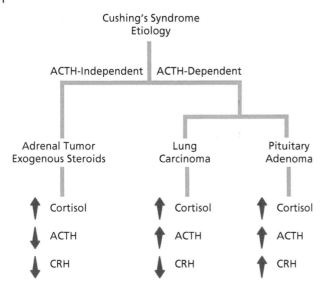

ACTH: Adrenocorticotropic Hormone
CRH: Corticotropin-Releasing hormone

Figure 6.37

- o Buffalo hump
- o ↑ BMI
- – Poor wound healing
- – Hyperglycemia
- – HTN
- – ↑ Risk of CAD
- – ↑ Risk of CHF [122]
- – ↑ Risk of osteoporosis
- – Metabolic derangements
  - o Hypokalemia
- – Musculoskeletal weakness/wasting
- Treatment
  - – See Daniel et al. [123]
  - – Discontinue exogenous corticoids
  - – Cabergoline
  - – Mifepristone
  - – Ketoconazole
  - – Metyrapone
  - – Mitotane
  - – Surgical removal of tumor
- Primary Concerns
  - – Electrolyte disturbances
  - – Musculoskeletal weakness
  - – Difficult airway
  - – Cardiovascular concerns
- Evaluation
  - – Consider endocrinologist consult
  - – Consider BMP
  - – Blood glucose
  - – HbA1c

- Anesthesia Management
  - – Monitor for hyperglycemia and treat it appropriately
  - – Avoid dexamethasone
  - – No specific contraindications to volatile agents or induction agents
  - – Consider etomidate induction as it does decrease cortisol secretion
    - o Uncertain clinical relevance
  - – Consider reducing NMB
    - o Skeletal muscle weakness baseline

Adrenal Insufficiency (Addison's Disease)

- Etiology/Risk Factors

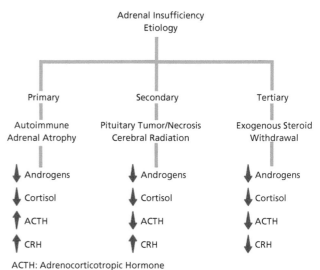

ACTH: Adrenocorticotropic Hormone
CRH: Corticotropin-Releasing hormone

Figure 6.38

- Pathophysiology
  - – ↓ Synthesis of adrenal hormones (Figure 6.38)
    - o Mainly androgens and cortisol
  - – Typically gradual onset, may go undetected until stress precipitates adrenal crisis
  - – Metabolic derangements
    - o Hyperkalemia
    - o Hyponatremia
  - – Hypoglycemia
  - – Cardiac pathology
- Treatment
  - – Steroid supplementation
- Primary Concerns
  - – Adrenal suppression
  - – ↑ Risk of cardiomyopathy
  - – Hyperkalemia

- Evaluation
  - Consider endocrinologist consult
  - Consider BMP
  - History
    - Last crisis
    - Hospitalization
- Anesthesia Management
  - Monitor blood glucose
  - Consider stress dose steroids
  - Avoid etomidate
  - Crisis presents as hypotensive shock
    - Fluid resuscitation with NS or D5NS
    - Administration of glucocorticoid – hydrocortisone or dexamethasone

6.15   Hematologic Disease

Sickle Cell Anemia

- Etiology/Risk Factors
  - Autosomal recessive
    - Point mutation in the gene HBB results in HgS
  - Homozygous HgS or heterozygous HgS and another HBB variant (e.g. coinheritance of β thalassemia) produce sickle cell disease
  - Sickle cell trait
    - Benign carrier state
- Pathophysiology
  - Polymerization of red blood cells into "sickle" shape under conditions of duress. Triggers include (Figure 6.39)
    - Stress
    - Hypovolemia
    - Infection
    - Hypoxia
    - Hypothermia

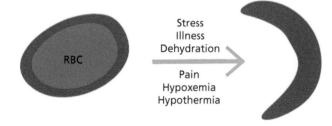

Figure 6.39

  - Vaso-occlusive pain
  - ↑ Risk of stroke/TIA
  - ↑ Risk of cardiac failure
  - ↑ Risk of ischemic heart disease
  - ↑ Risk of acute chest syndrome
  - ↑ Risk of pulmonary HTN
  - ↑ Risk of CKD [124]
  - ↑ Risk of hepatic dysfunction [125]
  - Hemolytic anemia

  - ↑ Risk of blood-borne pathogens especially if older
    - HIV
    - Hepatitis
  - Patients with sickle cell disease are more resistant to malarial infection
- Treatment [126]
  - Prevent crises
  - Hydroxyurea
  - Crizanlizumab
  - Blood transfusions
  - Gene therapy
  - Bone marrow transplant
- Primary Concerns
  - Sickle cell crisis
  - Microvascular occlusion and end-organ damage
- Evaluation
  - Consider hematology consult
  - Consider CBC
  - Consider LFTs
  - Consider BMP
  - Consider PT/PTT/INR
  - Consider echocardiogram
  - DASI/METs
  - History
    - Last crisis
    - Precipitating factors
    - Use of pain medication
  - Evaluate severity and frequency of crises by surveying end-organ damage
- Anesthesia Management
  - Patients undergoing low-risk procedures may not need a transfusion beforehand
  - Schedule patient early in the day
    - Avoid hypovolemia
  - Consider preoperative blood transfusion
  - Avoid sickle cell triggers
    - Dehydration
    - Acidosis
    - Hypothermia

- No specific contraindications to volatile agents or induction drugs [127]
- Consider multimodal analgesia due to likely high opioid tolerance
  - Dexmedetomidine
  - Ketamine
  - Gabapentin
  - Acetaminophen
  - NSAIDs
  - Lidocaine

Hemophilia

- Etiology/Risk Factors
  - X-linked recessive
- Pathophysiology
  - Bleeding disorder from a decrease in coagulation factors
  - Hemophilia A
    - Factor VIII deficiency
  - Hemophilia B
    - Factor IX deficiency
    - Also called Christmas disease
- Treatment
  - Hemophilia A
    - Desmopressin
    - Factor VIII infusions
  - Hemophilia B
    - Factor IX recombinant
    - Prothrombin complex
      - Factors II, IX, and X
- Primary Concerns
  - Perioperative bleeding
  - ↑ Risk of blood-borne pathogens, especially if older
    - HIV
    - Hepatitis
- Evaluation
  - Consider hematology consult
  - Hemophilia type
  - Recent labs for factor levels
  - Severity of factor deficiency

Severity classification	Factor VIII/IX activity
Mild	>5%
Moderate	1–5%
Severe	<1%

- Anesthesia Management
  - Coordinate with the surgeon
    - Evaluate the invasiveness of the procedure

- Preoperative factor infusion per hematology direction
  - Consider checking factor level after infusion, prior to surgery
- Attempt to avoid traumatic intubation
  - May choose to avoid nasal intubation
- Consider more aggressive local measures to promote hemostasis
  - Collagen plug [128]
  - Atraumatic extractions
  - Local anesthesia with vasoconstrictor
  - Suture placement
  - Consider tranexamic acid perioperatively
- Consider need for factor transfusion intraoperatively or postoperatively
- No specific contraindication to volatile agents or induction agents
- Avoid IM injections
- Postoperative coughing or vomiting could produce bleeding in posterior pharynx or floor of the mouth
  - Be prepared for emergent intubation if uncontrollable swelling causes impending obstruction [129]
- Avoid NSAIDs postoperatively [130, 131]

Von Willebrand Factor (vWF) Disease

- Etiology/Risk Factors
  - Most common inherited bleeding disorder
    - Variants in vWF gene can lead to impaired synthesis, secretion, clearance, or function of vWF
- Pathophysiology
  - ↓ Quality or quantity of vWF factor
  - ↑ Bleeding time
  - ↑ PTT
  - Normal PT
  - ↓ Factor VIII
    - vWF stabilizes factor VIII *in vivo*
- Treatment [132]
  - Desmopressin (DDAVP)
    - ↑ vWF release from Weibel–Palade bodies in endothelial cells
  - Factor VIII replacement
  - vWF factor replacement
  - Antifibrinolytics
- Primary Concerns
  - Perioperative bleeding
  - ↑ Risk of blood-borne pathogens, especially if older
    - HIV
    - Hepatitis
- Evaluation
  - Consider hematology consult
  - Consider PT/PTT/INR

– DDAVP trial to demonstrate response
– vWF disease type

Type 1	Partial quantitative deficiency
Type 2	Qualitative deficiency
Type 3	Complete quantitative deficiency

- Anesthesia Management
  – Preoperative DDAVP if patient has demonstrated adequate response
  – Preoperative infusion of vWF concentrates in patients with inadequate response to DDAVP
    ○ Plasma-derived vWF concentrates contain factor VIII
  – Attempt to avoid traumatic intubation
    ○ May choose to avoid nasal intubation
  – Coordinate with the surgeon
    ○ Evaluate the invasiveness of the procedure
  – Consider more aggressive local measures to promote hemostasis
    ○ Collagen plug [128]
    ○ Atraumatic extractions
    ○ Local anesthesia with vasoconstriction
    ○ Suture placement
    ○ Consider tranexamic acid postoperatively
  – No specific contraindication to volatile agents or induction agents
  – Be prepared for emergent intubation if uncontrollable swelling causes impending obstruction
  – Avoid NSAIDs postoperatively

Factor V Leiden

- Etiology/Risk Factors
  – Point mutation of F5 gene
  – Autosomal dominant
  – Most common in Scandinavian and northern European ethnicities
- Pathophysiology
  – Factor V rendered insensitive to activated protein C
  – Thrombophilia
  – Highly variable phenotype
  – For coagulation cascade, see page 59
- Treatment
  – Anticoagulation if Venous Thromboembolism (VTE) occurs
    ○ Maybe indefinite if VTE is unprovoked or recurring
- Primary Concerns
  – ↑ Risk of venous thromboembolism
    ○ Only 5–10% of heterozygous people will experience VTE
    ○ ↑ Risk by advanced age, coinheritance of other thrombophilias, homozygous inheritance, and hormonal alterations
  – Potential anticoagulation
- Evaluation
  – History
    ○ History of VTE and anticoagulation use
  – Consider hematology consult for patients with a history of VTE
- Anesthesia Management
  – No specific contraindications to volatile agents or induction agents
  – Discuss with surgeon avoidance of prolonged surgery (≥2 hours)
  – Pharmacologic DVT prophylaxis in conjunction with hematology consult, weighing surgical bleeding risk
  – Vigilance for signs and symptoms of DVT and PE, especially postoperatively
  – Encourage early and frequent ambulation
  – Consider having patient wear anti-embolism stockings or prescribed graduated compression stockings

6.16 Orthopedic Disease

Intervertebral Disk Disease

- Etiology/Risk Factors
  - ↑ Age
  - Trauma
- Pathophysiology
  - Anatomic changes and a loss of function of varying degrees of one or more intervertebral discs of the spine (Figure 6.40)

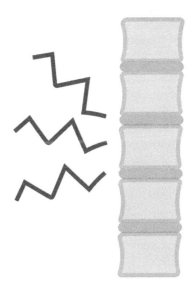

Figure 6.40

- Symptoms occur when nucleus pulposus herniates and compresses a nerve root
- Cervical disk herniates typically at C_5–C_6 or C_6–C_7
- Lumbar disk herniates typically at L_4–L_5 or L_5–S_1
- Treatment
  - Steroids
  - Opioids
  - Physical therapy
  - Surgical intervention

- Primary Concerns
  - Difficult positioning
  - Tolerance to opioids
  - Coughing or straining will exacerbate pain at any level
  - Adrenal axis suppression
- Evaluation
  - Imaging
  - Location and quality of pain, numbness, or weakness
  - Pain medication regimen
  - Baseline neuro exam
- Anesthesia Management
  - Consider video laryngoscope or fiberoptic intubation to reduce vertebral column manipulation in the setting of cervical disease
    - Stabilize affected portion to ensure comfort
  - Stress dose steroids may be required for high-risk patients
    - True adrenal insufficiency
    - Extensive surgical procedure
  - Consider multimodal analgesia as patient is likely
    - Dexmedetomidine
    - Ketamine
    - Gabapentin
    - Acetaminophen
    - NSAIDs
    - Lidocaine

Osteoarthritis

- Etiology/Risk Factors
  - Most common joint disease in US
  - Joint trauma
  - Biomechanical stresses
  - ↓ Joint support
  - Neuropathy
  - Ligamentous injury
  - Muscle atrophy

- Pathophysiology
  - Degenerative process that affects articular cartilage (Figure 6.41)

Osteoarthritis	Rheumatoid Arthritis
Degeneration Over Time	Autoimmune Component
Aggravated by Movement Relieved by Rest	Stress and Illness can Exacerbate

Figure 6.41

  - Most commonly affects weight-bearing joints
    - Hands
    - Lower back
    - Neck
- Treatment
  - Physical therapy
  - Exercise
  - Heat
  - Analgesics
    - NSAIDs
    - Opioids
    - Acetaminophen
  - Corticosteroid injection
  - Surgery
- Primary Concerns
  - Patient positioning
  - Adrenal axis suppression
- Evaluation
  - History
    - Location
    - Alleviating factors
    - Medication regimen including steroid history
- Anesthesia Management
  - Patient positioning
  - Pillow under legs prior to start
  - For patients who are wheelchair bound, careful consideration in succinylcholine administration as receptors could be upregulated

Osteogenesis Imperfecta

- Etiology/Risk Factors
  - Autosomal dominant in most cases
- Pathophysiology
  - Defective type I collagen synthesis
    - Short stature
    - Bone deformity

- Frequent fractures, often with minimal trauma
- Abnormal dentin
  - May also be associated with dentinogenesis imperfecta
- Blue sclera (Figure 6.42)

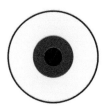

Blue Sclera

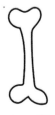

Bowing of Femur

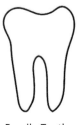

Fragile Teeth

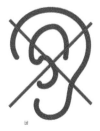

Deafness

Figure 6.42

- Facial dysmorphism
- Hearing loss
- Skin laxity
- Joint hypermobility
- Spectrum of clinical severity
- Treatment
  - Avoid physical trauma
  - Bisphosphonates
  - Physical therapy
  - Surgical intervention
- Primary Concerns
  - Teeth vulnerable to damage
  - Bone fragility
  - ↑ Bleeding time [133]
- Evaluation
  - Consider PT/PTT/INR
  - Check neck flexion
- Anesthesia Management
  - Difficult positioning and careful padding
  - Consider fiberoptic intubation
  - Succinylcholine contraindicated
    - Fasciculations may cause fractures
  - Caution with automated blood pressure cuff

6.17   Immune Disease

Acquired Immunodeficiency Syndrome (AIDS)

- Etiology/Risk Factors
  - Sexual transmission
  - Exposure to infected blood
  - Perinatal transmission
- Pathophysiology
  - Chronic infection with retrovirus HIV
  - Can be asymptomatic
  - Patients with HIV infection who are treated before significant immunosuppression occurs have close to normal life expectancy
  - Immune suppression may lead to opportunistic infections:
    - ○ Candidiasis
    - ○ MRSA
    - ○ Herpes simplex
    - ○ Molluscum contagiosum
- Treatment
  - Highly active antiretroviral therapy (HAART)
  - Nucleoside reverse transcriptase inhibitors
  - Non-nucleoside reverse transcriptase inhibitors
  - Protease inhibitors
  - Integrase strand transfer inhibitors
  - Entry inhibitors
  - Stem cell transplant
- Primary Concerns
  - Medications and effects on anesthetic agents
  - Immune suppression
- Evaluation
  - Current therapy
  - Current HIV/AIDs symptoms
  - Current staging (Figure 6.43)
  - Consider CBC
  - Consider BMP
  - Consider PT/PTT/INR
  - Consider LFTs
  - Consider echocardiogram, if cardiac abnormalities suspected

HIV/AIDS Classification

	CD4 Count (Cells/mm^3)	CD4 (%)	AIDS-Defining Condition?*
Stage 0	First 6 months of infection		
Stage 1	>500	>26	No
Stage 2	200–499	14–25	No
Stage 3	<200	<14	Yes

*Documentation of an AIDS-defining conditions automatically makes anyone Stage 3, regardless of CD4 count per HIV.va.gov:

Coccidioidomycosis, disseminated, or extrapulmonary
Cryptococcosis, extrapulmonary
Cytomegalovirus, extrapulmonary
Histoplasmosis, disseminated, or extrapulmonary
kaposi sarcoma
Lymphoma
Tuberculosis
Pneumocystis pneumonia

Figure 6.43

- Anesthesia Management
  - Universal standards for PPE do not change for patients with diagnosed blood-borne transmissible diseases
  - Typically, a well-controlled HIV-infected patient has little increased risk during surgical procedure [134]
  - No specific anesthetic technique favored
  - Autonomic neuropathy may be clinical
  - Consider immune suppression of anesthetics and perioperative stress response

Multiple Sclerosis

- Etiology/Risk Factors
  - Cause unclear
  - Female
  - Multifactorial

- o Genetic susceptibility
- o Environmental triggers
- o Viral infection serving as antigenic trigger through molecular mimicry
- Pathophysiology
  - Autoimmune inflammatory demyelinating disease of CNS (Figure 6.44)

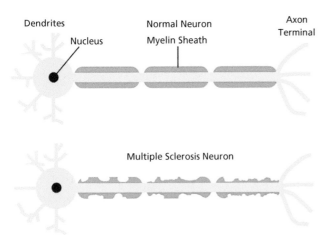

Figure 6.44

  - Chronic neurodegeneration, acute relapses.
  - Muscle weakness
    - o Will get progressively weak with use throughout the day
    - o Incoordination and gait imbalance
    - o Spasticity
  - Swallowing difficulties
    - o Aspiration
  - Cognitive impairment
  - Chronic pain
- Treatment
  - Symptom management
  - Corticosteroids
  - Anti-inflammatories
  - Interferon β
  - Glatiramer
    - o Simulates myelin basic protein
    - o Cardiac toxicity
  - Monoclonal antibody
- Primary Concerns
  - Muscle weakness
  - ↑ Risk of aspiration
  - Chronic pain
- Evaluation
  - History
    - o Last relapse
    - o Hospitalizations

- Anesthesia Management
  - Consider scheduling first case of the day when muscles are strongest
  - Avoid hyperthermia
    - o ↑ Body temperature blocks demyelinated nerve conduction
  - Avoid succinylcholine [135]
    - o ↑ K^+ release
  - Sensitivity to non-depolarizer NMB
  - Possible to exacerbate condition post operatively

Rheumatoid Arthritis

- Etiology/Risk Factors
  - 1% of adults
    - o Most common chronic inflammatory disease
  - Interaction between genetic predisposition, environment, and lifestyle
  - Female
  - Smoking
- Pathophysiology
  - Rheumatoid factor
    - o Autoantibody to IgG
  - Inflammation of one or more joints, typically symmetric
    - o Proximal interphalangeal and metacarpophalangeal joints of hand and wrists and small joints of the feet
  - Morning stiffness is a hallmark of rheumatoid arthritis
  - ↑ Inflammatory causes systemic issues:
    - o ↑ Coronary atherosclerosis
    - o Neuropathy
    - o Restrictive lung changes
    - o Keratoconjunctivitis
      - Lack of tear formation due to impaired lacrimal gland function
- Treatment
  - NSAIDs
    - o COX_2 inhibitors preferred
  - Corticosteroids
  - DMARDs
  - Methotrexate
  - Gold
  - Joint replacement surgery
- Primary Concerns
  - Difficult airway
    - o TMJ limitations
    - o Cervical spine involvement
    - o Potential atlantoaxial subluxation
  - Adrenal axis suppression

- Evaluation
  - Thorough airway evaluation
  - MRI
  - CT scan
  - Atlantoaxial subluxation evaluation
    - o Have patient demonstrate head movement or positioning that can be tolerated without discomfort or other symptoms
- Anesthesia Management
  - Potentially difficult airway
  - Consider fiberoptic intubation
  - C-spine precautions with atlantoaxial subluxation
  - Consider supplemental steroids

Systemic Lupus Erythematosus

- Etiology/Risk Factors
  - Unknown cause
  - Female
  - Catecholamines (stress)
  - Infection
  - Pregnancy
  - Drug-induced
    - o Procainamide
    - o Hydralazine
    - o Isoniazid
- Pathophysiology
  - Multisystem chronic autoimmune inflammatory disease that can affect any organ (Figure 6.45)
    - o Butterfly rash

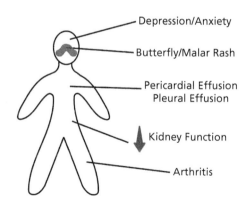

Depression/Anxiety

Butterfly/Malar Rash

Pericardial Effusion
Pleural Effusion

Kidney Function

Arthritis

Figure 6.45

- o Dermatitis
- o Polyarthritis
- o Proximal skeletal muscle weakness
- o Pericardial effusion
- o CAD
- o Pleural effusion
- o Hematologic abnormalities
  - Anemia
  - Thrombocytopenia
  - Lupus anticoagulant
- o Depression
- o Anxiety
- o Fatigue
  - Antinuclear antibodies
- Treatment
  - NSAIDs
  - Antimalarials
  - Hydroxychloroquine
  - Quinacrine
  - Sunscreens
  - Corticosteroids
  - Danazol
  - Vincristine
  - Cyclophosphamide
- Primary Concerns
  - ↓ Renal clearance
  - Adrenal axis suppression
  - Blood dyscrasias
  - Cardiac disease
  - Hypercoagulability
- Evaluation
  - Consider cardiologist consult
  - Consider rheumatologist consult
  - Consider the magnitude of organ system dysfunction and the medications taken
  - History of last flare up
  - Consider BMP
  - Consider CBC
- Anesthesia Management
  - Raynaud phenomenon is common and may interfere with pulse oximetry
  - Consider steroids
    - o *Consider stress dose (page 108)*
  - Be aware of potential laryngeal involvement
    - o Oral and nasal mucosal ulceration
    - o Cricoarytenoid arthritis

6.18 Connective Tissue Disease

Marfan Syndrome

- Etiology/Risk Factors
  - Autosomal dominant inheritance
- Pathophysiology
  - Mutation of gene encoding connective tissue protein fibrillin-1
  - Range of clinical severity
  - Excess growth of long bones and joint laxity
  - Cardiac dysfunction
    o Mitral valve prolapse
    o Aortic valve regurgitation
  - Aortic aneurysm
  - Aortic dissection
  - Emphysematous lung changes
  - Scoliosis
  - Retrognathia common
- Treatment
  - Avoid vigorous physical activity
  - β-blockers
  - ARBs
  - Elective surgical repair of aorta
- Primary Concerns
  - Cardiac dysfunction
  - May be anticoagulated if mitral valve replaced
  - Aortic root disease
  - Spontaneous pneumothorax
- Evaluation
  - Consider cardiology consultation
    o Monitoring of aortic disease should be done at least annually
  - Consider pulmonary consultation
  - PT/PTT/INR if anticoagulated
- Anesthesia Management
  - Careful positioning
  - Antibiotic prophylaxis for prosthetic valve, if applicable
  - Potentially difficult airway due to facial dysmorphism
  - Avoid high airway pressures
  - Avoid extremes of blood pressure

Ehlers–Danlos Syndrome

- Etiology/Risk Factors
  - Inherited genetic mutation affecting synthesis and processing of collagen
  - Autosomal dominant
- Pathophysiology
  - Skin hyperextensibility
  - Joint hypermobility
  - Tissue fragility
  - Premature degenerative arthritis and joint pain
  - Symptoms of mast cell activation
    o Asthma
    o Urticaria
    o Flushing
  - Scoliosis
- Treatment
  - Symptom management
  - Physical and occupational therapy
- Primary Concerns
  - May experience easy bruising and poor wound healing
  - Chronic pain
- Evaluation
  - Consider physician consultation
    o Periodic echocardiogram likely part of patient management
  - Pain medication regimen
  - Bleeding history
- Anesthesia Management
  - Careful positioning
  - Resistance to local anesthesia has been reported [136]
  - High suspicion for cervical spine instability and temporomandibular dysfunction
  - Avoid extremes of blood pressure

References

1 Corssen, G., Little, S.C., and Tavakoli, M. (1974). Ketamine and epilepsy. *Anesth. Analg.* 53 (2): 319–335.

2 Crozier, W.C. (1987). Upper airway obstruction in neurofibromatosis. *Anaesthesia* 42 (11): 1209–1211. https://doi.org/10.1111/j.1365-2044.1987.tb05232.x.

3 Richardson, M.G., Setty, G.K., and Rawoof, S.A. (1996). Responses to nondepolarizing neuromuscular blockers and succinylcholine in von Recklinghausen neurofibromatosis. *Anesth. Analg.* 82 (2): 382–385. https://doi.org/10.1097/00000539-199602000-00030.

4 Hirsch, N.P., Murphy, A., and Radcliffe, J.J. (2001). Neurofibromatosis: clinical presentations and anaesthetic implications. *Br. J. Anaesth.* 86 (4): 555–564. https://doi.org/10.1093/bja/86.4.555.

5 Ascherio, A. and Schwarzschild, M.A. (2016). The epidemiology of Parkinson's disease: risk factors and prevention. *Lancet Neurol.* 15 (12): 1257–1272. https://doi.org/10.1016/S1474-4422(16)30230-7.

6 Troche, M.S., Brandimore, A.E., Okun, M.S. et al. (2014). Decreased cough sensitivity and aspiration in Parkinson disease. *Chest* 146 (5): 1294–1299. https://doi.org/10.1378/chest.14-0066.

7 Izquierdo-Alonso, J.L., Jiménez-Jiménez, F.J., Cabrera-Valdivia, F., and Mansilla-Lesmes, M. (1994). Airway dysfunction in patients with Parkinson's disease. *Lung* 172 (1): 47–55. https://doi.org/10.1007/BF00186168.

8 Fasano, A., Visanji, N.P., Liu, L.W. et al. (2015). Gastrointestinal dysfunction in Parkinson's disease. *Lancet Neurol.* 14 (6): 625–639. https://doi.org/10.1016/S1474-4422(15)00007-1.

9 Krauss, J.K., Akeyson, E.W., Giam, P., and Jankovic, J. (1996). Propofol-induced dyskinesias in Parkinson's disease. *Anesth. Analg.* 83 (2): 420–422. https://doi.org/10.1097/00000539-199608000-00037.

10 Deogaonkar, A., Deogaonkar, M., Lee, J.Y. et al. (2006). Propofol-induced dyskinesias controlled with dexmedetomidine during deep brain stimulation surgery. *Anesthesiology* 104 (6): 1337–1339. https://doi.org/10.1097/00000542-200606000-00029.

11 Stirt, J.A., Frantz, R.A., Gunz, E.F., and Conolly, M.E. (1982). Anesthesia, catecholamines, and hemodynamics in autonomic dysfunction. *Anesth. Analg.* 61 (8): 701–704.

12 Paleacu, D., Anca, M., and Giladi, N. (2002). Olanzapine in Huntington's disease. *Acta Neurol. Scand.* 105 (6): 441–444. https://doi.org/10.1034/j.1600-0404.2002.01197.x.

13 Ciammola, A., Sassone, J., Colciago, C. et al. (2009). Aripiprazole in the treatment of Huntington's disease: a case series. *Neuropsychiatr. Dis. Treat.* 5: 1–4.

14 Paleacu, D. (2007). Tetrabenazine in the treatment of Huntington's disease. *Neuropsychiatr. Dis. Treat.* 3 (5): 545–551.

15 Melkani, G.C. (2016). Huntington's disease-induced cardiac disorders affect multiple cellular pathways. *React. Oxyg Species (Apex).* 2 (5): 325–338. https://doi.org/10.20455/ros.2016.859.

16 Reyes, A., Cruickshank, T., Ziman, M., and Nosaka, K. (2014). Pulmonary function in patients with Huntington's disease. *BMC Pulm. Med.* 14: 89. https://doi.org/10.1186/1471-2466-14-89.

17 van der Burg, J.M., Winqvist, A., Aziz, N.A. et al. (2011). Gastrointestinal dysfunction contributes to weight loss in Huntington's disease mice. *Neurobiol. Dis.* 44 (1): 1–8. https://doi.org/10.1016/j.nbd.2011.05.006.

18 Messmer, K. and Reynolds, G.P. (1998). Increased peripheral benzodiazepine binding sites in the brain of patients with Huntington's disease. *Neurosci. Lett.* 241 (1): 53–56. https://doi.org/10.1016/s0304-3940(97)00967-1.

19 Kivela, J.E., Sprung, J., Southorn, P.A. et al. (2010). Anesthetic management of patients with Huntington disease. *Anesth. Analg.* 110 (2): 515–523. https://doi.org/10.1213/ANE.0b013e3181c88fcd.

20 Mehdi, Z., Birns, J., Partridge, J. et al. (2016). Perioperative management of adult patients with a history of stroke or transient ischaemic attack undergoing elective non-cardiac surgery. *Clin. Med. (Lond.)* 16 (6): 535–540. https://doi.org/10.7861/clinmedicine.16-6-535.

21 Landercasper, J., Merz, B.J., Cogbill, T.H. et al. (1990). Perioperative stroke risk in 173 consecutive patients with a past history of stroke. *Arch. Surg.* 125 (8): 986–989. https://doi.org/10.1001/archsurg.1990.01410200044006.

22 Malamed, S.F. (2004). *Handbook of Local Anesthesia*, 5e, vol. xiii. Mosby, 399 p.

23 Borer, J.S. and Sharma, A. (2015). Drug therapy for heart valve diseases. *Circulation* 132 (11): 1038–1045. https://doi.org/10.1161/CIRCULATIONAHA.115.016006.

24 Elkayam, U. (1996). Nitrates in the treatment of congestive heart failure. *Am. J. Cardiol.* 77 (13): 41C–51C. https://doi.org/10.1016/s0002-9149(96)00188-9.

25 Bonow, R.O., Carabello, B.A., Kanu, C. et al. (2006). ACC/AHA 2006 guidelines for the management of patients with valvular heart disease: a report of the American College of Cardiology/American Heart Association Task Force on Practice Guidelines (writing committee to revise the 1998 Guidelines for the Management of Patients with Valvular Heart Disease): developed in collaboration with the Society of Cardiovascular Anesthesiologists: endorsed by the Society for Cardiovascular Angiography and Interventions and the Society of Thoracic Surgeons.

Circulation 114 (5): e84–e231. https://doi.org/10.1161/CIRCULATIONAHA.106.176857.

26 Sidhu, S. and Marine, J.E. (2020). Evaluating and managing bradycardia. *Trends Cardiovasc. Med.* 30 (5): 265–272. https://doi.org/10.1016/j.tcm.2019.07.001.

27 Khanna, S., Sreedharan, R., Trombetta, C., and Ruetzler, K. (2020). Sick sinus syndrome: sinus node dysfunction in the elderly. *Anesthesiology* 132 (2): 377–378. https://doi.org/10.1097/ALN.0000000000003004.

28 McCord, J. and Borzak, S. (1998). Multifocal atrial tachycardia. *Chest* 113 (1): 203–209. https://doi.org/10.1378/chest.113.1.203.

29 Scher, D.L. and Arsura, E.L. (1989). Multifocal atrial tachycardia: mechanisms, clinical correlates, and treatment. *Am. Heart J.* 118 (3): 574–580. https://doi.org/10.1016/0002-8703(89)90275-5.

30 Kim, L.K., Lee, C.S., and Jeun, J.G. (2010). Development of multifocal atrial tachycardia in a patient using aminophylline – a case report. *Korean J. Anesthesiol.* 59 (Suppl): S77–S81. https://doi.org/10.4097/kjae.2010.59.S.S77.

31 Arsura, E., Lefkin, A.S., Scher, D.L. et al. (1988). A randomized, double-blind, placebo-controlled study of verapamil and metoprolol in treatment of multifocal atrial tachycardia. *Am. J. Med.* 85 (4): 519–524. https://doi.org/10.1016/s0002-9343(88)80088-3.

32 Beach, S.R., Celano, C.M., Sugrue, A.M. et al. (2018). QT prolongation, Torsades de pointes, and psychotropic medications: a 5-year update. *Psychosomatics* 59 (2): 105–122. https://doi.org/10.1016/j.psym.2017.10.009.

33 Del Rosario, M.E., Weachter, R., and Flaker, G.C. (2010). Drug-induced QT prolongation and sudden death. *Mo. Med.* 107 (1): 53–58.

34 Yap, Y.G. and Camm, A.J. (1999). The current cardiac safety situation with antihistamines. *Clin. Exp. Allergy* 29 (Suppl 1): 15–24.

35 Stringer, J., Welsh, C., and Tommasello, A. (2009). Methadone-associated Q-T interval prolongation and torsades de pointes. *Am. J. Health-Syst. Pharm.* 66 (9): 825–833. https://doi.org/10.2146/ajhp070392.

36 Krantz, M.J., Lewkowiez, L., Hays, H. et al. (2002). Torsade de pointes associated with very-high-dose methadone. *Ann. Intern. Med.* 137 (6): 501–504. https://doi.org/10.7326/0003-4819-137-6-200209170-00010.

37 Kies, S.J., Pabelick, C.M., Hurley, H.A. et al. (2005). Anesthesia for patients with congenital long QT syndrome. *Anesthesiology* 102 (1): 204–210. https://doi.org/10.1097/00000542-200501000-00029.

38 Chang, D.J., Kweon, T.D., Nam, S.B. et al. (2008). Effects of fentanyl pretreatment on the QTc interval during propofol induction. *Anaesthesia* 63 (10): 1056–1060. https://doi.org/10.1111/j.1365-2044.2008.05559.x.

39 Gallagher, J.D., Weindling, S.N., Anderson, G., and Fillinger, M.P. (1998). Effects of sevoflurane on QT interval in a patient with congenital long QT syndrome. *Anesthesiology* 89 (6): 1569–1573. https://doi.org/10.1097/00000542-199812000-00038.

40 Medak, R. and Benumof, J.L. (1983). Perioperative management of the prolonged Q-T interval syndrome. *Br. J. Anaesth.* 55 (4): 361–364. https://doi.org/10.1093/bja/55.4.361.

41 Sun, Z.H., Swan, H., Viitasalo, M., and Toivonen, L. (1998). Effects of epinephrine and phenylephrine on QT interval dispersion in congenital long QT syndrome. *J. Am. Coll. Cardiol.* 31 (6): 1400–1405. https://doi.org/10.1016/s0735-1097(98)00104-1.

42 Xu, Y., Wang, Y., Chen, J. et al. (2020). The comorbidity of mental and physical disorders with self-reported chronic back or neck pain: results from the China Mental Health Survey. *J. Affect. Disord.* 260: 334–341. https://doi.org/10.1016/j.jad.2019.08.089.

43 Callaghan, M.L., Nichols, A.B., and Sweet, R.B. (1977). Anesthetic management of prolonged Q-T interval syndrome. *Anesthesiology* 47 (1): 67–69. https://doi.org/10.1097/00000542-197707000-00015.

44 Beccaria, E., Brun, S., Gaita, F. et al. (1989). Torsade de pointes during an atropine sulfate test in a patient with congenital long QT syndrome. *Cardiologia* 34 (12): 1039–1043.

45 Saarnivaara, L. and Simola, M. (1998). Effects of four anticholinesterase-anticholinergic combinations and tracheal extubation on QTc interval of the ECG, heart rate and arterial pressure. *Acta Anaesthesiol. Scand.* 42 (4): 460–463. https://doi.org/10.1111/j.1399-6576.1998.tb05142.x.

46 Hatta, K., Takahashi, T., Nakamura, H. et al. (2001). The association between intravenous haloperidol and prolonged QT interval. *J. Clin. Psychopharmacol.* 21 (3): 257–261. https://doi.org/10.1097/00004714-200106000-00002.

47 Collins, S., Widger, J., Davis, A., and Massie, J. (2012). Management of asthma in children with long QT syndrome. *Paediatr. Respir. Rev.* 13 (2): 100–105. https://doi.org/10.1016/j.prrv.2011.02.003.

48 Bengali, R., Wellens, H.J., and Jiang, Y. (2014). Perioperative management of the Wolff-Parkinson-White syndrome. *J. Cardiothorac. Vasc. Anesth.* 28 (5): 1375–1386. https://doi.org/10.1053/j.jvca.2014.02.003.

49 Page, R.L., Joglar, J.A., Caldwell, M.A. et al. (2015). ACC/AHA/HRS Guideline for the Management of Adult Patients With Supraventricular Tachycardia: a report of the American College of Cardiology/American Heart Association Task Force on Clinical Practice Guidelines and the Heart Rhythm Society. *Circulation* 133 (14): e506–e574. https://doi.org/10.1161/CIR.0000000000000311.

50 Gupta, A., Sharma, J., Banerjee, N., and Sood, R. (2013). Anesthetic management in a patient with Wolff-Parkinson-White syndrome for laparoscopic cholecystectomy. *Anesth. Essays Res.* 7 (2): 270–272. https://doi.org/10.4103/0259-1162.118988.

51 Hayward, R., Domanic, N., Enderby, G.E., and McDonald, L. (1982). Anaesthesia in first degree atrioventricular block. *Anaesthesia* 37 (12): 1190–1194. https://doi.org/10.1111/j.1365-2044.1982.tb01785.x.

52 Elayi, C.S., Lusher, S., Meeks Nyquist, J.L. et al. (2015). Interference between dental electrical devices and pacemakers or defibrillators: results from a prospective clinical study. *J. Am. Dent. Assoc.* 146 (2): 121–128. https://doi.org/10.1016/j.adaj.2014.11.016.

53 (2020). Practice advisory for the perioperative management of patients with cardiac implantable electronic devices: pacemakers and implantable cardioverter-defibrillators 2020: an updated report by the American Society of Anesthesiologists Task Force on Perioperative Management of Patients with Cardiac Implantable Electronic Devices: erratum. *Anesthesiology* 132 (4): 938. https://doi.org/10.1097/ALN.0000000000003217.

54 Andersen, C. and Madsen, G.M. (1990). Rate-responsive pacemakers and anaesthesia. A consideration of possible implications. *Anaesthesia* 45 (6): 472–476. https://doi.org/10.1111/j.1365-2044.1990.tb14339.x.

55 Finfer, S.R. (1991). Pacemaker failure on induction of anaesthesia. *Br. J. Anaesth.* 66 (4): 509–512. https://doi.org/10.1093/bja/66.4.509.

56 Chakravarthy, M., Prabhakumar, D., and George, A. (2017). Anaesthetic consideration in patients with cardiac implantable electronic devices scheduled for surgery. *Indian J. Anaesth.* 61 (9): 736–743. https://doi.org/10.4103/ija.IJA_346_17.

57 Kirklin, J.K., Naftel, D.C., Pagani, F.D. et al. (2015). Seventh INTERMACS annual report: 15,000 patients and counting. *J. Heart Lung Transplant.* 34 (12): 1495–1504. https://doi.org/10.1016/j.healun.2015.10.003.

58 Pisansky, A.J.B., Burbano-Vera, N., and Stopfkuchen-Evans, M.F. (2020). Anesthetic management of a patient with left ventricular assist device undergoing robotic laparoscopic prostatectomy: a case report. *JA Clin. Rep.* 6 (1): 57. https://doi.org/10.1186/s40981-020-00364-1.

59 Baker, P.R., Pavone, J., Teicher, R. et al. (2022). Management of the dental patient with an implanted left ventricular assist device (LVAD), a case report and suggested guidelines for care. *J. Dent. Oral Sci.* 4 (3): 1–10. https://doi.org/10.37191/Mapsci-2582-3736-4(3)-130.

60 Wilson, W.R., Gewitz, M., Lockhart, P.B. et al. (2021). Prevention of Viridans Group streptococcal infective endocarditis: a scientific statement from the American Heart Association. *Circulation* 143 (20): e963–e978. https://doi.org/10.1161/CIR.0000000000000969.

61 Hanada, S., Kawakami, H., Goto, T., and Morita, S. (2006). Hypertension and anesthesia. *Curr. Opin. Anaesthesiol.* 19 (3): 315–319. https://doi.org/10.1097/01.aco.0000192811.56161.23.

62 Hollmann, C., Fernandes, N.L., and Biccard, B.M. (2018). A systematic review of outcomes associated with withholding or continuing angiotensin-converting enzyme inhibitors and angiotensin receptor blockers before noncardiac surgery. *Anesth. Analg.* 127 (3): 678–687. https://doi.org/10.1213/ANE.0000000000002837.

63 Gill, R. and Goldstein, S. (2023). *Evaluation and Management of Perioperative Hypertension*. StatPearls.

64 Futier, E., Lefrant, J.Y., Guinot, P.G. et al. (2017). Effect of individualized vs standard blood pressure management strategies on postoperative organ dysfunction among high-risk patients undergoing major surgery: a randomized clinical trial. *JAMA* 318 (14): 1346–1357. https://doi.org/10.1001/jama.2017.14172.

65 McQuillan, B.M., Picard, M.H., Leavitt, M., and Weyman, A.E. (2001). Clinical correlates and reference intervals for pulmonary artery systolic pressure among echocardiographically normal subjects. *Circulation* 104 (23): 2797–2802. https://doi.org/10.1161/hc4801.100076.

66 Gille, J., Seyfarth, H.J., Gerlach, S. et al. (2012). Perioperative anesthesiological management of patients with pulmonary hypertension. *Anesthesiol. Res. Pract.* 2012: 356982. https://doi.org/10.1155/2012/356982.

67 Fox, C., Kalarickal, P.L., Yarborough, M.J., and Jin, J.Y. (2008). Perioperative management including new pharmacological vistas for patients with pulmonary hypertension for noncardiac surgery. *Curr. Opin. Anaesthesiol.* 21 (4): 467–472. https://doi.org/10.1097/ACO.0b013e3283007eb4.

68 Schulte-Sasse, U., Hess, W., and Tarnow, J. (1982). Pulmonary vascular responses to nitrous oxide in patients with normal and high pulmonary vascular resistance. *Anesthesiology* 57 (1): 9–13. https://doi.org/10.1097/00000542-198207000-00003.

69 Rich, G.F., Roos, C.M., Anderson, S.M. et al. (1994). Direct effects of intravenous anesthetics on pulmonary vascular resistance in the isolated rat lung. *Anesth. Analg.* 78 (5): 961–966. https://doi.org/10.1213/00000539-199405000-00022.

70 Keisler, B. and Carter, C. (2015). Abdominal aortic aneurysm. *Am. Fam. Physician* 91 (8): 538–543.

71 Twine, C.P. and Williams, I.M. (2011). Systematic review and meta-analysis of the effects of statin therapy on abdominal aortic aneurysms. *Br. J. Surg.* 98 (3): 346–353. https://doi.org/10.1002/bjs.7343.

72 Toskala, E. and Kennedy, D.W. (2015). Asthma risk factors. *Int. Forum Allergy Rhinol.* 5 (Suppl 1): S11–S16. https://doi.org/10.1002/alr.21557.

73 Warner, D.O., Warner, M.A., Barnes, R.D. et al. (1996). Perioperative respiratory complications in patients with asthma. *Anesthesiology* 85 (3): 460–467. https://doi.org/10.1097/00000542-199609000-00003.

74 Eisner, M.D., Klein, J., Hammond, S.K. et al. (2005). Directly measured second hand smoke exposure and asthma health outcomes. *Thorax* 60 (10): 814–821. https://doi.org/10.1136/thx.2004.037283.

75 Warner, M.E., Martin, D.P., Warner, M.A. et al. (2017). Anesthetic considerations for Angelman syndrome: case series and review of the literature. *Anesth. Pain Med.* 7 (5): e57826. https://doi.org/10.5812/aapm.57826.

76 Adamzik, M., Groeben, H., Farahani, R. et al. (2007). Intravenous lidocaine after tracheal intubation mitigates bronchoconstriction in patients with asthma. *Anesth. Analg.* 104 (1): 168–172. https://doi.org/10.1213/01.ane.0000247884.94119.d5.

77 Kim, E.S. and Bishop, M.J. (1999). Endotracheal intubation, but not laryngeal mask airway insertion, produces reversible bronchoconstriction. *Anesthesiology* 90 (2): 391–394. https://doi.org/10.1097/00000542-199902000-00010.

78 Jat, K.R. and Chawla, D. (2012). Ketamine for management of acute exacerbations of asthma in children. *Cochrane Database Syst. Rev.* 11 (11): CD009293. https://doi.org/10.1002/14651858.CD009293.pub2.

79 von Ungern-Sternberg, B.S., Boda, K., Chambers, N.A. et al. (2010). Risk assessment for respiratory complications in paediatric anaesthesia: a prospective cohort study. *Lancet* 376 (9743): 773–783. https://doi.org/10.1016/S0140-6736(10)61193-2.

80 Debley, J.S., Carter, E.R., Gibson, R.L. et al. (2005). The prevalence of ibuprofen-sensitive asthma in children: a randomized controlled bronchoprovocation challenge study. *J. Pediatr.* 147 (2): 233–238. https://doi.org/10.1016/j.jpeds.2005.03.055.

81 Austin, M.A., Wills, K.E., Blizzard, L. et al. (2010). Effect of high flow oxygen on mortality in chronic obstructive pulmonary disease patients in prehospital setting: randomised controlled trial. *BMJ* 341: c5462. https://doi.org/10.1136/bmj.c5462.

82 Abdo, W.F. and Heunks, L.M. (2012). Oxygen-induced hypercapnia in COPD: myths and facts. *Crit. Care* 16 (5): 323. https://doi.org/10.1186/cc11475.

83 Hausman, M.S., Jewell, E.S., and Engoren, M. (2015). Regional versus general anesthesia in surgical patients with chronic obstructive pulmonary disease: does avoiding general anesthesia reduce the risk of postoperative complications? *Anesth. Analg.* 120 (6): 1405–1412. https://doi.org/10.1213/ANE.0000000000000574.

84 Gramatica, L., Brasesco, O.E., Mercado Luna, A. et al. (2002). Laparoscopic cholecystectomy performed under regional anesthesia in patients with chronic obstructive pulmonary disease. *Surg. Endosc.* 16 (3): 472–475. https://doi.org/10.1007/s00464-001-8148-0.

85 Purugganan, R.V. (2011). Intravenous anesthesia for thoracic procedures. In: *Principles and Practice of Anesthesia for Thoracic Surgery* (ed. M.D.F.P. Slinger), 171–179. New York: Springer.

86 Giraud, M., Vandiedonck, C., and Garchon, H.J. (2008). Genetic factors in autoimmune myasthenia gravis. *Ann. N. Y. Acad. Sci.* 1132: 180–192. https://doi.org/10.1196/annals.1405.027.

87 Vachlas, K., Zisis, C., Rontogianni, D. et al. (2012). Thymoma and myasthenia gravis: clinical aspects and prognosis. *Asian Cardiovasc. Thorac. Ann.* 20 (1): 48–52. https://doi.org/10.1177/0218492311433189.

88 Farmakidis, C., Pasnoor, M., Dimachkie, M.M., and Barohn, R.J. (2018). Treatment of myasthenia gravis. *Neurol. Clin.* 36 (2): 311–337. https://doi.org/10.1016/j.ncl.2018.01.011.

89 Putman, M.T. and Wise, R.A. (1996). Myasthenia gravis and upper airway obstruction. *Chest* 109 (2): 400–404. https://doi.org/10.1378/chest.109.2.400.

90 Levitan, R. (2005). Safety of succinylcholine in myasthenia gravis. *Ann. Emerg. Med.* 45 (2): 225–226. https://doi.org/10.1016/j.annemergmed.2004.08.045.

91 Unterbuchner, C., Fink, H., and Blobner, M. (2010). The use of sugammadex in a patient with myasthenia gravis. *Anaesthesia* 65 (3): 302–305. https://doi.org/10.1111/j.1365-2044.2009.06236.x.

92 Kiran, U., Choudhury, M., Saxena, N., and Kapoor, P. (2000). Sevoflurane as a sole anaesthetic for thymectomy in myasthenia gravis. *Acta Anaesthesiol. Scand.* 44 (3): 351–353. https://doi.org/10.1034/j.1399-6576.2000.440324.x.

93 Hambly, P.R. and Martin, B. (1998). Anaesthesia for chronic spinal cord lesions. *Anaesthesia* 53 (3): 273–289. https://doi.org/10.1046/j.1365-2044.1998.00337.x.

94 Kazancioğlu, R. (2011). Risk factors for chronic kidney disease: an update. *Kidney Int. Suppl.* 3 (4): 368–371. https://doi.org/10.1038/kisup.2013.79.

95 Acedillo, R.R., Shah, M., Devereaux, P.J. et al. (2013). The risk of perioperative bleeding in patients with chronic kidney disease: a systematic review and meta-analysis. *Ann. Surg.* 258 (6): 901–913. https://doi.org/10.1097/SLA.0000000000000244.

96 Wagener, G. and Brentjens, T.E. (2010). Anesthetic concerns in patients presenting with renal failure. *Anesthesiol. Clin.* 28 (1): 39–54. https://doi.org/10.1016/j.anclin.2010.01.006.

97 Suparschi, V., Sigaut, S., and Paugam-Burtz, C. (2019). Prolonged muscle relaxation following succinylcholine administration in a cirrhotic patient: a case report. *Eur. J. Anaesthesiol.* 36 (11): 883–884. https://doi.org/10.1097/EJA.0000000000001057.

98 Benson, G.D., Koff, R.S., and Tolman, K.G. (2005). The therapeutic use of acetaminophen in patients with liver disease. *Am. J. Ther.* 12 (2): 133–141. https://doi.org/10.1097/01.mjt.0000140216.40700.95.

99 Nusrat, S., Khan, M.S., Fazili, J., and Madhoun, M.F. (2014). Cirrhosis and its complications: evidence based treatment. *World J. Gastroenterol.* 20 (18): 5442–5460. https://doi.org/10.3748/wjg.v20.i18.5442.

100 Wong F. Cirrhotic cardiomyopathy.

101 Blendis, L. and Wong, F. (2001). The hyperdynamic circulation in cirrhosis: an overview. *Pharmacol. Ther.* 89 (3): 221–231. https://doi.org/10.1016/s0163-7258(01)00124-3.

102 Gaude, G.S. (2009). Pulmonary manifestations of gastroesophageal reflux disease. *Ann. Thorac. Med.* 4 (3): 115–123. https://doi.org/10.4103/1817-1737.53347.

103 Cantillo, J., Cypel, D., Schaffer, S.R., and Goldberg, M.E. (1998). Difficult intubation from gastroesophageal reflux disease in adults. *J. Clin. Anesth.* 10 (3): 235–237. https://doi.org/10.1016/s0952-8180(98)00013-0.

104 Puig, I., Calzado, S., Suárez, D. et al. (2012). Meta-analysis: comparative efficacy of H2-receptor antagonists and proton pump inhibitors for reducing aspiration risk during anaesthesia depending on the administration route and schedule. *Pharmacol. Res.* 65 (4): 480–490. https://doi.org/10.1016/j.phrs.2012.01.005.

105 (2017). Practice Guidelines for Preoperative Fasting and the Use of Pharmacologic Agents to Reduce the Risk of Pulmonary Aspiration: application to healthy patients undergoing elective procedures: an updated report by the American Society of Anesthesiologists Task Force on Preoperative Fasting and the Use of Pharmacologic Agents to Reduce the Risk of Pulmonary Aspiration. *Anesthesiology* 126 (3): 376–393. https://doi.org/10.1097/ALN.0000000000001452.

106 Ehrenfeld, J.M., Cassedy, E.A., Forbes, V.E. et al. (2012). Modified rapid sequence induction and intubation: a survey of United States current practice. *Anesth. Analg.* 115 (1): 95–101. https://doi.org/10.1213/ANE.0b013e31822dac35.

107 Birenbaum, A., Hajage, D., Roche, S. et al. (2019). Effect of cricoid pressure compared with a sham procedure in the rapid sequence induction of anesthesia: the IRIS randomized clinical trial. *JAMA Surg.* 154 (1): 9–17. https://doi.org/10.1001/jamasurg.2018.3577.

108 Cook, W.P. and Schultetus, R.R. (1990). Lower esophageal sphincter integrity is maintained during succinylcholine-induced fasciculations in dogs with "full" stomachs. *Anesth. Analg.* 70 (4): 420–423. https://doi.org/10.1213/00000539-199004000-00013.

109 Felder, J.B., Korelitz, B.I., Rajapakse, R. et al. (2000). Effects of nonsteroidal antiinflammatory drugs on inflammatory bowel disease: a case-control study. *Am. J. Gastroenterol.* 95 (8): 1949–1954. https://doi.org/10.1111/j.1572-0241.2000.02262.x.

110 Hashim, K. and Thomas, M. (2014). Sensitivity of palm print sign in prediction of difficult laryngoscopy in diabetes: a comparison with other airway indices. *Indian J. Anaesth.* 58 (3): 298–302. https://doi.org/10.4103/0019-5049.135042.

111 Low, Y., White, W.D., and Habib, A.S. (2015). Postoperative hyperglycemia after 4- vs 8-10-mg dexamethasone for postoperative nausea and vomiting prophylaxis in patients with type II diabetes mellitus: a retrospective database analysis. *J. Clin. Anesth.* 27 (7): 589–594. https://doi.org/10.1016/j.jclinane.2015.07.003.

112 Tien, M., Gan, T.J., Dhakal, I. et al. (2016). The effect of anti-emetic doses of dexamethasone on postoperative blood glucose levels in non-diabetic and diabetic patients: a prospective randomised controlled study. *Anaesthesia* 71 (9): 1037–1043. https://doi.org/10.1111/anae.13544.

113 Joshi, G.P., Chung, F., Vann, M.A. et al. (2010). Society for Ambulatory Anesthesia consensus statement on perioperative blood glucose management in diabetic patients undergoing ambulatory surgery. *Anesth. Analg.* 111 (6): 1378–1387. https://doi.org/10.1213/ANE.0b013e3181f9c288.

114 Gerald S. Levey (1971). Catecholamine sensitivity, thyroid hormone and the heart: A reevaluation. *Am. J. Med.* 50 (4): 413–420, ISSN 0002-9343. https://doi.org/10.1016/0002-9343(71)90331-7.

115 Biondi, B., Palmieri, E.A., Lombardi, G., and Fazio, S. (2002). Subclinical hypothyroidism and cardiac function. *Thyroid* 12 (6): 505–510. https://doi.org/10.1089/105072502760143890.

116 Sadek, S.H., Khalifa, W.A., and Azoz, A.M. (2017). Pulmonary consequences of hypothyroidism. *Ann. Thorac. Med.* 12 (3): 204–208. https://doi.org/10.4103/atm.ATM_364_16.

117 Vanhaelst, L., Neve, P., Chailly, P., and Bastenie, P.A. (1967). Coronary-artery disease in hypothyroidism. Observations in clinical myxoedema. *Lancet* 2 (7520): 800–802. https://doi.org/10.1016/s0140-6736(67)92235-0.

118 Coulombe, P., Dussault, J.H., and Walker, P. (1976). Plasma catecholamine concentrations in hyperthyroidism and hypothyroidism. *Metabolism* 25 (9): 973–979. https://doi.org/10.1016/0026-0495(76)90126-8.

119 Little, J.W. (2006). Thyroid disorders. Part II: hypothyroidism and thyroiditis. *Oral Surg. Oral Med. Oral Pathol. Oral Radiol. Endod.* 102 (2): 148–153. https://doi.org/10.1016/j.tripleo.2005.05.070.

120 Sudha, P., Koshy, R.C., and Pillai, V.S. (2012). Undetected hypothyroidism and unexpected anesthetic complications. *J. Anaesthesiol. Clin. Pharmacol.* 28 (2): 276–277. https://doi.org/10.4103/0970-9185.94932.

121 Deb, S.J., Nichols, F.C., Allen, M.S. et al. (2005). Pulmonary carcinoid tumors with Cushing's syndrome: an aggressive variant or not? *Ann. Thorac. Surg.* 79 (4): 1132–1136; discussion 1132-6. https://doi.org/10.1016/j.athoracsur.2004.07.021.

122 Kamenický, P., Redheuil, A., Roux, C. et al. (2014). Cardiac structure and function in Cushing's syndrome: a cardiac magnetic resonance imaging study. *J. Clin. Endocrinol. Metab.* 99 (11): E2144–E2153. https://doi.org/10.1210/jc.2014-1783.

123 Daniel, E., Aylwin, S., Mustafa, O. et al. (2015). Effectiveness of Metyrapone in Treating Cushing's Syndrome: A Retrospective Multicenter Study in 195 Patients. *The Journal of Clinical Endocrinology & Metabolism* 100 (11): 4146–4154. https://doi.org/1033.1210/jc.2015-2616.

124 Ataga, K.I. and Orringer, E.P. (2000). Renal abnormalities in sickle cell disease. *Am. J. Hematol.* 63 (4): 205–211. https://doi.org/10.1002/(sici)1096-8652 (200004)63:4<205::aid-ajh8>3.0.co;2-8.

125 Ebert, E.C., Nagar, M., and Hagspiel, K.D. (2010). Gastrointestinal and hepatic complications of sickle cell disease. *Clin. Gastroenterol. Hepatol.* 8 (6): 483–489; quiz e70. https://doi.org/10.1016/j.cgh.2010.02.016.

126 Gardner, R.V. (2018). Sickle cell disease: advances in treatment. *Ochsner J.* 18 (4): 377–389. https://doi.org/10.31486/toj.18.0076.

127 Adjepong, K.O., Otegbeye, F., and Adjepong, Y.A. (2018). Perioperative management of sickle cell disease. *Mediterr J Hematol Infect Dis.* 10 (1): e2018032. https://doi.org/10.4084/MJHID.2018.032.

128 Cho, H., Jung, H.D., Kim, B.J. et al. (2015). Complication rates in patients using absorbable collagen sponges in third molar extraction sockets: a retrospective study. *J. Korean Assoc. Oral Maxillofac. Surg.* 41 (1): 26–29. https://doi.org/10.5125/jkaoms.2015.41.1.26.

129 Bogdan, C.J., Strauss, M., and Ratnoff, O.D. (1994). Airway obstruction in hemophilia (factor VIII deficiency): a 28-year institutional review. *Laryngoscope* 104 (7): 789–794. https://doi.org/10.1288/00005537-199407000-00002.

130 Laino, L., Cicciù, M., Fiorillo, L. et al. (2019). Surgical risk on patients with coagulopathies: guidelines on hemophiliac patients for oro-maxillofacial surgery. *Int. J. Environ. Res. Public Health* 16 (8): https://doi.org/10.3390/ijerph16081386.

131 Inwood, M.J., Killackey, B., and Startup, S.J. (1983). The use and safety of ibuprofen in the hemophiliac. *Blood* 61 (4): 709–711.

132 Mannucci, P.M. (2004). Treatment of von Willebrand's disease. *N. Engl. J. Med.* 351 (7): 683–694. https://doi.org/10.1056/NEJMra040403.

133 Keegan, M.T., Whatcott, B.D., and Harrison, B.A. (2002). Osteogenesis imperfecta, perioperative bleeding, and desmopressin. *Anesthesiology* 97 (4): 1011–1013. https://doi.org/10.1097/00000542-200210000-00039.

134 Horberg, M.A., Hurley, L.B., Klein, D.B. et al. (2006). Surgical outcomes in human immunodeficiency virus-infected patients in the era of highly active antiretroviral therapy. *Arch. Surg.* 141 (12): 1238–1245. https://doi.org/10.1001/archsurg.141.12.1238.

135 Levine, M. and Brown, D.F. (2012). Succinylcholine-induced hyperkalemia in a patient with multiple sclerosis. *J. Emerg. Med.* 43 (2): 279–282. https://doi.org/10.1016/j.jemermed.2011.06.062.

136 Honoré, M.B., Lauridsen, E.F., and Sonnesen, L. (2019). Oro-dental characteristics in patients with hypermobile Ehlers-Danlos syndrome compared to a healthy control group. *J. Oral Rehabil.* 46 (11): 1055–1064. https://doi.org/10.1111/joor.12838.

Section 7
Pediatric Disease and Syndromes

7.1 Pediatric Anatomy and Physiology

Airway

- External
  - Large occiput
  - ↓ BMI
  - ↑ Neck flexion and extension
- Oral Cavity
  - Small oral cavity
  - Relatively large tongue
  - Potentially loose primary dentition
- Pharynx
  - Waldeyer's ring
    - Enlarged adenoids
      - *See Figure 3.17 for Brodsky score*
    - Lingual, tubal, and palatine tonsils
    - Grow rapidly until age five to seven years, then physiological atrophy
- Larynx
  - Cephalad, anterior position
- Glottis
  - Vocal cord location
    - 0–12 months: at C_3
    - 1–2 years: at C_4
    - 3–10 years: at C_4–C_5
    - Adults: at mid C_5
  - Angled anterior-inferior to superior-posterior
    - May make insertion of endotracheal tube challenging
  - Broad, floppy, U-shaped epiglottis in young children
- Trachea
  - Flexibility of cartilaginous structures can predispose to dynamic obstruction with changes in airway pressure
  - Calcification of tracheal structures occurs in teenage years
  - Narrow tracheal diameter
    - *For ETT sizing, see page 299*

- In an emergency, diameter of patient's little finger can be used to guide ETT sizing
- Historically taught that the narrowest part of the pediatric airway was the circular cricoid cartilage
- Modern imaging studies demonstrate that the narrowest part is either at the vocal cords (as in adults) or the elliptical subglottic area
- Cuffed tubes could be used for patients >3 kg [1]

Fluid Management (Figure 7.1)

4-2-1 Rule

Weight (kg)	Hourly Maintenance Fluid Requirement
<10	4 ml/kg per hour
10–20	40 ml/h for first 10 kg PLUS 2 ml/kg/h for every kg above 10
20–80	60 ml/h for first 20 kg PLUS 1 ml/kg/h for every kg above 20

Maintenance rate should not exceed 100 ml/h

Figure 7.1

- ↑ Total body water results in higher volume of distribution of drugs
- Neonates have the highest total body water which gradually decreases over time
- Children have a relatively higher glucose requirement and may benefit from dextrose-containing maintenance fluids, especially after prolonged NPO times

Anesthesia for Dental and Oral Maxillofacial Surgery, First Edition. Spencer D. Wade, Caroline M. Sawicki, Megann K. Smiley, Michael A. Cuddy, Steven Vukas, and Paul J. Schwartz.

Cognitive Development (Piaget's Theory)

Birth–2 years Sensorimotor	Understanding the world through senses and actions
	Stranger anxiety
	Little meaningful verbal communication
	Follows single word direction
2–5 years Preoperational	Beginning to use language in ways similar to adults:
	Concrete and literal thinking
	Capable of pretend play
	Egocentric view of the world
6–11 years Concrete operational	Can see the world from different points of view
	Still benefits from concrete instructions
>11 years Formal operation	Can think about hypothetical concepts
	Capable of mature moral reasoning

Central Nervous System

- MAC Requirement
  - MAC is the highest at around six months of age and decreases by 6% per decade with a plateau/slight increase during puberty [2]
- Spinal Cord
  - Ends at L_3 in newborns
  - Migrates to L_1–L_2 by age three years and stays throughout adulthood
- FDA Warning
  - Issued in December 2016 about potential negative effects on developing brain
    - Based on animal studies
    - Risk remains unclear
  - Modified warning in April 2017 – medically necessary procedures should not be delayed

Cardiac

- Hypoxia most common cause of cardiac arrest
- ↑ Heart rate
  - Cardiac output more dependent on heart rate
- ↓ Blood pressure (Figure 7.2)
  - Stroke volume relatively fixed

Blood Pressure for Patients Ages 1–18 Years

MAP (50th percentile at 50th height percentile) = 1.5 × age in years + 55

Figure 7.2 Adapted from Haque and Zaritsky [3].

Pulmonary

- ↑ Respiratory Rate
  - Respiratory rate is inversely related to age
- ↑ Oxygen Consumption
  - 7–9 ml/kg/min in infants
  - 3–4 ml/kg/min in adults
  - Desaturation occurs more precipitously in pediatrics due to increased oxygen consumption
- Lung Volumes
  - Tidal volume 6–8 ml/kg
    - Similar to adults
  - Functional residual capacity ~30 ml/kg
- Musculoskeletal
  - Ribs more horizontally oriented
    - More difficult to elevate in order to increase thoracic volume
    - Cartilaginous costae make rib cage highly compliant
  - Flatter diaphragm with limited contractility
  - Intercostal muscles not well developed
- Alveoli Maturation
  - Incomplete until eight years of age
  - 85% of alveoli develop postnatally
  - Lung volume
    - Doubles by six months
    - Triples by one year
    - ↑ By a factor of ~13 by age seven years [4]

Other Systems

- Psychological
  - Patient may not be able to report NPO violation
    - ↑ Risk of aspiration
  - Difficulty cooperating
  - May have anxiety depending on age and demeanor
- Renal
  - Renal function similar to adults by around age two years
  - *Be conscious of medications and active metabolites cleared by the kidneys (see page 123)*
- Hepatic
  - Full maturity around two years after birth
  - ↑ Blood flow to vessel-rich organs results in generally higher rates of biotransformation and clearance of drugs
- Neuromuscular
  - Children are more prone to hypothermia
    - ↑ Body surface-to-weight ratio
    - ↓ BMI
    - ↓ Muscle mass
  - Routine use of succinylcholine contraindicated due to risk of hyperkalemia in children with undiagnosed muscular dystrophies (especially males)

7.2 Neonatal/Newborn Disorders

- This section covers basic medical management of neonatal disorders and long-term sequelae which may affect the patient and their anesthetic management into childhood and beyond

Premature Birth

- Live infant delivered before 37 weeks
- Gestational age (G_A) and birth weight (BW) are used to predict morbidity/mortality (Figure 7.3)

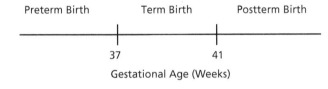

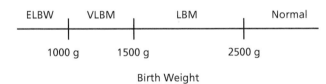

ELBW: Extremely Low Birth Weight
VLBW: Very Low Birth Weight
LBM: Low Birth Weight

Figure 7.3

- Etiology/Risk Factors
  - 70–80% result from preterm labor or premature rupture of membranes
  - 20–30% are initiated by health care providers because of health concerns for mother or child
  - Maternal risk factors:
    - Prior preterm birth
    - <17 or >35 years of age
    - Lower socioeconomic status
    - Short interpregnancy interval
    - Overweight
    - Underweight or low gestational weight gain
    - Conception by assisted reproductive technology
    - Pregnancy with multiples
    - Substance use, including smoking
- Prevalence
  - 5–18% of births worldwide
  - Varies by race and ethnicity in US. Below stats according to Center of Disease Control:
    - Non-Hispanic Blacks 14.1%
    - Hispanic 9.7%
    - Non-Hispanic White 9.1%
  - Associated with 30% of all infant deaths in US
- Treatment
  - Benign to symptomatic
  - Depends highly on BW and G_A
- Primary Concerns
  - ↑ Risk of bronchopulmonary dysplasia (BPD) and subsequent reactive airway disease
  - ↑ Risk of pulmonary hypertension
  - ↑ Risk of developmental disabilities
  - ↑ Risk of CHD
  - ↑ Risk intraventricular hemorrhage
- Evaluation
  - History
    - G_A at birth
    - Time in NICU
    - Need for supplemental oxygen, intubation, mechanical ventilation
    - Home use of apnea monitors
    - Persistent respiratory symptoms
  - Consider cardiologist consult if congenital heart defect is present
- Anesthesia Management
  - ↑ Suspicion for airway reactivity
    - *For bronchospasm management see page 260*
  - Consider tracheomalacia if prolonged intubation in NICU

Respiratory Distress Syndrome (RDS)

- Etiology/Risk Factors
  - Premature Birth
  - C-section
  - Maternal diabetes
  - Infection
  - Rare in infants born after 30 weeks
- Pathophysiology
  - Deficiency of pulmonary surfactant, which decreases alveoli surface tension, in immature lungs (Figure 7.4)

17–28 weeks G_A	Alveoli begin to form
28–36 weeks G_A	Pulmonary capillaries form: Beginning of alveolar-capillary barrier
32–34 weeks G_A	Surfactant production by type II pneumocytes

Laplace's Law

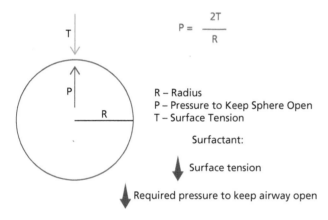

$$P = \frac{2T}{R}$$

R – Radius
P – Pressure to Keep Sphere Open
T – Surface Tension

Surfactant:

Surface tension

Required pressure to keep airway open

Figure 7.4

- Presents within minutes to hours of birth
  - Rapid and shallow breathing
  - Nasal flaring
  - Grunting
  - Tachypnea
  - Progressive cyanosis and dyspnea
  - Ultimately acidosis, hypotension, temperature instability, and apnea
- Treatment
  - Goal of maintaining $SpO_2 > 90\%$
  - Warm, humidified oxygen
  - Nasal CPAP
  - Exogenous surfactant via ETT
  - Mechanical ventilation

- If uncomplicated, will resolve in three to four days
- Chronic disease can develop if oxygen requirement persists
- Primary Concerns
  - Occurs in 75% infants born before 28 weeks G_A
  - May produce respiratory symptoms throughout childhood
- Evaluation
  - History
    - NICU course
    - Requirement for supplemental oxygen and mechanical ventilation
    - Persistent respiratory symptoms
- Anesthesia Management
  - ↑ Suspicion for airway reactivity
    - *For bronchospasm management see page 260*
  - Consider tracheomalacia if prolonged intubation

Bronchopulmonary Dysplasia (BPD)

- Etiology/Risk Factors
  - The main chronic complication of RDS
  - Preterm birth
    - Incidence ~40% in infants born before 28 weeks
  - Prolonged ventilation and oxygen therapy
  - Male gender
  - Some evidence for maternal smoking
- Pathophysiology
  - Exposure to mechanical ventilation and requirement of supplemental oxygen beyond 28 days of life
    - Disrupts pulmonary development and causes lung injury
  - Elevated oxygen requirement
  - ↓ Lung compliance
  - Reversible airway obstruction
- Treatment
  - Adequate nutrition
  - Respiratory support as required
  - Diuretics
  - Inhaled and systemic corticosteroids
  - Bronchodilators
  - Most patients improve gradually as growth continues and healing occurs
- Primary Concerns
  - Pulmonary symptoms persist for months to years
  - Children who survive BPD have double the incidence of motor and cognitive delays [5]

- Evaluation
  - Records
    - Patient may have been followed by BPD clinic
  - History
    - Persistent respiratory symptoms
    - NICU course
    - Requirement for supplemental oxygen and mechanical ventilation
    - Persistent respiratory symptoms
- Anesthesia Management
  - ↑ Suspicion for airway reactivity
    - *For bronchospasm management see page 260*
  - Consider tracheomalacia in younger children who required mechanical ventilation

Apnea of Prematurity (AOP)

- Cessation of breathing for more than 20 seconds or shorter pauses associated with desaturation and/or bradycardia
- Etiology/Risk Factors
  - Underdeveloped diaphragm
  - Premature birth
  - Hypoglycemia
  - Hypoxia
  - Anemia
  - Hypothermia
  - Sepsis
- Pathophysiology
  - Blunted chemoreceptor response to hypercarbia and/or hypoxia (Figure 7.5)
- Treatment
  - Treat and rule out possible underlying issues
    - Anemia
    - Infection

Types of Apnea of Prematurity

Central	No inspiratory effort
Obstructive	Inspiratory effort is present but ineffective due to upper airway obstruction
Mixed	Upper airway obstruction with inspiratory effort that precedes or follows central apnea

Most apnea of prematurity episodes are central or mixed

Figure 7.5

- Hypoglycemia
- Drugs
- IVH
- NEC
- Upper airway anomalies
- Seizures
- Feeding difficulty
  - Head and neck positioning
  - Prone positioning
  - Supplemental oxygen
  - CPAP
  - IV or oral caffeine or theophylline administration
  - Can be discharged to home without monitoring after 7–10 days free of apneic episodes
  - Not a risk factor for SIDS
- Primary Concerns
  - Almost all infants born before 28 weeks G_A are affected
  - Usually resolves by 36–37 weeks G_A
- Evaluation
  - History
    - Perinatal course
    - Requirement for supplemental oxygen and mechanical ventilation
    - Home apnea monitor use
- Anesthesia Management
  - Incidence of postoperative apnea drops significantly after 35 weeks G_A
  - Consider tracheomalacia in younger children who required mechanical ventilation
  - No known data/literature to guide perioperative management once AOP resolves.

Retinopathy of Prematurity (ROP)

- Visual impairment beginning in the neonatal period
- Etiology/Risk Factors
  - Injury or premature birth disrupts normal angiogenesis
  - Premature birth
  - Hypotension
  - Hypoxia
  - Hyperoxia
- Pathophysiology
  - 15–18 weeks G_A
    - Retinal vascularization begins
  - 36–40 weeks G_A
    - Vascular development complete
  - AAP guidelines suggest screening for all infants BW < 1500 g or G_A < 30 weeks

- Treatment
  - Based on disease severity
- Primary Concerns
  - ↑ Risk of retinal detachment
- Evaluation
  - History
  - Consider ophthalmology consult
- Anesthesia Management
  - May be noted on history
  - For patients with long-term retinal deformity/blindness, best to reasonably explain all actions and surroundings to avoid startling patient

Neonatal Abstinence Syndrome (NAS)

- Infant born to a woman with substance use disorder and is at risk for withdrawal
- Etiology/Risk Factors
  - Most commonly associated with opioids [6]
  - Often details of exposure are uncertain or there are multiple exposures
- Pathophysiology
  - Effects presumed to be due to altered levels of neurotransmitters
    - Sleep/wake cycle disturbance
    - Altered muscle tone
      - Tremors or jitteriness

Autonomic Dysfunction	
Sympathetic	Sweating
	Tachycardia
	Crying
	Hyper arousal
Parasympathetic	Nasal congestion
	Frequent yawning

- Treatment
  - Infant is kept in NICU at least four to five days to avoid onset of NAS after discharge
  - More severe opioid withdrawals may need to be managed pharmacologically
    - Buprenorphine [7]
    - Methadone [8]
- Primary Concerns
  - Long-term effects are not well understood due to confounding socioeconomic and social challenges

- Evaluation
  - History
- Anesthesia Management
  - Families may express concerns about exposure to anesthetic agents and opioids
  - No data/literature to support needing to avoid perioperative opioids once NAS resolved

Esophageal Atresia/Tracheoesophageal Fistula (EA/TEF)

- Etiology/Risk Factors
  - Generally presents during infant's first feedings as significant regurgitation and/or aspiration
  - 50% have other congenital anomalies
  - Often a component of VACTERL association
    - Vertebral defects
    - Anal atresia
    - Cardiac defects
    - TEF
    - Renal anomalies
    - Limb abnormalities
- Pathophysiology
  - Defect in septation and/or connection between esophagus, trachea, and stomach (Figure 7.6)
  - Feeding difficulties
  - Aspiration
- Treatment
  - Surgical
- Primary Concerns
  - After repair patients still may experience dysphagia, gastroesophageal reflux disease (GERD), RAD
- Evaluation
  - History
    - NICU course
    - Surgical history
    - Persistent respiratory and GI symptoms
    - Consultations if cardiac and renal anomalies are present
- Anesthesia Management
  - ↑ Suspicion for airway reactivity
    - *For bronchospasm management see page 260*
  - Consider RSI as may have higher aspiration risk
  - Consider tracheomalacia in younger children who required mechanical ventilation

Tracheoesophageal Fistula Classifications

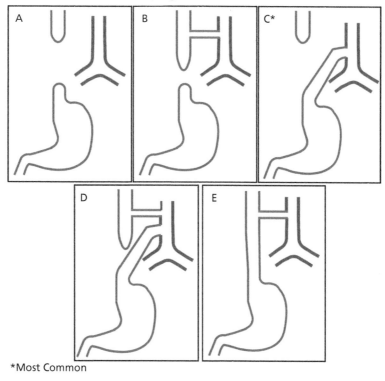

*Most Common

Figure 7.6

Tracheomalacia

- Etiology/Risk Factors
  - Congenital
  - Acquired
    - ○ Prolonged intubation at birth
    - ○ Surgical repair of EA/TEF
- Pathophysiology
  - Upper airway anomaly causing dynamic collapse of the trachea during respiration
    - ○ Categorized as either intrathoracic or extrathoracic (Figure 7.7)
- Treatment
  - Most patients will improve spontaneously by one year of age as child grows
- Primary Concerns
  - Depends on location and severity
  - Croup-like cough
  - Inspiratory stridor
  - Respiratory distress
  - Frequent respiratory illness
- Evaluation
  - ENT consult
    - ○ Records may be obtained from ENT follow up
  - Monitor for stridor at baseline

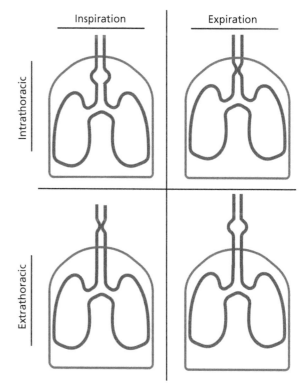

Tracheomalacia

Figure 7.7

- Anesthesia Management
  - Consider smaller ETT
  - ↑ Risk of airway obstruction

Diaphragmatic Hernia

- Etiology/Risk Factors
  - Can be diagnosed on prenatal ultrasound
  - Idiopathic
  - Genetic
  - Environmental triggers
- Pathophysiology
  - Failure of closure of pleuroperitoneal folds in utero creating a defect in diaphragm
    - ○ Allows abdominal viscera to herniate into the thoracic cavity
    - ○ Most commonly herniates through Foramen of Bochdalek
  - Presents within first few hours of life with significant respiratory depression
  - Size of hernia predicts severity of cardiorespiratory compromise and prognosis
  - 20% have associated cardiac defects
- Treatment
  - Medical management
    - ○ Stabilize patient's oxygenation, blood pressure, and acid–base balance
    - ○ Typically involves intubation soon after delivery
  - Surgical correction
- Primary Concerns
  - CHD
  - Patients may have restrictive lung disease from thoracic deformities
    - ○ Pectus excavatum
    - ○ Pectus carinatum
    - ○ Scoliosis
    - ○ Pulmonary hypoplasia
- Evaluation
  - Medical records from follow up
  - NICU course
  - Cardiology consult for CHD
- Anesthesia Management
  - Consider RSI for increased risk of GERD
  - ↑ Inspiratory pressures and cuffed ETT may be required due to restrictive lung disease
  - Consider tracheomalacia in younger children who required mechanical ventilation

Omphalocele

- Etiology/Risk Factors
  - Typically diagnosed on prenatal ultrasound
  - Only 25% are preterm or LBW
- Pathophysiology
  - Midline abdominal wall defect involving omphalos (Greek: navel)
- Treatment
  - Small defects surgically closed soon after birth
  - Large defects covered with a silo
    - ○ Gradual reduction of silo over three to seven days
    - ○ Delayed surgical closure
- Primary Concerns
  - Associated with other anomalies
    - ○ CHD
    - ○ Bladder
    - ○ Cloaca
    - ○ Craniofacial
- Evaluation
  - History
    - ○ Other anomalies
    - ○ Respiratory function
      - ● ↑ Risk of pulmonary hypoplasia
      - ● Requirement for prolonged mechanical ventilation
- Anesthesia Management
  - ↑ Risk of compromised pulmonary function
    - ○ ↑ Inspiratory pressures may be required due to lung hypoplasia

Gastroschisis

- Etiology/Risk Factors
  - Typically diagnosed on prenatal ultrasound
  - Preterm birth
- Pathophysiology (Figure 7.8)
  - Paraumbilical defect in the abdominal wall, usually to the right of midline
  - Intestines herniate through abdominal wall

Gastroschisis vs. Omphalocele

Gastroschisis	Omphalocele
Paraumbilical Herniation No Surrounding Membrane Not Associated with Syndromes or Cardiac Defects	Umbilical Herniation Membranous Surrounding Associated with Syndromes and Cardiac Defects

Figure 7.8

- Treatment
  - Surgical closure as soon as feasible
  - Sometimes silo covering required
- Primary Concerns
  - ↑ Risk of pathology related to intestinal adhesions:
    o Malrotation
    o Atresia
    o Stenosis
    o Perforation
    o Necrosis
- Evaluation
  - History
- Anesthesia Management
  - Surgical outcomes generally good and may be noted on history
  - Consider RSI for patients with continued GERD

Pyloric Stenosis

- Etiology/Risk Factors
  - Unclear but probably multifactorial
  - More common in males 5:1
- Pathophysiology (Figure 7.9)
  - Hypertrophy of the pylorus which can progress and constitute a near complete obstruction of the gastric outlet
  - Infants feed well at first, but at 2–12 weeks present with relentless, progressive, non-bilious projectile vomiting after feeding

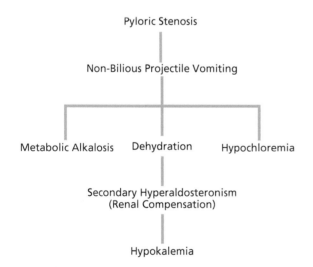

Figure 7.9

- Treatment
  - Medical management of electrolyte abnormalities
  - Surgical management via pyloromyotomy
    o More typical and definitive

- Primary Concerns
  - GERD is common
- Evaluation
  - History
- Anesthesia Management
  - Prognosis is good and may be noted on surgical history
  - Once surgical correction is resolved, many patients are asymptomatic with no special perioperative concerns

Necrotizing Enterocolitis (NEC)

- Etiology/Risk Factors
  - 90% of cases occur in preterm infants
  - Multifactorial cause
    o Ischemic insult to gut
    o Bacterial colonization of bowel
    o Substrate
      • Typically milk or formula
- Pathophysiology
  - Most common GI emergency of newborn
  - Ischemic necrosis of intestinal mucosa
- Treatment
  - Medical management with antibiotics
  - Sepsis
    o Coagulopathies requiring transfusion
  - Surgery
    o Laparotomy with resection
    o Peritoneal drainage
- Primary Concerns
  - Long-term sequelae
    o Malnutrition
    o GI obstruction
    o Strictures
    o Failure to thrive
- Evaluation
  - History
    o GI function
    o Patient growth and development
- Anesthesia Management
  - ~50% of survivors have no long-term sequelae [9]
  - Consider RSI for patients with ongoing GI symptoms

Gastroesophageal Reflux Disease (GERD)

- Etiology/Risk Factors
  - Common in infancy and typically resolves in first year of life [10]
    o 1.8–8.2% of children in US report symptoms suggestive of GERD
    o 3–5% of adolescents use antacid medication

- Prematurity
- Neuromuscular disorders
  o CP
  o Down syndrome
  o Muscular dystrophy
- Obesity
- Pathophysiology
  - Frequent regurgitation of gastric contents into the esophagus secondary to an underdeveloped and incompetent lower esophageal sphincter
  - May present as respiratory symptoms
  - Characteristic erosion of dentition
- Treatment
  - Lifestyle changes
    o Diet
    o Weight management
  - Acid suppressing medication
- Primary Concerns
  - Respiratory
    o Recurrent pneumonia and bronchiectasis
  - Barrett's esophagus
- Evaluation
  - History
    o Children may be able to describe symptoms of heartburn and "spicy burps"
- Anesthesia Management
  - ↑ Risk of dysphagia
  - ↑ Risk of related asthma symptoms
  - ↑ Risk of chronic cough
  - Consider RSI

Germinal Matrix Hemorrhage and Intraventricular Hemorrhage (GMH-IVH)

- Etiology/Risk Factors
  - Prematurity
  - Incidence and severity inversely related to G_A
  - Fragile microvasculature
  - Fluctuation in cerebral blood flow
    o Anemia
    o Hypercarbia
    o Acidemia
    o Hypoglycemia
    o Asphyxia
    o Abrupt elevation in systemic blood pressure
  - Traumatic delivery
  - Diagnosed via cranial ultrasound
- Pathophysiology
  - Leading cause of acquired infantile hydrocephalus
    o Incidence declining since 1980s but survivability improving for extremely preterm infants

- Bleeding in the small blood vessels of the germinal matrix secondary to disturbed vascular autoregulation or rapid fluid shifts
- Presenting symptoms
  o Seizures
  o Apnea
  o Cardiovascular instability
  o Acidosis
- Treatment
  - Management of symptoms
  - Supportive and directed to preserving cerebral perfusion
  - Ventriculoperitoneal shunt (VPS) to prevent increased intracranial pressure (ICP)
- Primary Concerns
  - Outcomes range from normal neuro exam to motor and cognitive deficits (cerebral palsy) to death
- Evaluation
  - History
  - Evaluate neurologic defects
  - Neurology consult
- Anesthesia Management
  - Depends on degree and severity
  - Patients with a VPS will be followed by Neurology and those clinic notes may be obtained for review

Cerebral Palsy (CP)

- Etiology/Risk Factors [11]
  - Diagnosis typically made between ages of 12–24 months
  - Anomaly or insult to immature CNS
  - Prematurity
  - Low birth weight
  - Trauma
- Pathophysiology
  - Non-progressive encephalopathy manifested as permanent motor dysfunction affecting muscle tone, posture, and movement (Figure 7.10)
  - Cognitive impairment is NOT a consistent feature

Cerebral Palsy Classification

Distribution	Type
Monoplegia One Extremity Affected	Spastic Muscles Constantly Contracted
Hemiplegia One Side Affected	Dyskinetic Involuntary Movements
Diplegia Legs Affected	Ataxic Uncoordinated Movements
Quadriplegia Whole Body Affected	Mixed Combination of the Above

Figure 7.10

- Treatment
  - Physical therapy
  - Bracing
  - Targeted botulinum neurotoxin
  - Oral or intrathecal baclofen to decrease spasticity
  - Surgical intervention for contractures
  - Anticonvulsants
  - Stimulants
  - PEG tube for nutrition
- Primary Concerns
  - Behavioral concerns
  - Impaired oral motor function increases risk of aspiration
  - ~45% of patients also have seizures
  - Restrictive lung disease secondary to scoliosis
- Evaluation
  - History
    o Seizures
    o GERD
    o Aspiration
    o Pneumonia
  - Record neurologic deficiencies
  - Consultation with patient's specialists
- Anesthesia Management
  - Continue antiepileptics, stimulants, and spasmolytic medications
  - Behavioral concerns may warrant premedication
  - Careful positioning and padding
    o May consider leaving wheelchair bound patients in their wheelchair if chair has adequate functionality
  - Potentially difficult IV access
  - ↓ MAC requirement for inhalation agents
  - Chronic anticonvulsants may increase resistance to non-depolarizing neuromuscular blockade
  - Prone to hypothermia due to low BMI
  - ↓ Exercise tolerance
  - Weak cough reflex
    o Concerns postoperatively
  - Difficult pain assessment
    o Can be aided by family members familiar with indicators
  - Succinylcholine use is OK as comparable serum potassium increase noted in patients with and without CP [12]

Cleft Lip and Cleft Palate

- Types
  - Cleft lip (CL)
    o Unilateral
    o Bilateral

    o With or without cleft palate
  - Cleft palate (CLP)
    o May involve hard and soft palate or hard palate only
    o Bifid uvula may indicate submucous cleft palate
  - 85% of bilateral CL and 70% of unilateral CL are associated with CLP [13]
- Etiology/Risk Factors
  - Assessment of upper lip component of standard prenatal ultrasound
  - When not syndrome-related, likely due to gene–gene and gene–environment interactions
    o More clearly illustrated in animal models
  - More common in Native American, Japanese, and Chinese populations
- Pathophysiology
  - Cleft lip
    o Failure of any of the lateral nasal, median nasal, or maxillary mesodermal processes to merge at around 35 days postconception
  - Cleft palate
    o Abnormalities in programmed cell death contribute to failure of palatal shelves to fuse at 56–58 days postconception
  - Associated with:
    o Otitis media (OM)
    o Feeding difficulty
    o Misaligned teeth
    o Phonation problems
- Treatment
  - Adaptive equipment needed for feeding initially
  - Surgical correction
    o CL around three months of age
    o CLP around six months of age
  - Revisions, orthodontics, speech therapy as needed
- Primary Concerns
  - Dependent on cleft and stage of treatment
- Evaluation
  - History
  - ENT consultation
  - Cleft Team records
- Anesthesia Management
  - Use of pharyngeal flap post CLP repair to improve nasal speech may make nasal intubation difficult
  - Consider oral intubation or smaller, softened ETT and/or fiberoptic bronchoscope assistance for nasal intubation

7.3 Congenital Heart Defects

- *Antibiotics prophylaxis covered on pages 83–84*
- Typical circulatory system flow (Figure 7.11)

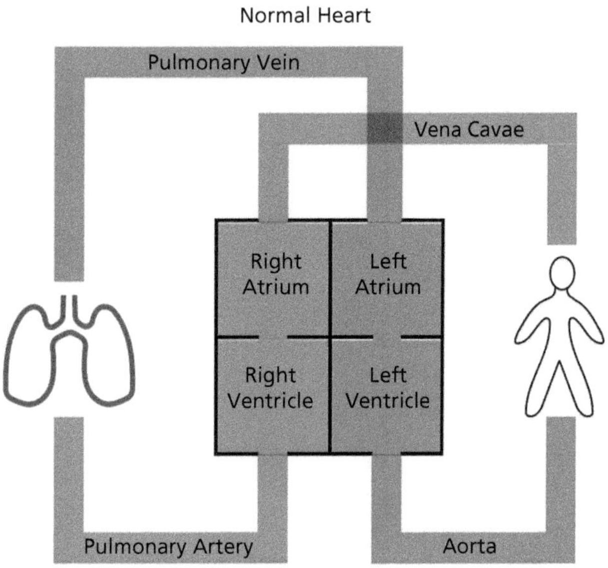

Normal Heart

Figure 7.11

Innocent Murmur

- Also known as Still's murmur
- Etiology/Risk Factors
  - Benign finding in ~30% of children ages two to seven years
- Pathophysiology
  - High-pitched, vibratory, short systolic murmur heard at left mid-sternal border
  - Frequently silent in supine position
  - Turbulent blood flow
    - o Fever
    - o Anemia
    - o Rapid growth
- Treatment
  - Generally none indicated
  - Evaluation for true valvular dysfunction
- Primary Concerns
  - Distinguishing from other murmurs

- Evaluation
  - Auscultation
  - History
    - o Exercise tolerance
    - o Chest pain
  - Consider cardiologist consult
    - o ECG
    - o Echo
- Anesthesia Management
  - Patients are generally asymptomatic with no special perioperative concerns

Patent Ductus Arteriosus (PDA)

- Etiology/Risk Factors
  - Premature birth [14]
  - Chromosomal abnormalities
- Pathophysiology
  - In fetal circulation, the ductus arteriosus allows blood to flow from the pulmonary artery to the aorta, bypassing the nonfunctioning lungs
  - Typically closes soon after birth in response to:
    - o ↑ PaO_2
    - o ↓ PGE2
  - Small lesions are asymptomatic, while large lesions may lead to significant left-to-right shunting, cardiomegaly, and CHF (Figure 7.12)
  - Continuous "mechanical" murmur (much like a Russian submarine) heard at midclavicular line between first and second interspace
- Treatment
  - Spontaneous closure beyond infancy is rare
  - COX inhibitor
  - Surgical or catheter closure
- Primary Concerns
  - Risk for infective endocarditis low
- Evaluation
  - Auscultation
  - Review past records for documentation of normal function
  - Cardiology consult

Patent Ductus Arteriosus

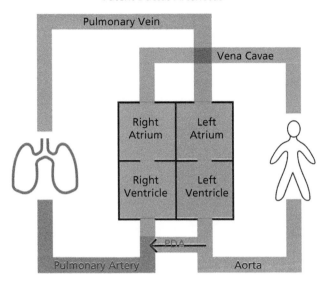

Figure 7.12

Ventricular Septal Defect

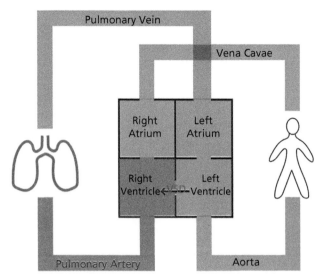

Figure 7.13

- Anesthesia Management
  - Antibiotic prophylaxis generally NOT necessary unless there is other associated unrepaired cyanotic heart disease, recent device closure, or device closure with residual adjacent defect
  - Post closure, patients are generally asymptomatic with no special perioperative concerns

Ventricular Septal Defect (VSD)

- Etiology/Risk Factors
  - Most common CHD in term infants
    o 25% of all congenital heart defects
  - Unknown cause
- Pathophysiology (Figure 7.13)
  - Failure of closure of the interventricular foramen
  - Diagnosed at one to three months of age as pulmonary vascular resistance decreases
  - Murmur is holosystolic and harsh, heard at lower sternal border

- Treatment
  - ~25% of cases close spontaneously
  - Small
    o VSD that persist into adulthood are usually benign
  - Large/symptomatic
    o Surgery
- Primary Concerns
  - Risk for infective endocarditis low
  - Avoid reversing shunt to right-to-left cyanotic physiology
  - Exacerbating left-to-right shunt

- Evaluation
  - Auscultation
  - Consider cardiologist consult
    o ECG
    o Echo
- Anesthesia Management
  - Surgical closure typically has good outcome and patients are generally asymptomatic with no special perioperative concerns
  - Antibiotic prophylaxis generally NOT necessary unless there is other associated unrepaired cyanotic heart disease, recent device closure, or device closure with residual adjacent defect
  - If unrepaired, hemodynamic goals are to maintain or slightly decrease SVR and avoid changes in PVR
    o Avoid agents that increase PVR
      • N_2O
    o Avoid decreasing PVR
      • High FiO_2
      • Hypocarbia
    o It should also be known that excessively lowering SVR will reverse the shunt and many common anesthetic agents decrease SVR. Be judicious with their use

Atrial Septal Defect (ASD)

- Types
  - Ostium primum
  - Ostium secundum
    o Most common
  - Coronary sinus defects
  - Sinus venosus defects
  - Patent foramen ovale (PFO)

- Etiology/Risk Factors
  - 10–15% of CHDs
- Pathophysiology
  - Failure of fusion of the septum primum, septum secundum, or AV canal septum
  - PFO
    - In fetal circulation foramen ovale is held open by pressure gradient allowing right-to-left shunt to bypass nonfunctioning lungs (Figure 7.14)
    - At birth lungs expand and systemic vascular resistance increases, pushing septum primum against septum secundum, which typically fuse
    - If they do not fuse, a PFO can be opened by a reversal of pressure gradients
  - Midsystolic pulmonary flow murmur with fixed splitting of S2 heard at left upper sternal border

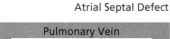

Atrial Septal Defect

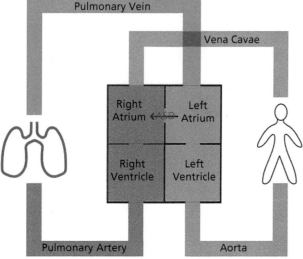

Figure 7.14

- Treatment
  - Small defect likely to close spontaneously or not pose any significant hemodynamic compromise
  - Surgical closure reserved for symptomatic patients with significant shunt
    - RV enlargement
    - Pulmonary hypertension
- Primary Concerns
  - Right-sided volume overload typically well tolerated into adulthood but later may lead to heart failure, arrhythmia, and pulmonary hypertension
  - Avoid reversing shunt to right-to-left cyanotic physiology

- Evaluation
  - Auscultation
  - Consider cardiologist consult
    - ECG
    - Echo
- Anesthesia Management
  - Patients may have cardiac evaluation but may not require follow up for trivial or clinically insignificant defects
  - Surgical closure typically has good outcome and patients are generally asymptomatic with no special perioperative concerns
  - Antibiotic prophylaxis generally NOT necessary unless there is other associated unrepaired cyanotic heart disease, recent device closure, or device closure with residual adjacent defect
  - For patients with a small ASD, consider avoiding agents that exacerbate a left-to-right shunt
    - Avoid increases in SVR
    - Avoid decreases in PVR
      - High FiO_2
      - Hyperventilation leading to hypocarbia
    - Hypotension may be treated with phenylephrine
      - Increases both SVR and PVR

Tetralogy of Fallot

- Etiology/Risk Factors
  - Many diagnosed prenatally on ultrasound
  - Unknown
  - Typically occurs sporadically but can be associated with syndromes
    - Down syndrome
    - Alagille syndrome
    - DiGeorge syndrome
- Pathophysiology (Figure 7.15)

Pulmonary Valve Stenosis

Ventricular Septal Defect

Overriding Aorta

Right ventricular hypertrophy (RVH) with right ventricular outflow tract (RVOT) obstruction

Figure 7.15

- Severity of symptoms depends on degree of RVOT obstruction
- "Tet" spells
  - o Right-to-left shunting leading to cyanosis due to exacerbation of dynamic component of RVOT obstruction during high catecholamine states
    - Crying/agitation
    - Stress
    - Dehydration
- Treatment
  - Surgical repair
    - o May be staged with palliative shunts or stenting of ductus arteriosus before definitive repair
    - o Complete repair is typically performed by one year of age

- Primary Concerns
  - Post-surgery
    - o May have pulmonary valve regurgitation
    - o Prone to arrhythmias with right bundle branch block very common
    - o May have ICD
- Evaluation
  - Auscultation
  - Cardiologist consult
    - o ECG
    - o Echo
- Anesthesia Management
  - Patients should have long-term cardiac follow up
  - Any treatment should be in close consultation with cardiologist
  - *For ICD management see pages 175–176*

7.4 Childhood Disorders

- For disorders associated with reactive airway disease consider supraglottic airway or natural guarded airway (NGA) instead of an ETT, if indicated. Intubation and airway instrumentation are strongly associated with bronchospasm
- *For intraoperative bronchospasm see page 260*

Secondhand Smoke (SHS) Exposure

- Types
  - Secondhand smoke
    - Mixture of side stream smoke given off by the smoking material and exhaled mainstream smoke
  - Thirdhand smoke
    - Smoke components that have settled on surfaces and can be absorbed through the skin, ingested, or inhaled when they become resuspended dust
- Etiology/Risk Factors
  - Based on serum cotinine levels, 37.9% of children aged 3–11 years in the US are exposed to SHS [15]
  - Low socioeconomic status
- Pathophysiology
  - ↑ Frequency of respiratory symptoms
  - ↑ Risk and severity of asthma and wheezing
  - ↑ Caries rate in primary teeth [16]
- Treatment
  - Counsel parents on creating smoke-free homes and vehicles
  - Smoking outside or only when children are not present is less effective
  - Limited evidence on passive e-cigarette "vaping" aerosol exposure
- Primary Concerns
  - Prone to reactive airway
- Evaluation
  - History
  - Presence of smoke in the preoperative room
- Anesthesia Management
  - ↑ Risk of reactive airway
  - ↑ Risk of intraoperative bronchospasm

- ↑ Risk of excess secretions
- Consider lower threshold for case deferment for patients who have had recent upper respiratory tract infection (URTI) depending on other risk factors
- Keep patient at deeper level of anesthesia to avoid bronchospasm

Upper Respiratory Tract Infection (URTI) (Common Cold)

- Etiology/Risk Factors
  - Most commonly caused by rhinoviruses
  - Most successful means of transmission is contaminated hands to mucus membranes of nose and eyes
  - Fall and winter months
  - Incidence highest in six to eight years olds
  - Toddler and school-age children may get six to nine URTIs per year
- Pathophysiology
  - Acute self-limiting viral infection of upper respiratory tract
  - Associated symptoms
    - Sneezing
    - Congestion
    - Rhinorrhea
    - Sore throat
    - Low-grade fever
    - Headache
    - Malaise
  - Common trigger for wheezing in susceptible children
- Treatment
  - Symptomatic support
- Primary Concerns
  - Exacerbating factors
    - History of reactive airway disease
    - Premature birth
    - SHS exposure
    - Plan for endotracheal intubation

- Mucociliary dysfunction and airway hyperreactivity present for weeks after recovery
  o Data are conflicting but may be two to four weeks for bronchial recovery
- Evaluation
  - History
  - Physical exam
- Anesthesia Management
  - Children with current and recent URTIs at increased risk of perioperative respiratory events
  - Decision to proceed should be based on local resources and clinical experience
  - Keep patient at deeper level of anesthesia to avoid bronchospasm
  - COLDS tool developed by Lee and August for risk stratification [17]:
    o Score 5–25
    o Points assigned to identify range of perioperative risk

	1	2	5
Current symptoms	None	Mild Parent confirms URTI Congestion Rhinorrhea Sore throat Low fever Dry cough	Moderate/severe Purulent congestion Wet cough Abnormal lung sounds Lethargy Toxic appearance High fever
Onset	>4 weeks	2–4 weeks	<2 weeks
Lung disease	None	Mild	Moderate/severe
Airway device	None or facemask	Supraglottic airway	Endotracheal tube
Surgery	Other	Minor airway T&A Flexible bronchoscopy Dental	Major airway Cleft repair Rigid bronchoscopy Maxillofacial

Respiratory Syncytial Virus (RSV)

- Etiology/Risk Factors
  - Transmission similar to URTI
  - Annual epidemic from November through April in northern hemisphere
  - Infects >1 million children annually
  - ↑ Risk for morbidity
    o <6 months of age
    o Premature birth
    o Chronic lung disease
    o Congenital heart disease
    o SHS exposure
    o Immunocompromised
- Pathophysiology
  - Most common cause of lower respiratory tract infection in children
  - Associated symptoms
    o URTI
    o Fever
    o OM
    o Bronchiolitis
    o Pneumonia
  - Previous infection does not appear to protect from reinfection
- Treatment
  - Supportive care
  - Humidified oxygen
  - Inhaled bronchodilators
  - May require hospitalization in severe cases
  - CDC RSV vaccination recommendations
    o Mothers at 32–36 weeks of pregnancy during RSV season
    o Infants <8 months of age born during RSV season or entering their first RSV season if mother was not vaccinated
    o Some children 8–24 months of age at higher risk
- Primary Concerns
  - Patients with a history of RSV are more likely to have wheezing later in life
  - ↑ Risk of reactive airway
- Evaluation
  - History
  - Physical exam
- Anesthesia Management
  - Acute illness
    o Delay elective procedure
  - Recovering
    o Delay depending on severity and timing of symptoms in conjunction with patient risk factors
    o ↑ Risk of reactive airway
    o ↑ Risk of intraoperative bronchospasm
    o Keep patient at deeper level of anesthesia to avoid bronchospasm

Croup (Laryngotracheobronchitis)

- Etiology/Risk Factors
  - Most commonly caused by parainfluenza viruses
  - Congenital narrowing of the airway

- Hyperreactive airway
- Peak incidence 18 months to 3 years of age
- Fall or early winter
- Pathophysiology
  - Inflammation of the larynx and subglottic airway (Figure 7.16)

Croup

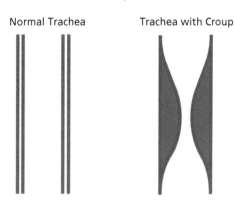

Normal Trachea   Trachea with Croup

Figure 7.16

- Barking cough
- Hoarseness
- Inspiratory stridor
- Symptoms last four to six days and are typically worse while lying flat
- Exacerbated by agitation and crying
- Treatment
  - Humidity
  - Hydration
  - Fever reduction
  - May require hospitalization
    - Inhaled racemic epinephrine
    - Systemic steroids
    - Monitoring for impending respiratory failure
- Primary Concerns
  - History of frequent croup may predispose to post-intubation croup
- Evaluation
  - History
- Anesthesia Management
  - Acute Illness
    - Delay elective procedure
  - Recovering
    - Delay depending on severity and timing of symptoms in conjunction with patient risk factors
    - Consider smaller ETT
    - Ensure appropriate cuff leak
    - Consider longer PACU recovery to monitor for post-intubation croup symptoms

Acute Otitis Media (OM)

- Etiology/Risk Factors
  - Bacterial
  - Viral
  - Fall and winter months
  - Peak incidence 6–12 months of age
- Pathophysiology
  - Inflammation of the middle ear
  - Pain
  - Ear rubbing
  - Hearing loss
  - Drainage
  - Fever
  - On otoscopy:
    - Red tympanic membrane
    - Immobile
    - Bulging
    - Loss of landmarks
  - Typically resolves in ~3 days with or without antibiotics
- Treatment
  - Oral antibiotics
  - May be referred for myringotomy and tube placement after repeated episodes
- Primary Concerns
  - Tube placement commonly reported on surgical histories
- Evaluation
  - History
- Anesthesia Management
  - Active infection considered a contraindication to N_2O
  - No current literature on increased perioperative morbidity with patient who has active OM infection

Asthma

- Etiology/Risk Factors
  - Approximately 5.5 million children in US
  - 80% of asthmatics diagnosed by fourth birthday
  - 50% of asthmatics are symptom free by age 20
    - Resolution rare in steroid dependent disease
  - Preterm birth
  - African American ethnicity
  - Polluted environment
    - Urban environment
    - SHS exposure
  - Strong association with poor socioeconomic status [18]
  - Obesity
- Pathophysiology
  - Reversible, nonuniform airway obstruction and V/Q mismatch
    - ↑ Smooth muscle tone

o Hyperplasia

o Mucus hypersecretion

o Mucosal edema

o Cellular infiltration

- Episodic expiratory wheezing and coughing

  o Typically nocturnal dry cough

- Difficulty exhaling due to increased resistance of the smaller airways (Figure 7.17)

• Poiseuille's Law

$$Q = \frac{\Delta P \pi r^4}{8 \eta l}$$

Q – Flow Rate
ΔP – Pressure Difference
η – Fluid Viscosity
l – Length
r – Radius

Figure 7.17

• Exacerbating factors

- URTI
- Exercise
- Weather
- SHS exposure
- Environmental allergens
- Noncompliance with medication regimens

• Treatment

- Acute therapy

  o Inhaled β_2 agonists

  o Severe bronchospasm – IM or titrated IV epinephrine

- Chronic therapy

  o Antihistamines

  o Inhaled and oral glucocorticoids

  o Antimuscarinics

- Short-term systemic corticosteroids for asthma flare ups

• Primary Concerns

- Airway reactivity

• Evaluation

- History

  o Current symptoms

  o Typical symptom patterns

  o Triggering factors

  o Maintenance medication use

  o Rescue medication use

  o Recent exacerbations

  o Systemic steroid use

  o Hospitalization and emergency room admissions for exacerbation

- Auscultation

- May obtain records if patient is followed by pulmonologist or allergist

• Anesthesia Management

- Continue regular medications

- Consider having patients bring their albuterol MDI and administering prior to induction

- Anticholinergics

  o ↓ Volume but does not thicken secretions

  o Bronchodilatory properties

- Most IV and inhalation anesthetic agents blunt airway reflexes and bronchodilate to varying degrees

  o Opioids blunt cough reflex

  • Studies of histamine releasing effects have variable findings and conclusions

  • Morphine may not be desirable due to histamine-releasing effects

  • Consider fentanyl or hydromorphone

  o Avoid desflurane

  • Airway resistance increased at higher MAC

  o Avoid histamine-releasing muscle relaxants

  • Atracurium

  • Mivacurium

  o Avoid thiopental

  • Wheezing documented in asymptomatic asthmatics and nonasthmatics [19]

  o Keep patient at deeper level of anesthesia to avoid bronchospasm (Figure 7.18)

- Weigh risks of deep versus awake extubation

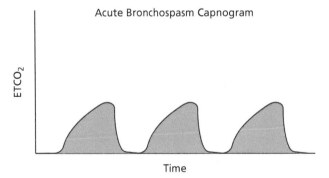

Acute Bronchospasm Capnogram

ETCO₂ / Time

Figure 7.18

Diabetes Mellitus (DM) Type 1 (Insulin-Dependent DM)

• Etiology/Risk Factors

- Bimodal peak of presentation

  o 4–6 years old

  o 10–14 years old

- Genetic susceptibility

- Pathophysiology (Figure 7.19)

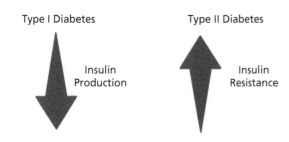

Figure 7.19

- Autoimmune destruction of pancreatic beta cells leading to insulin production deficiency
  - *Diabetes mellitus type 2 covered on pages 231–232*
- Increased circulating glucose leads to:
  - Polyuria from osmotic diuresis
  - Polydipsia
  - Weight loss
  - Hyperglycemia
  - Ketonuria
- 30% present in diabetic ketoacidosis (DKA) as initial presentation
- Treatment
  - Glycemic control
    - Frequent blood glucose testing
    - Insulin administration
    - Dietary control
    - Carbohydrate containing meals and snacks
  - Long-term glycemic control monitored regularly via glycated hemoglobin (HbA1c)
    - *Blood glucose and HbA1c covered on page 73*
  - Common insulin regimen
    - Long-acting insulin given once or twice a day
    - Rapid-acting insulin administered as premeal bolus
    - Insulin pumps increasingly used for pediatric patients with or without continuous glucose sensor
- Primary Concerns
  - Avoiding hypoglycemia from NPO and insulin administration
  - Avoiding hyperglycemia from withholding too much insulin
- Evaluation
  - HbA1c
  - Normal blood glucose readings
  - Amount of exogenous insulin usage
  - Endocrinology consult
  - Pump settings, if applicable
- Anesthesia Management
  - Patient should ideally be first case of the day to reduce fluctuations in blood glucose

- Goal is to perioperatively maintain blood glucose levels 90–180 mg/dl
- Insulin regimen day of surgery can be altered and is based on patient's glycemic control, preferably in consultation with patient's endocrinologist but generally:
  - Long-acting insulin
    - Maintain regular schedule
  - Intermediate-acting insulin
    - Take ½ to ⅔ of their regular dose morning of procedure
  - Rapid-acting insulin
    - Hold rapid-acting insulin bolus while fasting
  - Insulin pump
    - Maintain lowest basal rate
- Test preoperative blood glucose level
- Subsequent glucose readings as needed perioperatively
  - At least every one to two hours
- Dextrose administration
  - Children up to 12 years
    - 0.25–0.5 g/kg (Maximum single dose 25 g)
  - Adults
    - Blood glucose increases ~4–6 mg/dL for every gram of dextrose administered
  - Remeasure blood glucose 15–30 minutes after bolus dextrose
- Avoid dextrose containing IV solutions unless used in conjunction with insulin infusion
- Check blood glucose levels prior to discharge
- Insulin regimen restarts as soon as patient can resume eating, using sliding scale

Cystic Fibrosis (CF)

- Etiology/Risk Factors
  - Most patients diagnosed on newborn screening
  - Genetic
    - Autosomal recessive
    - CF gene is most commonly carried by northern central Europeans
- Pathophysiology
  - Abnormal transport of sodium and chloride across secretory membranes (Figure 7.20)
    - Thickened secretions in airway, GI tract, sweat glands, and GU system
  - Obstruction and chronic infection of airways
  - Bronchiolitis progressing to bronchiectasis progressing to fibrosis
  - Characteristic pulmonary function tests (PFTs)
    - Obstructive pattern
      - ↑ Residual volume
      - ↑ Airway resistance

Cystic Fibrosis Airway

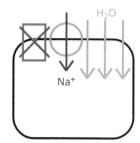

Figure 7.20

- ↓ Vital capacity
- ↓ Expiratory flow rate
- ↓ FEV_1
- Right ventricular hypertrophy and cor pulmonale in advanced disease
- Malabsorption secondary to exocrine pancreatic insufficiency
  o By age 10 years, 85% will develop DM type 1 secondary to endocrine pancreatic insufficiency
- Males are almost always infertile, but not sterile
- Treatment
  - High-calorie diet
  - Vitamin supplements
  - Pancreatic enzyme replacement
  - Antibiotics
  - Anti-inflammatory agents
  - Nebulized medications
  - Airway clearance therapies
  - Supplemental oxygen in advanced cases
- Primary Concerns
  - Compromised pulmonary function
  - Coagulopathy secondary to decreased synthesis of clotting factors and impaired vitamin K absorption
  - DM Type 1
  - Electrolyte imbalances
    o Malabsorption
- Evaluation
  - History
  - INR
  - CMP
  - Physician consult
  - Pulmonologist consult

- Anesthesia Management
  - Due to the chronic and debilitating nature of the disease the patient's physicians should be closely consulted
  - Avoid general anesthesia (GA), if possible
  - Preoperative optimization
    o Daily physiotherapy
    o Continue nebulized medications
    o Consider obtaining baseline ABG
  - Consider arterial line for monitoring blood gases
  - Careful positioning and protection from hypothermia as patients may be cachectic
  - Avoid nasal intubation because of high incidence of nasal polyps
  - May require prolonged postoperative ventilation
  - *If applicable, see Type 1 Diabetes section*

Adenotonsillar Hypertrophy/Sleep Disordered Breathing (SDB)

- Etiology/Risk Factors
  - Obesity
  - Reactive airway disease
  - Craniofacial anomalies
  - Conditions associated with hypotonia
- Pathophysiology
  - Enlarged tonsils and adenoids
  - ↑ Upper airway resistance and work of breathing at night
  - Loud snoring
  - Mouth breathing
  - Gasping/choking/coughing
  - Periods of apnea
    o Hypoxia and hypercarbia
  - Sleep disruption
    o Restlessness
    o Unusual sleep positions
  - Morning headaches
  - Long-term complications
    o Pulmonary hypertension
    o Systemic hypertension
    o Morphometric facial changes
    o Behavioral symptoms
- Treatment
  - Weight loss measures
  - T&A
- Primary Concerns
  - ↑ Risk of upper airway obstruction
- Evaluation
  - History
  - ENT consultation
  - Referral for diagnostic sleep study

- Anesthesia Management
  - Many screening tools available
    - *See figure 3.17 for Brodsky score*
  - Have a variety of airway adjuncts immediately available
  - Having a definitive airway may be beneficial over an NGA if significant obstruction is expected
  - Symptoms may not immediately resolve after T&A
    - Usually improves over a few weeks
    - No common consensus on wait time for nasal intubation post-T&A

Duchene Muscular Dystrophy (DMD)

- Etiology/Risk Factors
  - X-linked recessive inheritance
  - Defect in DMD gene which codes for protein dystrophin
    - Stabilizes and protects skeletal muscle and cardiac smooth muscle fibers
- Pathophysiology
  - Progressive skeletal muscle weakness secondary to muscle fiber degeneration
  - Onset of symptoms by two to three years of age
  - Wheel chair bound by 12 years of age
  - ↑ Risk of developing dilated cardiomyopathy
  - Patients rarely survive beyond third decade of life
- Treatment
  - Supportive
  - Glucocorticoids improve motor and lung function
  - Physical therapy and orthopedic interventions
  - ICD for patients with cardiomyopathy
- Primary Concerns
  - Hypotonia
  - Poor lung function
  - Inability to manage secretions with forceful cough
  - Cardiac arrhythmias
- Evaluation
  - History
  - Physician consult
  - Cardiologist consult
    - ECG
    - Echo
- Anesthesia Management
  - Many will have PPM/ICD/LVADs for cardiomyopathy
    - *Covered on pages 175–177.*
  - Due to the chronic and debilitating nature of the disease the patient's physicians should be closely consulted
  - ↑ Risk from rhabdomyolysis when exposed to inhalation agents

Figure 7.21

- Avoid paralytics, if possible
  - ↑ Sensitivity to non-depolarizing NMB
- Depolarizing NMB can tear plasma membranes leading to life-threatening hyperkalemia and myoglobinemia causing asystole and renal failure, respectively (Figure 7.21)
- Careful titration of anesthetic medications in patients with cardiomyopathy
- Consider avoiding non-depolarizing paralytics due to residual weakness
- May have ICD
  - Myocardial fibrosis
  - LV dysfunction
- Malignant hyperthermia is not a coexisting condition
- Postoperative ventilation may be required

Autism Spectrum Disorder (ASD)

- Etiology/Risk Factors
  - Not well understood
    - Likely epigenetic factors and exposure to environmental modifiers
  - Three to four times more common in males
- Pathophysiology
  - Neurodevelopmental disorder characterized by atypical communication and social interaction
  - Restricted, repetitive, and inflexible patterns of behavior, interests, and activities
  - Broad range of manifestations
    - Speech/language delays
    - Failure to make eye contact
    - Little interest in social interaction
    - Motor mannerisms that can be self-stimulating (e.g. hand flapping) or self-injurious (e.g. head banging)
    - Frequently associated with:
      - Anxiety
      - ADHD (30–50%)
      - Oppositional defiant disorder (ODD)
      - Tic disorders
    - Some patients may be nonverbal

- Treatment
  - Individualized depending on patient need
    o Behavioral therapy
    o Pharmacologic therapy
      • Stimulants
      • Antipsychotics
      • Anxiolytics
  - Families may pursue alternative therapies
    o Supplements
    o Special diets
    o Chelation
- Primary Concerns
  - Difficult following instructions
  - Behavior management
    o Caregivers are great resource for how to approach patient
- Evaluation
  - History
- Anesthesia Management
  - Parental/guardian support will be your biggest ally in letting you know what they like and dislike
    o To help understand if patient has an aversion to noises, touch, and odors, and visual stimulation can contribute to anxiety and to avoid those preoperatively
  - Even if the patient is nonverbal, many can still follow instructions
  - Continue patient's normally scheduled behavior-modifying medications
  - Consider additional preoperative medication in uncooperative/anxious patients
  - Consider making first case of the day due to:
    o Cognitive rigidity makes deviation from routine frustrating
    o Snacks/foods cravings at certain times
    o Day-of-surgery alterations like NPO guidelines difficult
    o Less "office traffic" as may overstimulate the patient
    o Generalized anxiety which may worsen as day progresses
  - Patient may not be able to report NPO violation
    o ↑ Risk of aspiration
  - May exhibit indifference to pain postoperatively, but still important to manage
  - Consider having family and caregivers at bedside once patient is medically safe in PACU
  - No current literature on increased perioperative morbidity with patient who has ASD

Attention Deficit Disorder With or Without Hyperactivity

- Etiology/Risk Factors
  - Not definitively known
  - Premature birth
  - Male
  - Head injuries
- Pathophysiology
  - Likely genetic imbalance of catecholamines in the cerebral cortex
  - Affects cognitive, academic, behavioral, emotional, and social functioning
  - Predominately hyperactive/impulsive subtype
    o Inability to sit still or inhibit behaviors
    o Typically presents by four years of age
    o Behaviors peak at seven to eight years of age
    o Observable hyperactive symptoms decline into adolescence, but impulsivity persists throughout life
  - Predominantly inattentive subtype
    o ↓ Ability to focus
    o ↓ Speed of cognitive processing
    o Typically presents by eight to nine years of age
  - Frequently associated with:
    o ODD
    o Conduct disorders
    o Anxiety
    o Learning disabilities
    o ASD
- Treatment
  - Behavioral therapy
  - Pharmacotherapy
    o Stimulants
      • First-line agents
      • Methylphenidate
      • Amphetamines
    o Non-stimulants
      • Selective norepinephrine reuptake inhibitors
      • α_2 adrenergic agonists
- Primary Concerns
  - Behavior management
    o Caregivers are great resource for how to approach patient
  - Difficulty following instructions
- Evaluation
  - History
  - Physician consultation
    o Should have frequent pediatrician follow-ups to monitor for medication adverse effects and manage refills
- Anesthesia Management
  - Parental/guardian support will be your biggest ally in letting you know what they like and dislike
  - May withhold or continue medications day of surgery for GA. Continue for moderate sedation
    o Family may prefer patient to have meds if surgery is later in the day
  - Consider additional preoperative medication in uncooperative/anxious patients
  - No current literature on increased perioperative morbidity with patient who has ADHD

7.5 Syndromes

Klinefelter Syndrome

- Etiology/Risk Factors
  - Genetic
  - Mean age of diagnosis is 30 years old
    - Only 25–50% are diagnosed during their lifetimes
- Pathophysiology
  - Supernumerary X chromosome in an XY male: XXY
  - Either maternal or paternal meiotic nondisjunction of X chromosome during ova or sperm production
  - Infants may present with:
    - Micropenis
    - Hypospadias
    - Cryptorchidism
  - Teenage boys may present with
    - Delayed puberty
    - Behavioral abnormalities
    - Learning disabilities
  - Progressive fibrosis and destruction of seminiferous tubules and Leydig cells
    - ↓ Sperm
    - ↓ Testosterone production
    - Small testes
    - Infertility
  - Associated dentofacial abnormalities
    - Taurodontism
    - Mandibular prognathism
    - Agenesis of permanent teeth
- Treatment
  - Dependent on age of diagnosis and severity of phenotype
  - Often includes testosterone therapy
- Primary Concerns
  - Related health issues
- Evaluation
  - May not be noted on history
  - Genetics consultation
- Anesthesia Management
  - Patients not treated with testosterone may be obese and develop type 2 diabetes
  - ↑ Risk of osteoporosis secondary to androgen deficiency
  - No current literature on increased perioperative morbidity with patient who has Klinefelter syndrome

Rett Syndrome

- Etiology/Risk Factors
  - Mutation of the MECP2-encoding gene located on the X chromosome
    - Expressed in all tissues
    - Most abundant in the brain
    - Only affects females
  - Mechanism of symptomology unknown but may be due to failure of synaptic maturation and maintenance in the cortex
  - Sporadic in almost all cases
- Pathophysiology
  - Normal development first 6–18 months of life, then loss of speech and purposeful use of hands
  - Hypotonia
  - Stereotypical hand movement
  - Gait abnormality
  - Deceleration of head growth
  - Seizures
  - Autistic features
  - Disordered breathing pattern
  - Bruxism
  - Excessive drooling
- Treatment
  - Behavioral medications
  - Antiepileptics
  - Management of associated conditions
- Primary Concerns
  - Disordered breathing with alternating hyperventilation and apneic episodes
  - Associated with long QT syndrome
  - Hypotonia
  - Behavioral concerns
- Evaluation
  - History
  - Physician consultation
  - Cardiac consultation
    - ECG
- Anesthesia Management
  - Consider additional preoperative medication in uncooperative/anxious patients

- Continue antiepileptic medications day of surgery
- Insensitivity or hypersensitivity to pain
- ↑ Risk of respiratory complications [20]
- Often develop scoliosis
  - Positioning
- Avoid non-depolarizing neuromuscular blocking agents as patient is likely sensitive

Pierre Robin Sequence

- Etiology/Risk Factors
  - Multifactorial
  - Associated syndromes:
    - Fetal alcohol syndrome
    - Stickler syndrome
    - Velocardiofacial syndrome
    - Treacher Collins syndrome
- Pathophysiology
  - First branchial arch embryologic defect
  - Respiratory distress
  - Feeding difficulties
  - Cleft palate
  - Micrognathia
  - Glossoptosis
    - Posterior inferior displacement of the tongue base with possible occlusion of the airway (Figure 7.22)

Pierre Robin Sequence

Unaffected

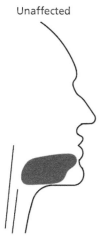 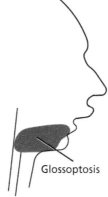

Glossoptosis

Figure 7.22

- Treatment
  - Facial growth improves airway problems
  - Surgical correction
    - Glossopexy
    - Mandibular distraction osteogenesis
    - Palatoplasty

- Primary Concerns
  - Airway
- Evaluation
  - Physician consult
- Anesthesia Management
  - Anticipate difficult airway even after corrective surgery
    - Difficult airway covered on page 258
  - ↑ Risk of OSA
  - ↑ Risk of swallowing disorders and GER
  - May have history of tracheostomy to manage airway obstruction
    - Possible subglottic stenosis

Down Syndrome

- Etiology/Risk Factors
  - Most common chromosomal abnormality in live births
  - Meiotic nondisjunction error
  - Advanced maternal age is a risk factor
- Pathophysiology
  - Trisomy 21, an additional part of or whole chromosome 21
  - Characteristics features:
    - Upslanting palpebral fissures
    - Almond-shaped eyes
    - Flat nasal bridge
    - Low-set ears
    - Brachycephaly
    - Protruding tongue
    - Lingual tonsil hypertrophy
    - Short neck
    - Short stature
  - Mild to moderate cognitive impairment
    - Associated with ADHD and ASD
  - CHD in 40% of patients
    - Endocardial cushion defect
    - VSD
  - Associated morbidities:
    - Subglottic stenosis
    - TEF
    - Seizures
    - Hypothyroidism
- Treatment
  - Antileptics
  - Behavior medications
  - Evaluation for associated comorbidities
  - Supportive
- Primary Concerns
  - Airway
  - Atlantoaxial instability
    - 13% of patients affected
    - May lead to subluxation of C_1/C_2 and compression of spinal cord

- o Radiographic exam is not routinely done unless symptomatic
  - o If children have participated in the Special Olympics they will have had screening radiographs
  - Endocrinology
  - Behavioral concerns
- Evaluation
  - Auscultation
  - Physician consult
  - Cardiologist consult
    - o ECG
    - o Echo
  - Endocrinologist consult
    - o For possible hypothyroidism
  - Radiologist consult
    - o Evaluate for atlantoaxial instability
- Anesthesia Management
  - Potential difficult airway, especially mask airway
  - Cardiologist consultation strongly recommended
  - Continue patient's normally scheduled behavior-modifying and antiepileptics medications
  - Consider additional preoperative medication in uncooperative/anxious patients
  - Often require smaller than expected ETT, especially for nasal intubation
  - ↑ Rate of OSA
  - ↑ Sensitivity to cardiodepressive effects of inhalation agents
    - o Manifested as bradycardia on mask induction
    - o Consider making first patient of the day to avoid dehydration

Angelman Syndrome

- Etiology/Risk Factors
  - Microdeletion of maternally derived chromosome 15 between 15q11 and 15q13 (Figure 7.23)

Angelman Syndrome	Prader–Willi Syndrome
Microdeletion of Maternally Derived Chromosome 15	Microdeletion of Paternally Derived Chromosome 15

Figure 7.23

- Pathophysiology
  - "Happy Puppet" – apparent happy demeanor with emotional lability
  - Severe developmental delay
  - Fascination with water
  - Seizures

- Spasticity, gait ataxia, and tremulous movement of limbs
- Disordered swallowing
  - o Aspiration
  - o GER
  - o Cyclic vomiting
  - o Excessive drooling
- Microcephaly
- Prognathia
- Wide mouth
- Treatment
  - Antileptics
  - Behavior medications
  - Evaluation for associated comorbidities
  - Supportive
- Primary Concerns
  - Behavioral concerns
  - Seizures
  - GABA$_A$ receptor abnormalities
    - o Both increased and decreased sensitivity to hypnotics have been reported
  - ↑ Vagal tone
    - o Cases of bradydysrhythmias under anesthesia are reported [21]
- Evaluation
  - Physician consult
- Anesthesia Management
  - Potential difficult airway
  - Continue patient's normally scheduled behavior-modifying and antiepileptics medications
  - Consider additional preoperative medication in uncooperative/anxious patients
  - Intellectual disability and happy demeanor may make pain assessment challenging

Prader–Willi Syndrome

- Etiology/Risk Factors
  - Genetic (Figure 7.23)
  - Majority occur sporadically
- Pathophysiology
  - Microdeletion of paternally derived chromosome 15 between 15q11 and 15q13
  - Hypotonia
  - Hyperphagia
  - Obesity
  - Genital hypoplasia
  - Small hands and feet
  - 25% have focal seizures (staring spells)
  - Behavioral problems
    - o ASD
  - Mild to moderate cognitive impairment

- Treatment
  - Obesity control through diet
  - Screening and management of comorbidities
- Primary Concerns
  - Behavioral concerns
  - Hypotonia
  - Obesity-related complications
    - OSA
    - DM
    - Cor pulmonale
    - Cardiovascular disease
    - Difficult IV access
- Evaluation
  - Physician consult
  - LFTs in obese patients
  - Consider polysomnogram
- Anesthesia Management
  - Consider making first patient of the day due to strong food cravings
  - Continue patient's normally scheduled behavior-modifying medications
  - Consider additional preoperative medication in unco-operative/anxious patients
  - ↑ Risk of aspiration
    - Hypotonia
    - ↓ GI motility
  - ↑ Risk of obstructive sleep apnea
  - Ensure facility can be kept warm as hypothermia can be problematic

Treacher Collins Syndrome

- Etiology/Risk Factors
  - Mutation in the gene TCOF1 on chromosome 5
  - Autosomal dominant with variable penetrance
- Pathophysiology
  - Abnormal bilateral first and second branchial arch development
  - Characteristic appearance:
    - Downward slanting eyes
    - Underdeveloped midface
    - Convex profile with micrognathia
  - Cleft lip and palate and choanal atresia in up to 35% of patients
  - Dental abnormalities including hypoplasia and malocclusion
  - External and middle ear abnormalities with hearing loss
- Treatment
  - Early surgery
    - Address airway and feeding problems

  - Later surgery
    - Improve function and facial appearance
- Primary Concerns
  - Airway
- Evaluation
  - Physician consult
- Anesthesia Management
  - Potential difficult airway
  - May have a gastrostomy tube secondary to weak, uncoordinated swallowing

Beckwith–Wiedemann Syndrome

- Etiology/Risk Factors
  - 85% genetic mutations occur sporadically
- Pathophysiology
  - Alterations of chromosome 11
  - ↑ Variable presentation
  - Pediatric overgrowth
    - Macroglossia
    - Gigantism
    - Hemihyperplasia
    - Organomegaly
    - Omphalocele
    - Predisposition to tumor development
  - Characteristic features
    - Hypoplastic midface
    - Infraorbital creases
- Treatment
  - Tumor surveillance
  - Management of airway and feeding concerns secondary to macroglossia
- Primary Concerns
  - Airway
    - Macroglossia
  - Organomegaly
    - ↑ Risk of cardiomyopathy
    - ↑ Risk of hypoglycemia
      - Islet cell hyperplasia and hyperinsulinemia
    - ↑ Risk of hepatoblastoma
- Evaluation
  - Physician consult
  - Cardiac consultation
    - ECG
    - Echo
  - CMP
  - LFTs
- Anesthesia Management
  - Careful airway assessment
    - May be followed by craniofacial team and may have had palliative procedures

o Patient may have had tongue reduction surgery
  • Typically addresses length not thickness
- Hepatic dysfunction may decrease metabolism and clearance of some medications
- Preoperative blood glucose and monitor perioperatively

Cornelia de Lange Syndrome

- Etiology/Risk Factors
  - Genetically heterogeneous causation
  - Sporadic
- Pathophysiology
  - Severe growth retardation
  - Variable severity
  - Distinctive features
    o Microcephaly
    o Highly arched eyebrows
    o Flat midface
    o Mandibular micrognathia
    o High arched palate
    o 30% have cleft palate
  - Profound intellectual disability
  - 20–30% have CHD
    o VSD
    o ASD
    o Pulmonic stenosis
    o Tetralogy of Fallot
    o Hypoplastic left heart syndrome
    o Tricuspid aortic valve
  - ↑ Incidence GI defect
    o GERD
    o Malrotation
    o Diaphragmatic hernia
  - Limb abnormalities
  - Hirsutism
- Treatment
  - Management of associated symptoms
- Primary Concerns
  - Behavioral concerns
  - Difficult IV access
  - Airway
  - CHD
- Evaluation
  - Physician consult
  - Cardiologist consult
    o ECG
    o Echo
- Anesthesia Management
  - Potential difficult airway
  - Continue patient's normally scheduled behavior-modifying medications

- Consider additional preoperative medication in uncooperative/anxious patients
- Aspiration risk

Mitochondrial Disorders

- Etiology/Risk Factors
  - Mitochondria responsible for intracellular oxidative phosphorylation
  - Once thought to be rare but now evidence suggests relatively common (Figure 7.24)

Mitochondrial Defect

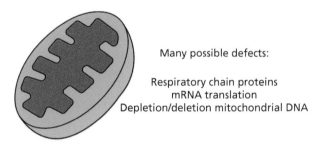

Many possible defects:

Respiratory chain proteins
mRNA translation
Depletion/deletion mitochondrial DNA

Figure 7.24

- Pathophysiology
  - Organs with highest energy requirement most affected
    o Heart
    o Nervous system
    o Skeletal muscle
    o GI tract
  - Wide range of clinical expression
    o Myopathy
    o Multisystem illness
  - Symptoms present during physiologic stress
    o Prolonged recovery
    o Rhabdomyolysis
  - Severe forms present early in life and are debilitating
  - Developmental delays
- Treatment
  - Supportive
  - Supplemental vitamins, coenzyme-Q, L-carnitine
- Primary Concerns
  - Connection between mitochondrial function and anesthetic response not well understood
    o Case reports of adverse events
  - ↑ Risk for respiratory depression
  - ↑ Risk for metabolic disturbance
  - ↑ Risk for neurologic injury
  - ↑ Risk for arrhythmias/cardiovascular instability

- Evaluation
  - History
  - Physician consult
  - Cardiologist consult
    o ECG
    o Echo
- Anesthesia Management
  - Consider referral to hospital for care
  - First case of the day
    o Avoid metabolic burden of prolonged fasting, postoperative nausea and vomiting, shivering
  - Consider additional preoperative medication in uncooperative/anxious patients
  - May require smaller anesthetic doses
  - Abnormal lactate metabolism
    o Avoid Lactated Ringer's
  - Many, if not all, anesthetic agents affect the mitochondria to varying degrees
    o Propofol seems to have a more profound effect on the mitochondria
      • Avoid infusion
      • Induction boluses reported to be well tolerated [22]
  - Attempt to avoid paralytics
  - May require postoperative intubation

Glucose-6-phosphate Dehydrogenase (G6PD) Deficiency

- Etiology/Risk Factors
  - X-linked recessive disorder
- Pathophysiology
  - Deficiency in G6PD enzyme resulting in hemolysis induced by exposure to oxidative stress (Figure 7.25):
    o Certain drugs
      • Most anesthetic drugs are considered safe
      • Lidocaine should be avoided
    o Certain foods
      • Fava beans
    o Infection
    o Metabolic abnormalities
  - Often asymptomatic with episodic anemia
  - Develops 24–72 hours after exposure
    o Headache
    o Fatigue
    o Jaundice
    o Cyanosis
    o Tachycardia
    o Dyspnea
    o Hemoglobinuria

Glucose-6-phosphate Dehydrogenase (G6PD) Deficiency

NADP/NADPH: Nicotinamide Adenine Dinucleotide Phosphate
GSH/GSSG: Glutathione

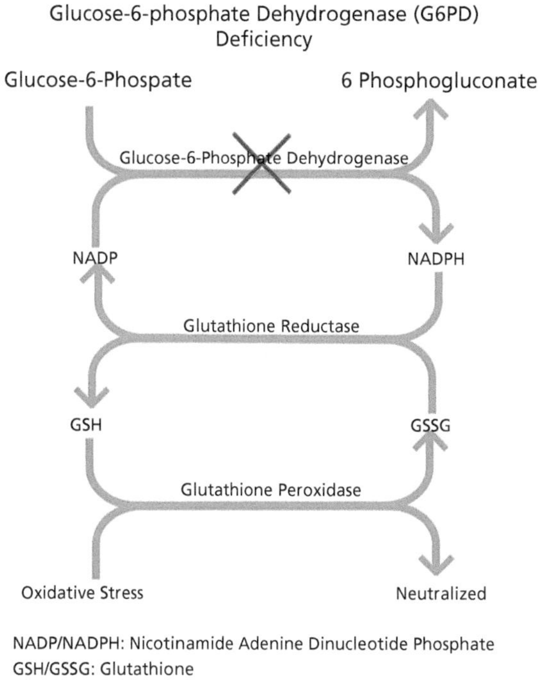

Figure 7.25

- Treatment
  - Avoid inciting substances
- Primary Concerns
  - ↑ Risk for methemoglobinemia
    o Methylene blue is ineffective treatment in this case as it is itself an oxidant which can precipitate hemolysis
- Evaluation
  - History
  - CBC
- Anesthesia Management
  - Avoid inciting substances
    o Sulfas
    o Aspirin
    o Methylene blue
    o Procainamide
  - Extensive list of drugs to be avoided can be found at www.g6pd.org

Methylenetetrahydrofolate Reductase (MTHFR) Mutation

- Etiology/Risk Factors
  - Genetic
  - ~30% US population heterozygous for MTHFR variant gene
  - ~10% homozygous

- Pathophysiology
  - Error of metabolism in folate cycle leading to (Figure 7.26):
    - ↓ Myelin

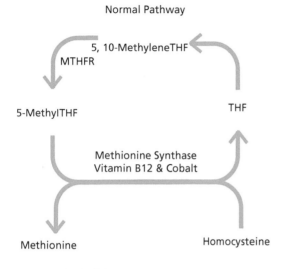

Normal Pathway

THF: Tetrahydrofolate

Figure 7.26

- Myelin is essential for assembly of myelin sheath, methyl substitutions in neurotransmitters, DNA synthesis
  - ↑ Homocysteine
    - ↑ Risk for atherosclerotic vascular disease
    - ↑ Risk for venous thromboembolism
- Treatment
  - Folic acid
  - Vitamin B12
- Primary Concerns
  - N_2O contraindicated
    - Irreversibly oxidizes cobalt atom of B12 and inhibits methionine synthase
    - Exposure to N_2O increases homocysteine levels in homozygous patients
    - Case reports of catastrophic neurological outcomes in children with MTHFR gene mutations after exposure to N_2O- "double hit" [23]
- Evaluation
  - Homocysteine levels not routinely checked
  - Young patients may be aware of deficiency because of family history
- Anesthesia Management
  - N_2O contraindicated

References

1 Klabusayová, E., Klučka, J., Kratochvíl, M. et al. (2022). Airway management in pediatric patients: cuff-solved problem? *Children (Basel)* 9 (10): https://doi.org/10.3390/children9101490.

2 Cameron, C.B., Robinson, S., and Gregory, G.A. (1984). The minimum anesthetic concentration of isoflurane in children. *Anesth. Analg.* 63 (4): 418–420.

3 Haque, I.U. and Zaritsky, A.L. (2007). Analysis of the evidence for the lower limit of systolic and mean arterial pressure in children. *Pediatr. Crit. Care Med.* 8 (2): 138–144. https://doi.org/10.1097/01.PCC.0000257039.32593.DC.

4 Merkus, P.J., ten Have-Opbroek, A.A., and Quanjer, P.H. (1996). Human lung growth: a review. *Pediatr. Pulmonol.* 21 (6): 383–397. https://doi.org/10.1002/(SICI)1099-0496(199606)21:6<383::AID-PPUL6>3.0.CO;2-M.

5 Doyle, L.W. and Anderson, P.J. (2009). Long-term outcomes of bronchopulmonary dysplasia. *Semin. Fetal Neonatal Med.* 14 (6): 391–395. https://doi.org/10.1016/j.siny.2009.08.004.

6 Hirai, A.H., Ko, J.Y., Owens, P.L. et al. (2021). Neonatal abstinence syndrome and maternal opioid-related diagnoses in the US, 2010–2017. *JAMA* 325 (2): 146–155. https://doi.org/10.1001/jama.2020.24991.

7 Kraft, W.K., Adeniyi-Jones, S.C., Chervoneva, I. et al. (2017). Buprenorphine for the treatment of the neonatal abstinence syndrome. *N. Engl. J. Med.* 376 (24): 2341–2348. https://doi.org/10.1056/NEJMoa1614835.

8 Davis, J.M., Shenberger, J., Terrin, N. et al. (2018). Comparison of safety and efficacy of methadone vs morphine for treatment of neonatal abstinence syndrome: a randomized clinical trial. *JAMA Pediatr.* 172 (8): 741–748. https://doi.org/10.1001/jamapediatrics.2018.1307.

9 Jones, I.H. and Hall, N.J. (2020). Contemporary outcomes for infants with necrotizing enterocolitis-a systematic review. *J. Pediatr.* 220: 86–92.e3. https://doi.org/10.1016/j.jpeds.2019.11.011.

10 Dent, J., El-Serag, H.B., Wallander, M.A., and Johansson, S. (2005). Epidemiology of gastro-oesophageal reflux disease: a systematic review. *Gut* 54 (5): 710–717. https://doi.org/10.1136/gut.2004.051821.

11 Nelson, K.B. (2003). Can we prevent cerebral palsy? *N. Engl. J. Med.* 349 (18): 1765–1769. https://doi.org/10.1056/NEJMsb035364.

12 Fleisher, L.A., Fleischmann, K.E., Auerbach, A.D. et al. (2015). 2014 ACC/AHA guideline on perioperative cardiovascular evaluation and management of

patients undergoing noncardiac surgery: executive summary: a report of the American College of Cardiology/American Heart Association Task Force on practice guidelines. Developed in collaboration with the American College of Surgeons, American Society of Anesthesiologists, American Society of Echocardiography, American Society of Nuclear Cardiology, Heart Rhythm Society, Society for Cardiovascular Angiography and Interventions, Society of Cardiovascular Anesthesiologists, and Society of Vascular Medicine Endorsed by the Society of Hospital Medicine. *J. Nucl. Cardiol.* 22 (1): 162–215. https://doi.org/10.1007/s12350-014-0025-z.

13 Milerad, J., Larson, O., Hagberg, C., and Ideberg, M. (1997). Associated malformations in infants with cleft lip and palate: a prospective, population-based study. *Pediatrics* 100 (2 Pt 1): 180–186. https://doi.org/10.1542/peds.100.2.180.

14 Tanner, K., Sabrine, N., and Wren, C. (2005). Cardiovascular malformations among preterm infants. *Pediatrics* 116 (6): e833–e838. https://doi.org/10.1542/peds.2005-0397.

15 Tsai, J., Homa, D.M., Gentzke, A.S. et al. (2018). Exposure to secondhand smoke among nonsmokers - United States, 1988–2014. *MMWR Morb. Mortal. Wkly Rep.* 67 (48): 1342–1346. https://doi.org/10.15585/mmwr.mm6748a3.

16 Aligne, C.A., Moss, M.E., Auinger, P., and Weitzman, M. (2003). Association of pediatric dental caries with passive smoking. *JAMA* 289 (10): 1258–1264. https://doi.org/10.1001/jama.289.10.1258.

17 Lee, B.J. and August, D.A. (2014). COLDS: a heuristic preanesthetic risk score for children with upper respiratory tract infection. *Paediatr. Anaesth.* 24 (3): 349–350. https://doi.org/10.1111/pan.12337.

18 Kuruvilla, M.E., Vanijcharoenkarn, K., Shih, J.A., and Lee, F.E. (2019). Epidemiology and risk factors for asthma. *Respir. Med.* 149: 16–22. https://doi.org/10.1016/j.rmed.2019.01.014.

19 Pizov, R., Brown, R.H., Weiss, Y.S. et al. (1995). Wheezing during induction of general anesthesia in patients with and without asthma. A randomized, blinded trial. *Anesthesiology* 82 (5): 1111–1116. https://doi.org/10.1097/00000542-199505000-00004.

20 Kako, H., Martin, D.P., Cartabuke, R. et al. (2013). Perioperative management of a patient with Rett syndrome. *Int. J. Clin. Exp. Med.* 6 (5): 393–403.

21 Warner, M.E., Martin, D.P., Warner, M.A. et al. (2017). Anesthetic considerations for Angelman syndrome: case series and review of the literature. *Anesth. Pain Med.* 7 (5): e57826. https://doi.org/10.5812/aapm.57826.

22 Hsieh, V.C., Niezgoda, J., Sedensky, M.M. et al. (2021). Anesthetic hypersensitivity in a case-controlled series of patients with mitochondrial disease. *Anesth. Analg.* 133 (4): 924–932. https://doi.org/10.1213/ANE.0000000000005430.

23 Nagele, P., Zeugswetter, B., Wiener, C. et al. (2008). Influence of methylenetetrahydrofolate reductase gene polymorphisms on homocysteine concentrations after nitrous oxide anesthesia. *Anesthesiology* 109 (1): 36–43. https://doi.org/10.1097/ALN.0b013e318178820b.

Section 8

Perioperative Emergencies and Urgencies

This section is courtesy of and adapted from the American Dental Society of Anesthesiology (ADSA) Ten Minutes Saves a Life app.

This guide attempts to present an algorithmic approach for recognizing and treating specific emergent conditions. However, every situation and patient is different, and care may require escalation sooner than anticipated. Furthermore, treatment options may also vary by location. For example, in a mobile practice setting, "calling for help" will likely mean "Call 911" where as "calling for help" in a hospital/ASC may get you more personnel to assist you.

Anesthesia for Dental and Oral Maxillofacial Surgery, First Edition. Spencer D. Wade, Caroline M. Sawicki, Megann K. Smiley, Michael A. Cuddy, Steven Vukas, and Paul J. Schwartz.
© 2024 John Wiley & Sons, Inc. Published 2024 by John Wiley & Sons, Inc.

8.1 Cardiac

- Cardiac Arrest (Figure 8.1)
- Hypotension (Figure 8.2)
- Bradycardia Symptomatic (Figure 8.3)
- Tachycardia with a Pulse (Figure 8.4)
- Hypertension (Emergency/Urgency) (Figure 8.5)
- Chest Pain (Figure 8.6)

8.2 Respiratory

- Airway Differential (Figure 8.7)
- Upper Airway Obstruction (Figure 8.8)
- Apnea (Figure 8.9)
- Cannot Ventilate; Cannot Intubate (Figure 8.10)
- Laryngospasm (Figure 8.11)
- Bronchospasm (Figure 8.12)
- Allergic Reaction (Mild) Figure 8.13)
- Anaphylaxis (Figure 8.14)
- Foreign Body Airway Obstruction (Figure 8.15)
- Aspiration (Figure 8.16)
- Post-intubation Laryngeal Edema (Figure 8.17)
- Pulmonary Edema Figure 8.18)
- Chest Wall Rigidity (Figure 8.19)
- Hyperventilation/Tachypnea (Figure 8.20)
- Airway Fire (Figure 8.21)

8.3 Neuro

- Seizure (Figure 8.22)
- Syncope/Altered Mental Status (Figure 8.23)
- Local Anesthesia Toxicity (Figure 8.24)
- Delayed Emergence (Figure 8.25)
- Stroke (Figure 8.26)

8.4 Metabolic

- Hypoglycemia (Figure 8.27)
- Hyperkalemia (Figure 8.28)
- Malignant Hyperthermia (Figure 8.29)
- Neuroleptic Malignant Syndrome (Figure 8.30)

8.5 Other

- Nausea and Vomiting (Figure 8.31)
- Incapacitated Provider (Figure 8.32)

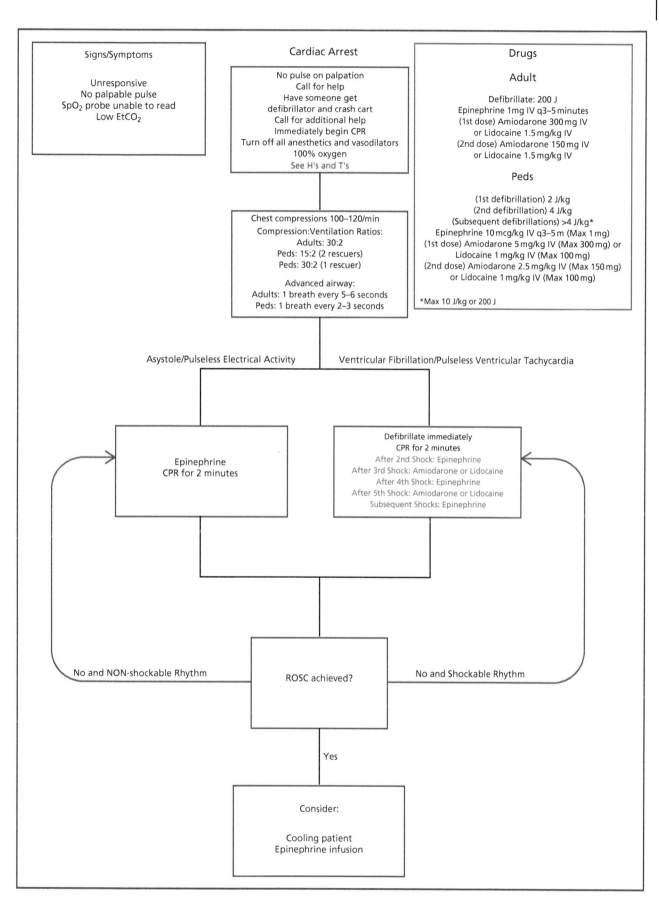

Figure 8.1

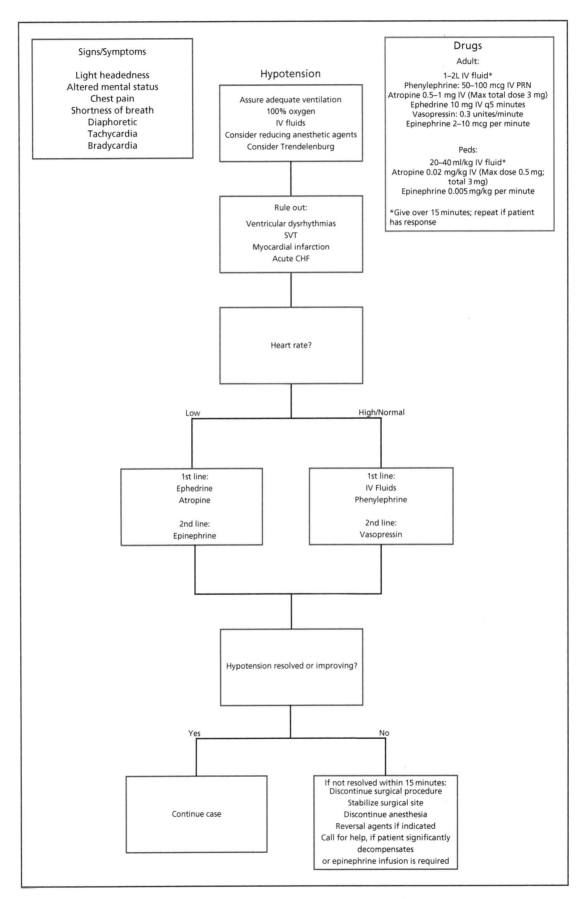

Figure 8.2

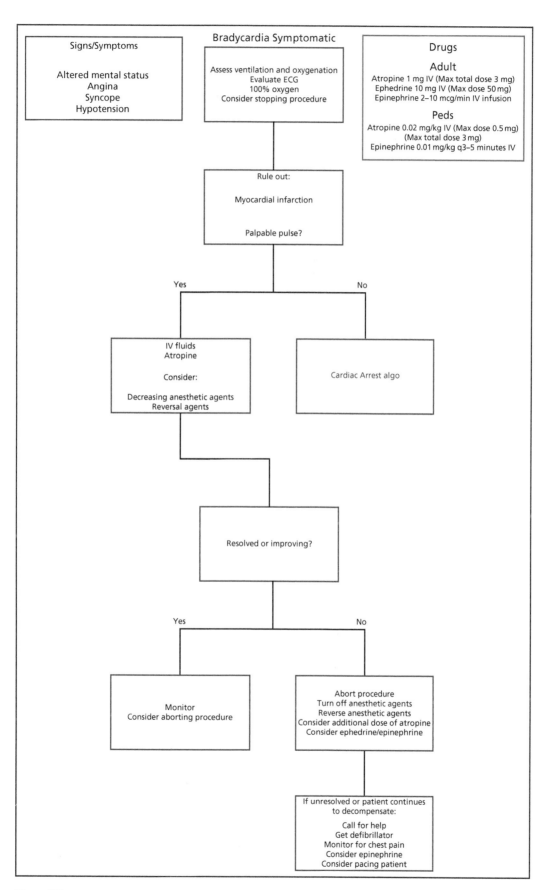

Figure 8.3

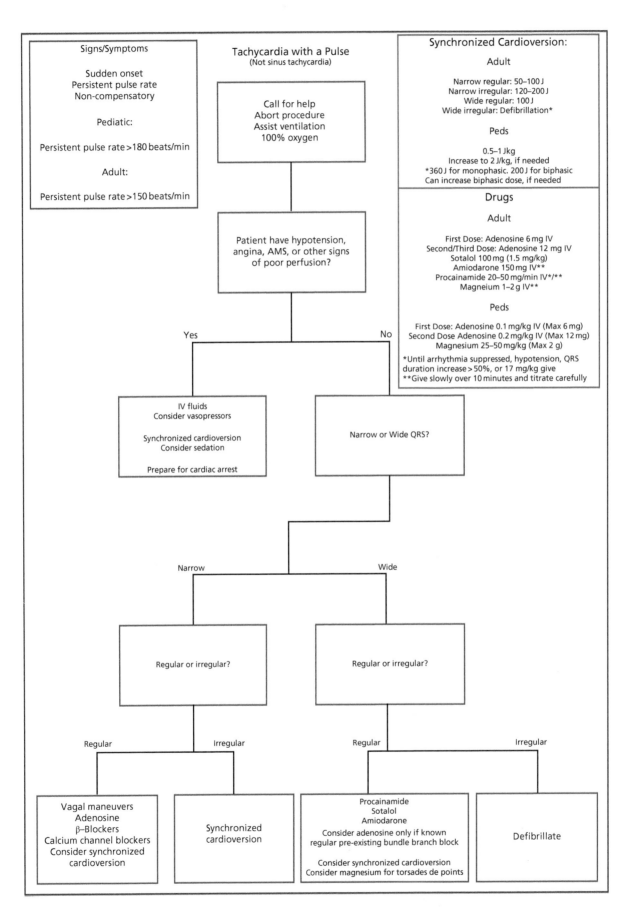

Figure 8.4

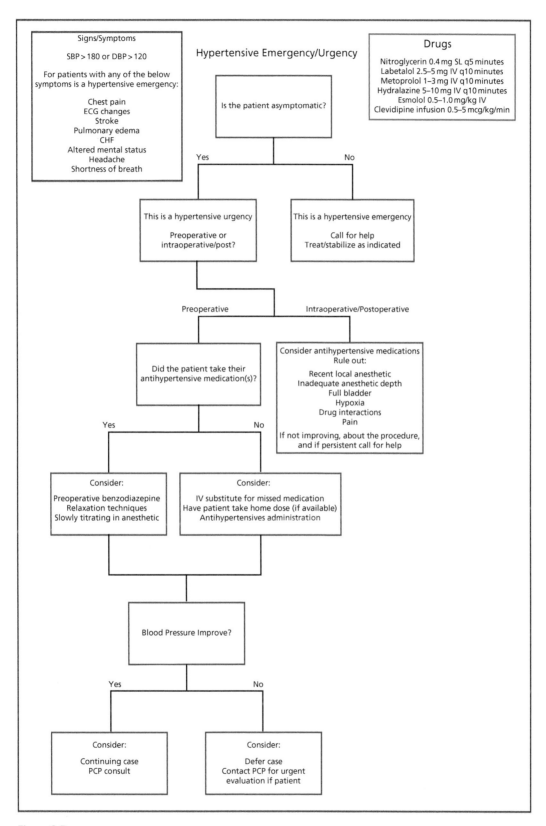

Figure 8.5

254

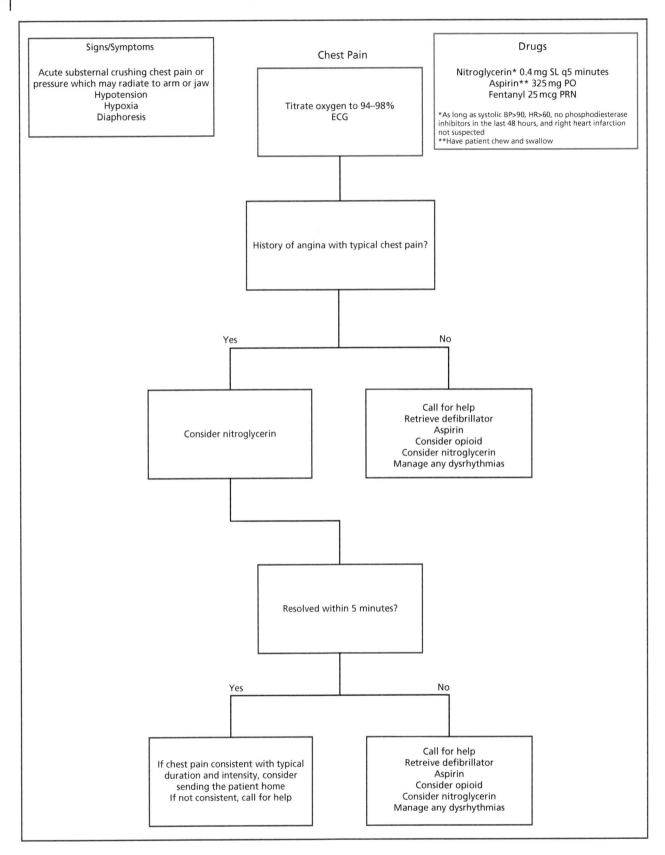

Figure 8.6

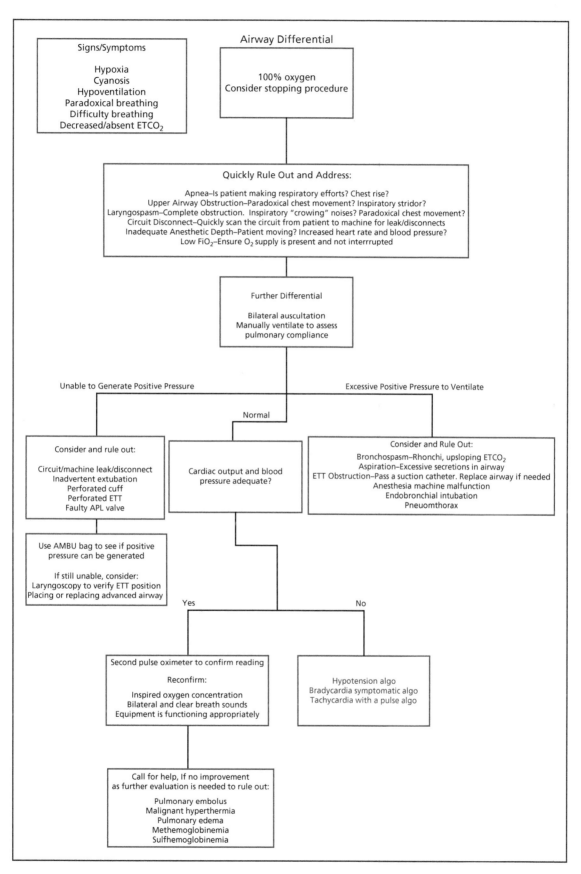

Figure 8.7

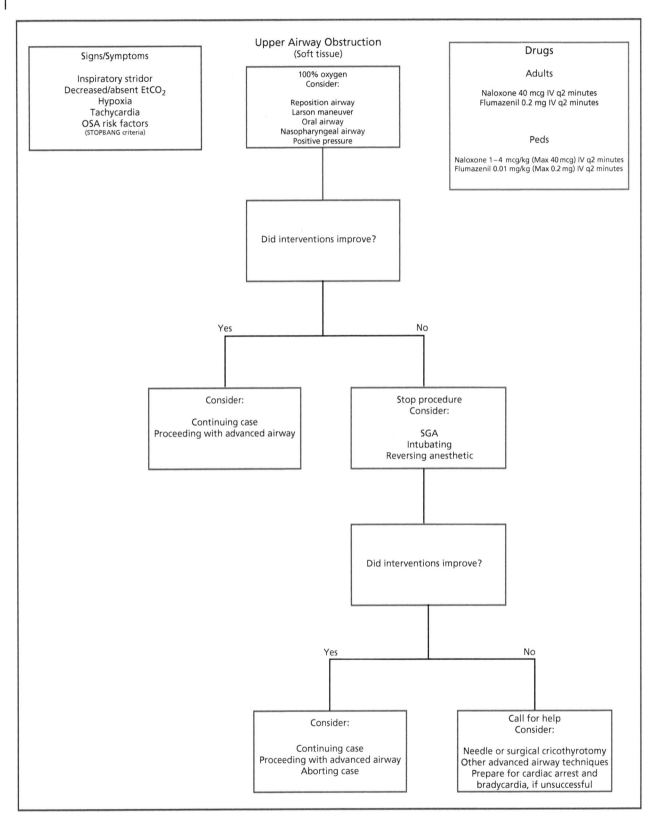

Figure 8.8

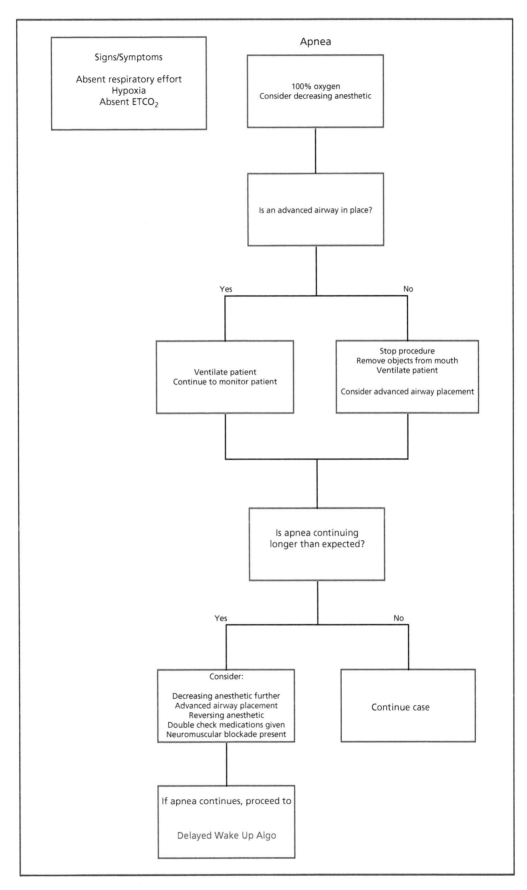

Figure 8.9

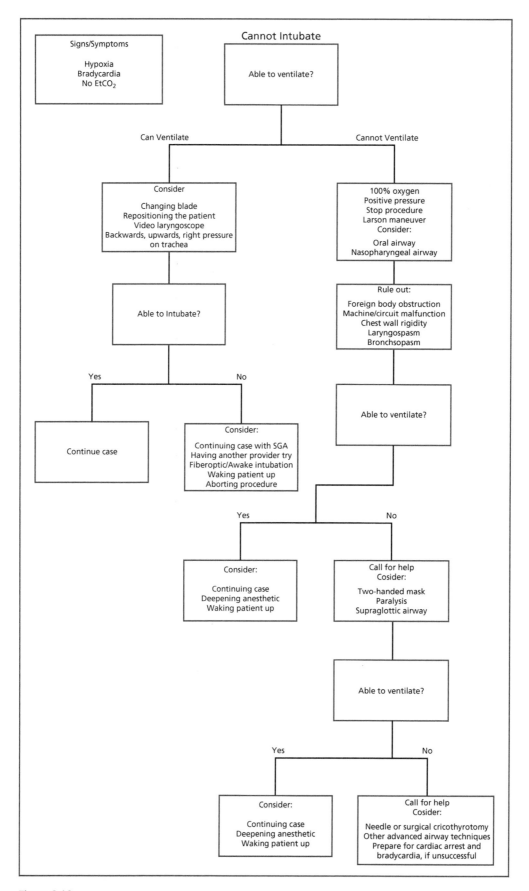

Figure 8.10

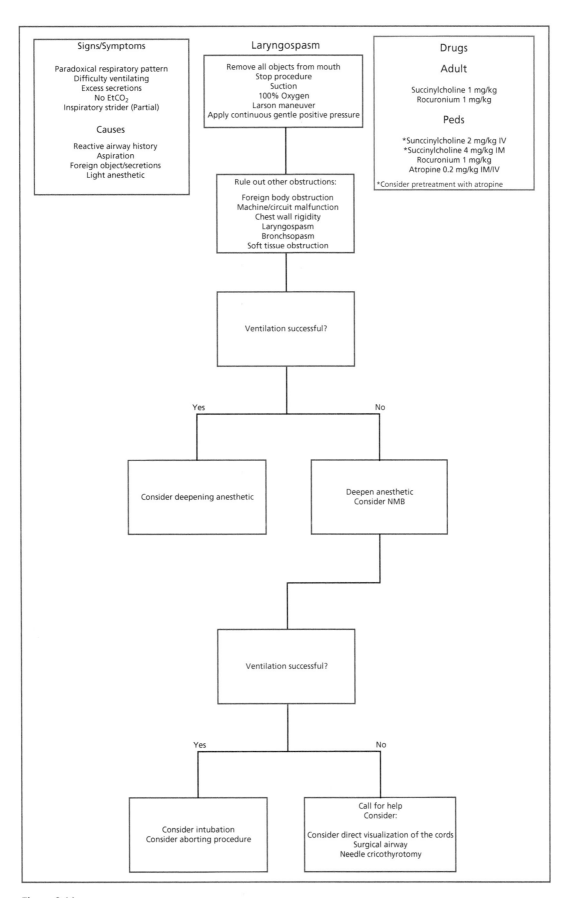

Figure 8.11

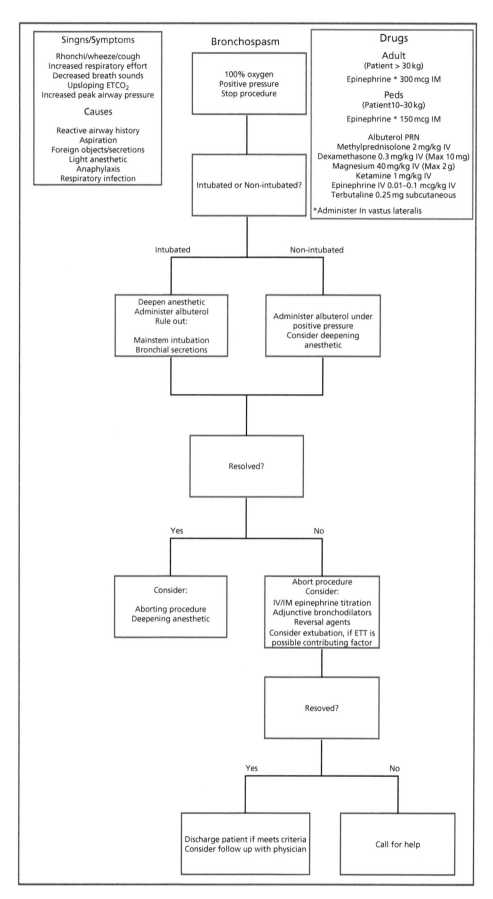

Figure 8.12

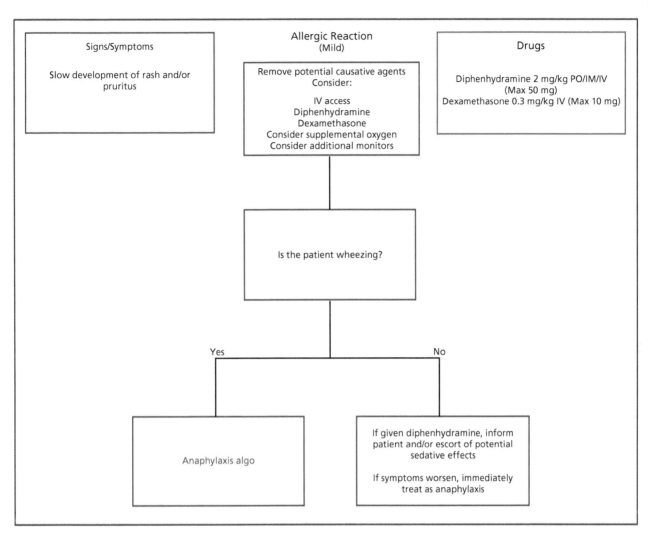

Figure 8.13

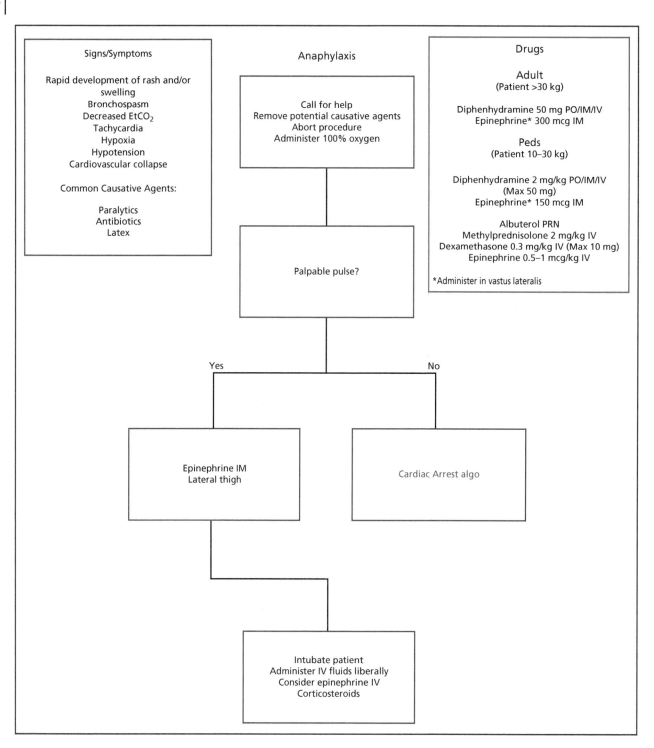

Signs/Symptoms

Rapid development of rash and/or
swelling
Bronchospasm
Decreased EtCO$_2$
Tachycardia
Hypoxia
Hypotension
Cardiovascular collapse

Common Causative Agents:

Paralytics
Antibiotics
Latex

Anaphylaxis

Call for help
Remove potential causative agents
Abort procedure
Administer 100% oxygen

Palpable pulse?

Yes   No

Epinephrine IM
Lateral thigh

Cardiac Arrest algo

Intubate patient
Administer IV fluids liberally
Consider epinephrine IV
Corticosteroids

Drugs

Adult
(Patient >30 kg)

Diphenhydramine 50 mg PO/IM/IV
Epinephrine* 300 mcg IM

Peds
(Patient 10–30 kg)

Diphenhydramine 2 mg/kg PO/IM/IV
(Max 50 mg)
Epinephrine* 150 mcg IM

Albuterol PRN
Methylprednisolone 2 mg/kg IV
Dexamethasone 0.3 mg/kg IV (Max 10 mg)
Epinephrine 0.5–1 mcg/kg IV

*Administer in vastus lateralis

Figure 8.14

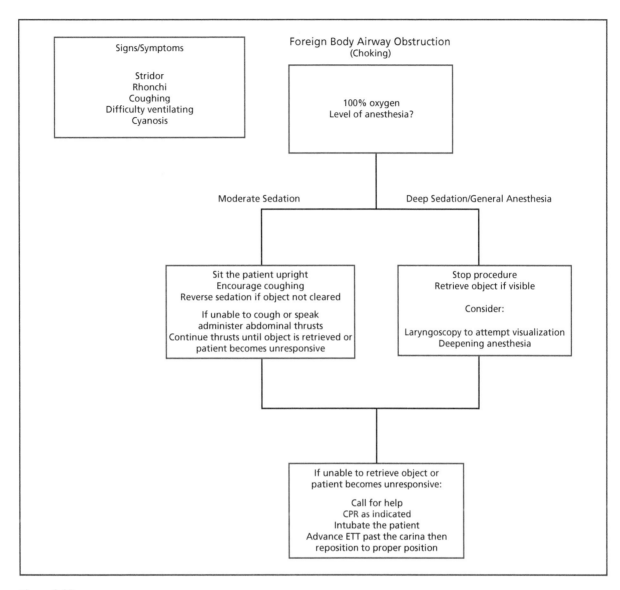

Figure 8.15

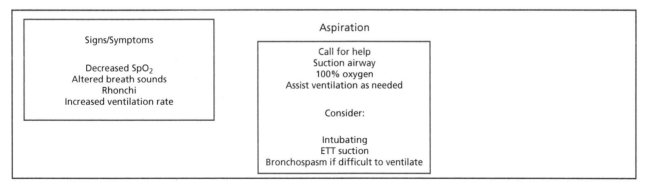

Figure 8.16

264

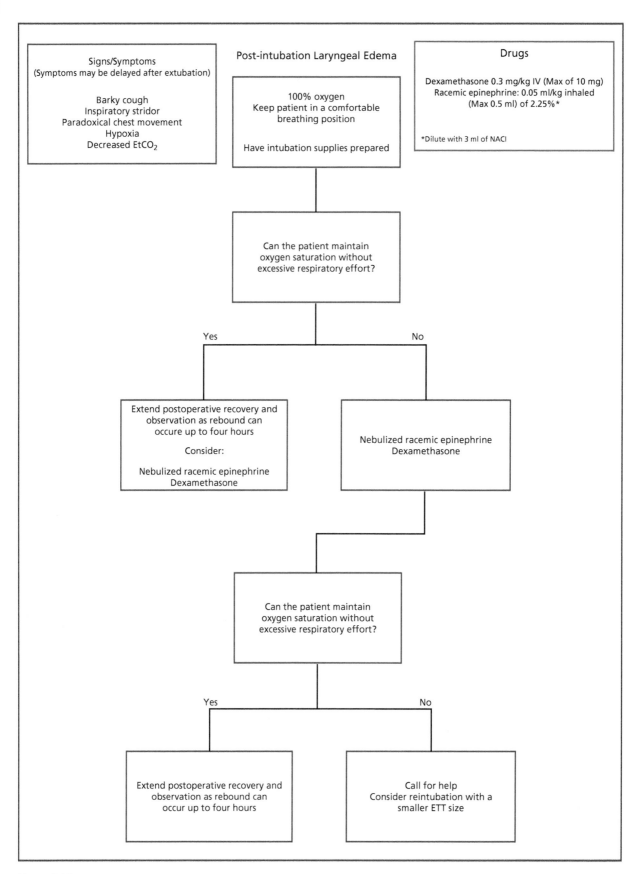

Post-intubation Laryngeal Edema

Signs/Symptoms
(Symptoms may be delayed after extubation)

Barky cough
Inspiratory stridor
Paradoxical chest movement
Hypoxia
Decreased EtCO$_2$

Drugs

Dexamethasone 0.3 mg/kg IV (Max of 10 mg)
Racemic epinephrine: 0.05 ml/kg inhaled
(Max 0.5 ml) of 2.25%*

*Dilute with 3 ml of NACl

100% oxygen
Keep patient in a comfortable
breathing position

Have intubation supplies prepared

Can the patient maintain
oxygen saturation without
excessive respiratory effort?

Yes

No

Extend postoperative recovery and
observation as rebound can
occure up to four hours

Consider:

Nebulized racemic epinephrine
Dexamethasone

Nebulized racemic epinephrine
Dexamethasone

Can the patient maintain
oxygen saturation without
excessive respiratory effort?

Yes

No

Extend postoperative recovery and
observation as rebound can
occure up to four hours

Call for help
Consider reintubation with a
smaller ETT size

Figure 8.17

Signs/Symptoms

Hypoxia
Recent laryngospasm/obstruction
Rales
Frothy pink sputum
Respiratory distress
Tachycardia
Acute congestive heart failure

Pulmonary Edema

Call for help
Administer 100% oxygen
Abort procedure
Intubate
Consider furosemide

Drugs

Furosemide 1 mg/kg IM/IV (Max of 40 mg)

Figure 8.18

Signs/Symptoms

Chest wall is stiff and patient
unable to be ventilated
Generally after opioid administration

Chest Wall Rigidity

Administer succinylcholine
Remove all objects from mouth
Triple airway maneuver
100% oxygen
Positive pressure

Consider naloxone
Consider differential if ventilation
is still inadequate

Drugs

Adult

Succinylcholine 1.2 mg/kg IV
Rocuronium 1 mg/kg IV
Naloxone 0.4–2 mg IV

Peds

Succinylcholine 2 mg/kg IV
Rocuronium 1 mg/kg IV
Naloxone 0.1 mg/kg IV (Max dose 2 mg)
Atropine 0.2 mg/kg IV

*Consider pretreatment with atropine

Figure 8.19

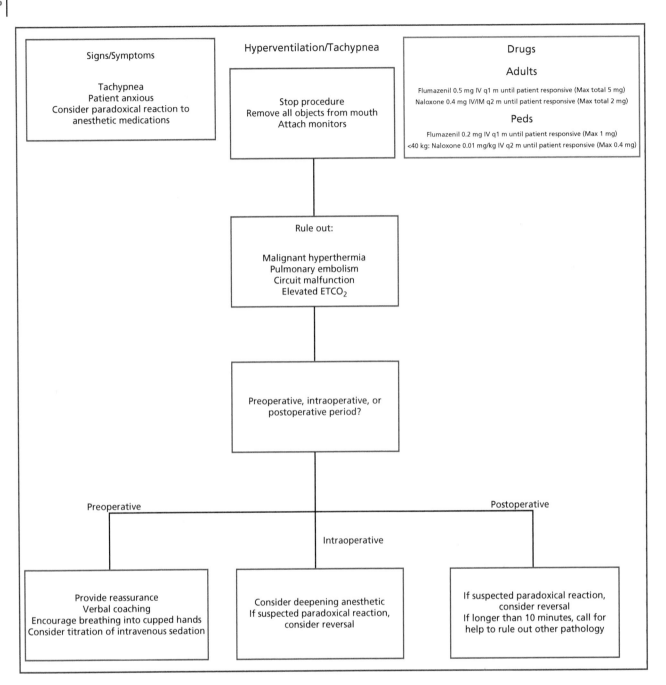

Figure 8.20

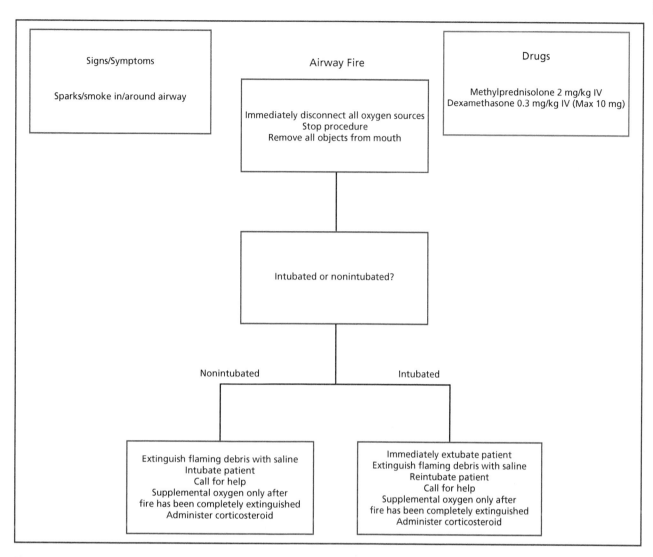

Figure 8.21

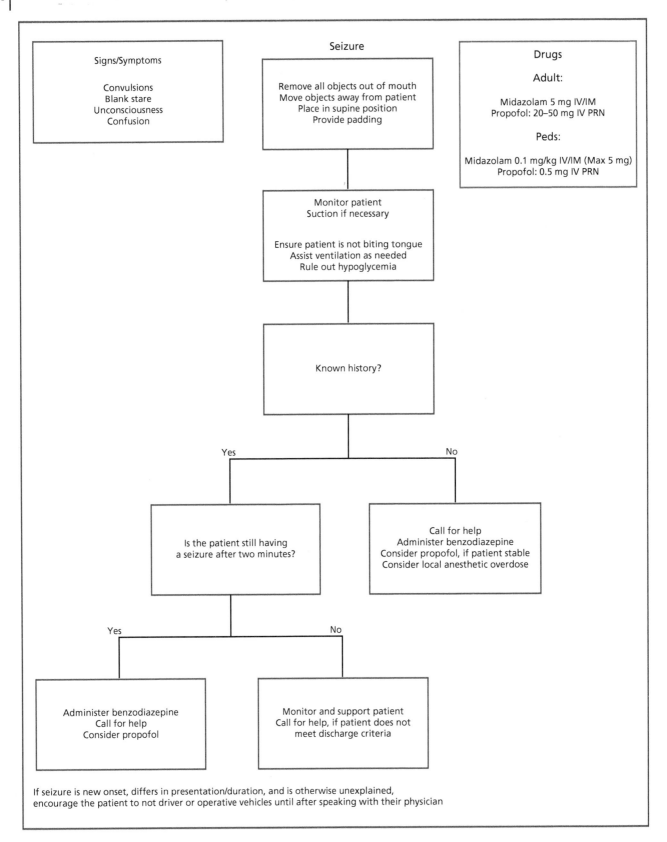

Figure 8.22

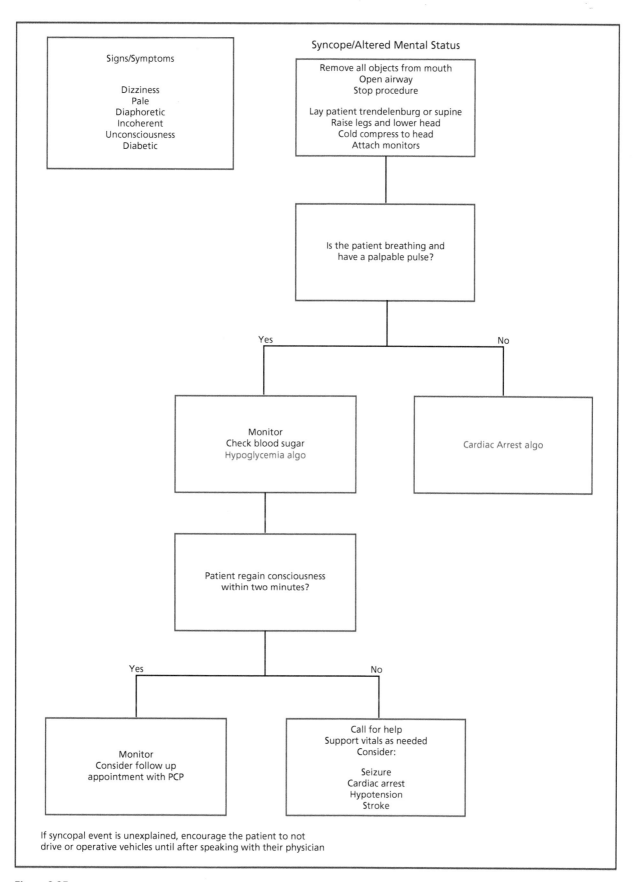

Figure 8.23

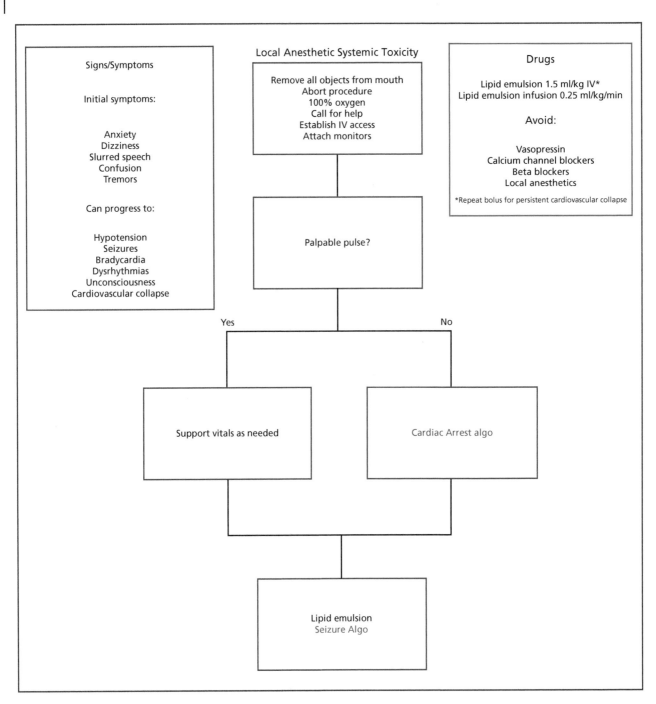

Figure 8.24

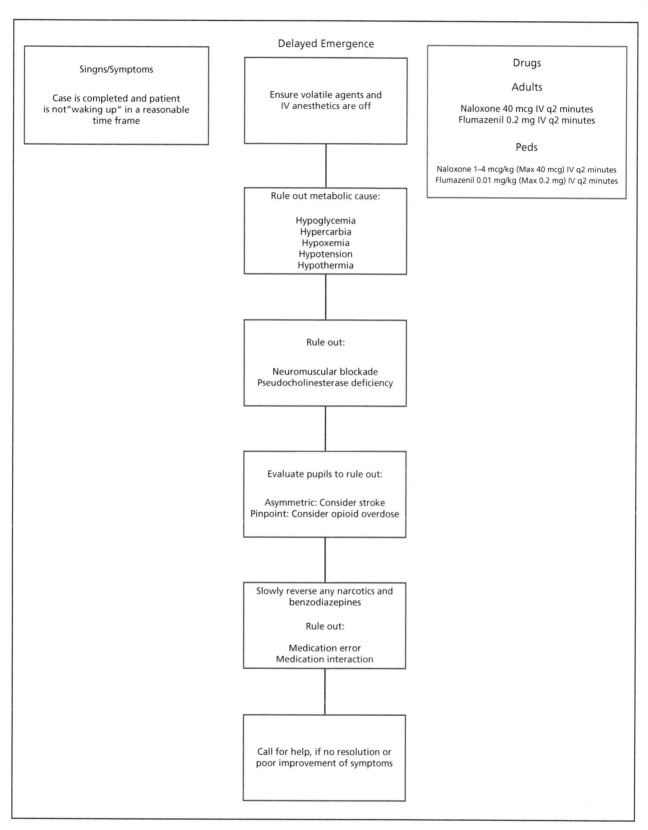

Delayed Emergence

Singns/Symptoms

Case is completed and patient is not"waking up" in a reasonable time frame

Ensure volatile agents and IV anesthetics are off

Rule out metabolic cause:

Hypoglycemia
Hypercarbia
Hypoxemia
Hypotension
Hypothermia

Rule out:

Neuromuscular blockade
Pseudocholinesterase deficiency

Evaluate pupils to rule out:

Asymmetric: Consider stroke
Pinpoint: Consider opioid overdose

Slowly reverse any narcotics and benzodiazepines

Rule out:

Medication error
Medication interaction

Call for help, if no resolution or poor improvement of symptoms

Drugs

Adults

Naloxone 40 mcg IV q2 minutes
Flumazenil 0.2 mg IV q2 minutes

Peds

Naloxone 1–4 mcg/kg (Max 40 mcg) IV q2 minutes
Flumazenil 0.01 mg/kg (Max 0.2 mg) IV q2 minutes

Figure 8.25

Signs/Symptoms

Facial droop
Speech difficulties
Muscle weakness on one side of the body
Headache
Blurred vision
Delayed awakening or unable to awaken

Stroke

Call for help
Monitor and support as needed
Titrate oxygen to 98% SpO$_2$
Check glucose levels
Transfer to stroke center

Figure 8.26

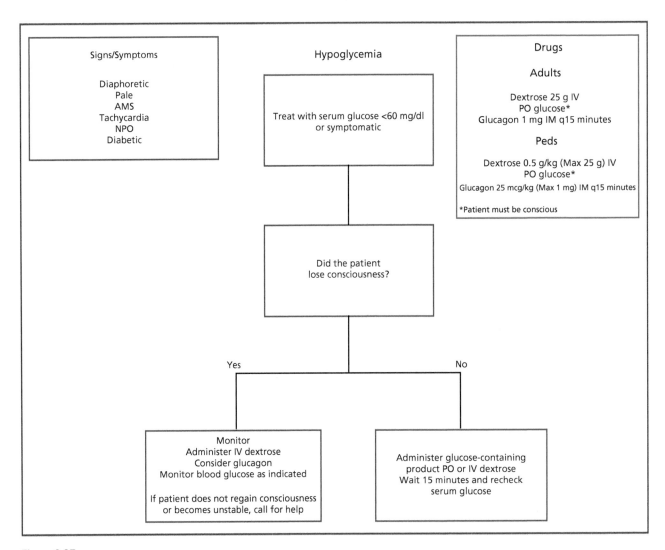

Signs/Symptoms

Diaphoretic
Pale
AMS
Tachycardia
NPO
Diabetic

Hypoglycemia

Treat with serum glucose <60 mg/dl
or symptomatic

Drugs

Adults

Dextrose 25 g IV
PO glucose*
Glucagon 1 mg IM q15 minutes

Peds

Dextrose 0.5 g/kg (Max 25 g) IV
PO glucose*
Glucagon 25 mcg/kg (Max 1 mg) IM q15 minutes

*Patient must be conscious

Did the patient
lose consciousness?

Yes

No

Monitor
Administer IV dextrose
Consider glucagon
Monitor blood glucose as indicated

If patient does not regain consciousness
or becomes unstable, call for help

Administer glucose-containing
product PO or IV dextrose
Wait 15 minutes and recheck
serum glucose

Figure 8.27

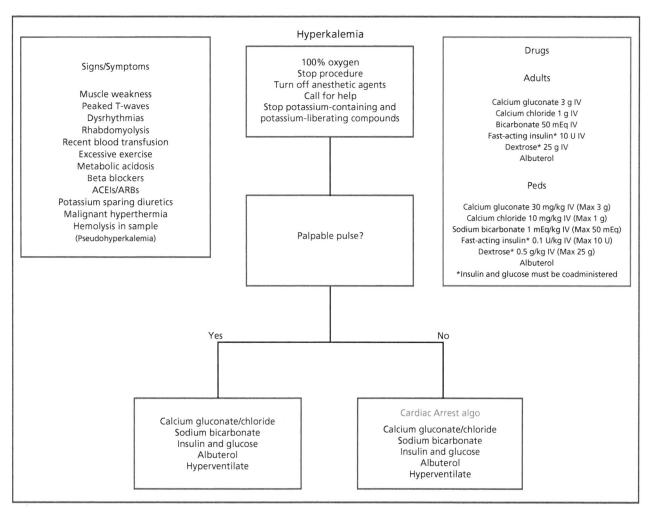

Figure 8.28

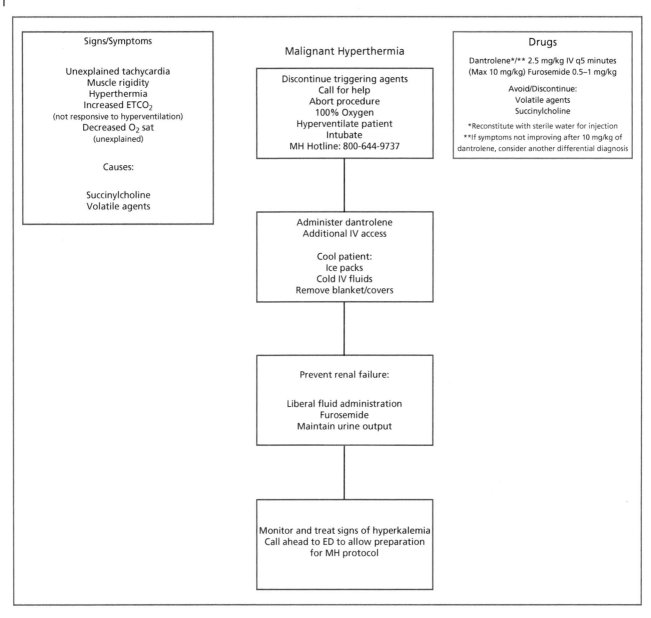

Signs/Symptoms

Unexplained tachycardia
Muscle rigidity
Hyperthermia
Increased ETCO$_2$
(not responsive to hyperventilation)
Decreased O$_2$ sat
(unexplained)

Causes:

Succinylcholine
Volatile agents

Malignant Hyperthermia

Discontinue triggering agents
Call for help
Abort procedure
100% Oxygen
Hyperventilate patient
Intubate
MH Hotline: 800-644-9737

Drugs

Dantrolene*/** 2.5 mg/kg IV q5 minutes
(Max 10 mg/kg) Furosemide 0.5–1 mg/kg

Avoid/Discontinue:
Volatile agents
Succinylcholine

*Reconstitute with sterile water for injection
**If symptoms not improving after 10 mg/kg of
dantrolene, consider another differential diagnosis

Administer dantrolene
Additional IV access

Cool patient:
Ice packs
Cold IV fluids
Remove blanket/covers

Prevent renal failure:

Liberal fluid administration
Furosemide
Maintain urine output

Monitor and treat signs of hyperkalemia
Call ahead to ED to allow preparation
for MH protocol

Figure 8.29

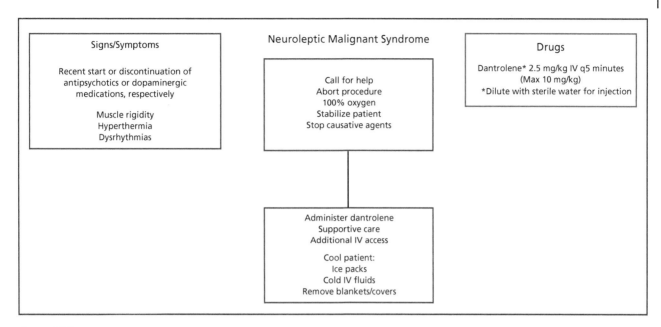

Figure 8.30

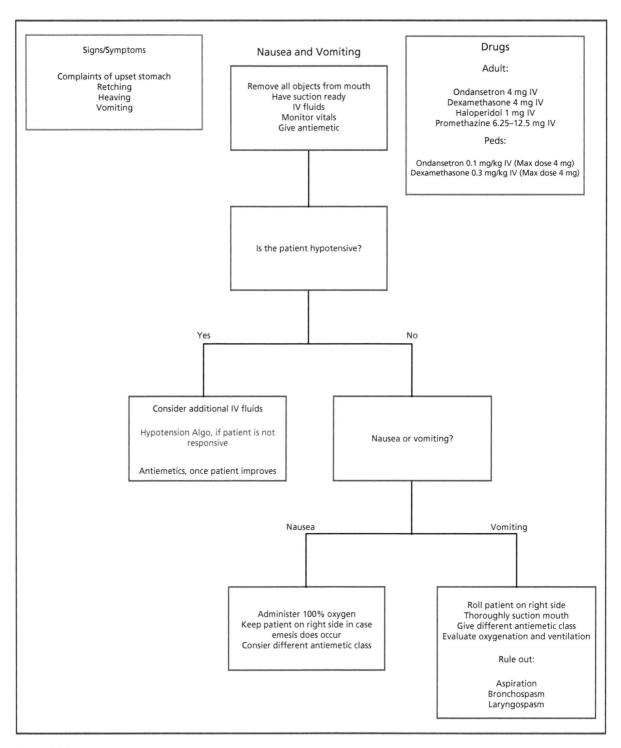

Figure 8.31

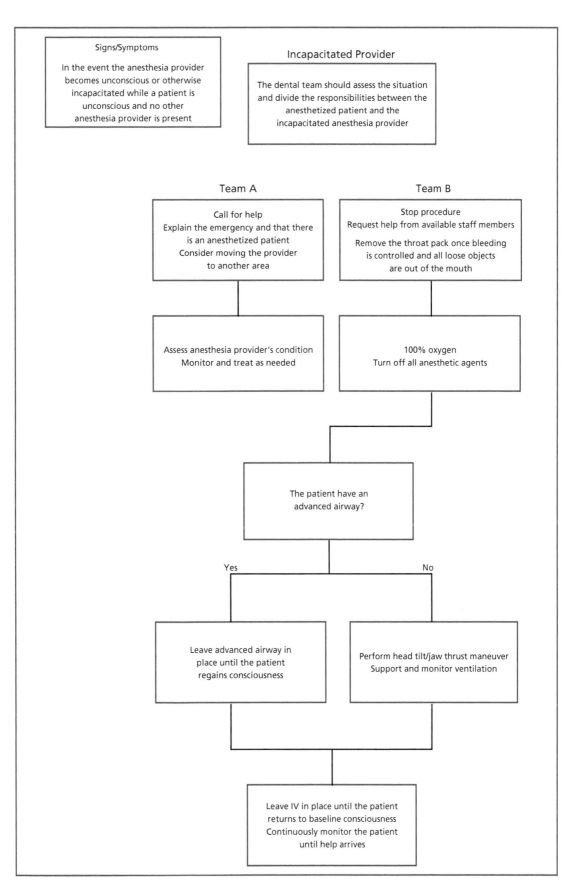

Figure 8.32

Section 9
Dental Specifics

9.1 Common Drug Dosing

- The following drug dosing ranges are an approximation based on a healthy adult patient, unless otherwise specified. This does not consider extremes in BMI, age, nor comorbidities
- Sedation level is never based on a specific dose or dosing schedule, but rather the patient's response
  - *Sedation levels covered on page 64*
- The anesthesia provider should check with their state dental board and sedation/general anesthesia regulations to confirm the level of sedation, patient age, and drugs allowed

Minimal Sedation

- Mainly a single drug technique
- Indications
  - Age two years and above
  - Must be able to cooperate
  - Mild to moderate adult anxiety
  - Mild to moderate invasive procedure with effective local anesthesia
  - Preoperative anxiolysis prior to IV placement
  - Medically compromised
- Contraindications
  - Uncooperative
  - Severe anxiety
  - Local anesthesia may be incomplete

Nitrous oxide	Most effective range is usually 30–50%
Midazolam	IV – 1–3 mg Peds PO – 0.2–0.5 mg/kg (max 10 mg)
Lorazepam	PO – 1–2 mg At least an hour prior to procedure
Triazolam	PO/SL – 0.125–0.5 mg 30–45 minutes prior to procedure
Meperidine	Peds PO – 1–2 mg/kg Several black box warnings [1]

| Hydroxyzine | PO – 50 mg
Peds PO – 1–2 mg/kg (max dose 50 mg) |
| Tizanidine | PO – 4–8 mg |

Moderate Sedation

- Multiple drugs may be used in this technique
- May be obtained via PO, IV, IM, inhalation, or IN
- Previously referred to as "conscious" sedation
- Indications
  - Generally, must have some degree of cooperation
  - Longer appointment times
  - Mild to moderate adult anxiety
  - Mild to moderate invasive procedure
  - Excessive gag reflex
- Contraindications
  - Poor results likely for pre-cooperative and younger children
  - Uncooperative/combative older children and adults
  - Severe anxiety
  - Highly invasive procedure

Midazolam	IV – 2–4 mg q3–5 minutes additional doses as needed during procedure, be careful with elderly PO – 0.5–1 mg/kg (max 20 mg) IM – 0.07–0.08 mg/kg IN – 0.2–0.3 mg/kg (max 10 mg)
Fentanyl	IV – 25–50 mcg q3–5 minutes for analgesia Usually not used as a sole sedative agent Additional doses may be needed
Propofol	Infusion range will vary Not a medication for moderate sedationists May not be permitted in many states, should only be used by DS/GA permit holders
Remimazolam	5 mg bolus over 2 minutes 2.5 mg q5 minutes as needed

Anesthesia for Dental and Oral Maxillofacial Surgery, First Edition. Spencer D. Wade, Caroline M. Sawicki, Megann K. Smiley, Michael A. Cuddy, Steven Vukas, and Paul J. Schwartz.
© 2024 John Wiley & Sons, Inc. Published 2024 by John Wiley & Sons, Inc.

Deep Sedation/General Anesthesia

- Indications
  - Uncooperative patients
  - Pediatric patients
  - Severe anxiety
  - Moderate to highly invasive procedure
- Contraindications
  - Medical history
    - Especially advanced cardiovascular and pulmonary disease
  - Airway concerns
  - Age extremes
  - Concurrent medications
    - Anticoagulation with nasal intubation
    - Lithium with succinylcholine
  - Procedure can be reasonably performed under moderate or minimal sedation

Fentanyl	IV – 1–2 mcg/kg Additional doses as needed
Sufentanil	IV – 0.1–0.2 mcg/kg Additional doses as needed
Remifentanil	IV – infusion rates will vary Commonly 0.02–0.1 mcg/kg/h
Propofol	IV Induction – 1–2 mg/kg Maintenance infusion doses will vary Commonly 50–200 mcg/kg/h
Dexmedetomidine	IV – 4–8 mcg q10 minutes Infusion – 1 mcg/kg loading dose over 10 minutes, then 0.2–0.7 mcg/kg/h IN – 2–4 mcg/kg
Ketamine	IV induction – 1–2 mg/kg IM induction – 4–8 mg/kg IM – 1–3 mg/kg in a larger muscle mass for managing uncooperative patient

9.2   Local Anesthetics

- Structure
  - Ester or amide linkage (Figure 9.1)

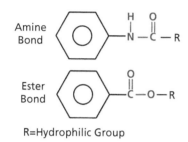

Figure 9.1

  - Esters have one I in their name
    - ○ Procaine
    - ○ Benzocaine
  - Amides have two I's in their name
    - ○ Lidocaine
    - ○ Articaine
    - ○ Mepivacaine
- Mechanism of Action (Figure 9.2)
  - Antagonize neuronal Na⁺ channels to prevent signal transmissions
  - Must cross the cell membrane and inactivate the channel intracellularly

Pharmacokinetics

- ↑ Potency
  - ↑ Lipid solubility
- ↓ Onset of Action
  - ↑ Concentration
  - ↑ Lipid solubility
    - ○ Easier to diffuse through cellular membranes
  - pKa closer to physiologic pH

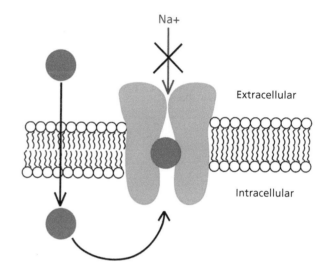

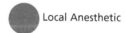

Figure 9.2

- ↑ Duration
  - Presence of vasoconstrictors
  - ↑ Protein binding

Physiologic Effects

- Cerebral
  - IV
    - ○ ↓ ICP on intubation
    - ○ ↓ MAC
      - Except cocaine
- Cardiovascular
  - Lidocaine
    - ○ Class 1B antidysrhythmic

- Bupivacaine
  o Complete cardiac conduction block with overdose or accidental intravascular injection
- Regional
  o If vasoconstrictors are included, may transiently increase CO, MAP, and HR
- Pulmonary
  - IV
    o May block reflexive bronchoconstriction [2]
- Renal
  - Minimal
- Hepatic
  - Amides
    o Primary site of metabolism
    o Metabolites are commonly active and may contribute to toxicity
- Contraindications
  - True documented allergy
  - No "real" contraindication but caution in pediatric patients and those with special health care needs as it may result in trauma-induced lip bite [3–5]

- Board Facts
  - *For more details on vasoconstrictors see page 287*
  - Esters are metabolized by pseudocholinesterase
  - Para-aminobenzoic acid (PABA) metabolite of ester local anesthetics has been implicated in allergic reactions
  - Analgesic duration can be shortened with phentolamine (Oraverse®)
    o α_1 adrenergic receptor antagonist leading to vasodilation and increased uptake of local anesthetic from tissues
    o May be useful in shortening duration for pediatric and special needs populations to prevent self-inflicted perioral trauma
  - Bupivacaine is not recommended for children under 12 years of age
  - Articaine is not recommended for children under than four years of age
  - For easier mg calculations, see figure 9.3

Max dose table for adult and pediatric patients based on weight.

Wgh (kg)	Wgh (lb)	Lidocaine Max = 7 mg/kg 2%, 1:100 k epi	Articaine Max = 7 mg/kg 4% 1:100 k or 1:200 k epi	Mepivacaine Max = 6.6 mg/kg 3% plain	Prilocaine Max = 8.8 mg/kg 4% w or w/o epi	Bupivacaine Max = 1.3 mg/kg 0.5% 1:200 k epi
		# Cartridges				
10	22	1.9	1.0	1.2	1.1	N/A
15	33	2.9	1.5	1.8	1.7	N/A
20	44	3.9	1.9	2.4	2.2	N/A
25	55	4.9	2.4	3.1	2.8	N/A
30	66	5.8	2.9	3.7	3.3	N/A
35	77	6.8	3.4	4.3	3.9	N/A
40	88	7.8	3.9	4.9	4.4	N/A
45	99	8.8	4.4	5.5	5.0	6.6
50	110	9.7	4.9	6.1	5.6	7.3
55	121	10.7	5.3	6.7	6.1	8.1
60	132	11.1	5.8	7.3	6.7	8.8
65	143	11.1	6.3	7.4	7.2	9.5
>70	>154	11.1	6.9	7.4	8.3	10.0

Source: Reprinted with permission from Joseph A. Giovannitti Jr. *Moderate Sedation and Emergency Medicine for Periodontists.*

2% = 20 mg/ml
0.5% = 5 mg/ml

Figure 9.3

- *Local anesthetic toxicity covered on page 270*
- Complications
  - Methemoglobinemia
    - ○ Triggered by benzocaine and prilocaine metabolite O-toluidine
    - ○ Blood will appear chocolate-brown in color
    - ○ Iron (Fe^{2+}) of hemoglobin is oxidized to ferric form (Fe^{3+}) (Figure 9.4)
      - Ferric iron is unable to bind oxygen

Common Oxidizers

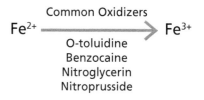

$$Fe^{2+} \longrightarrow Fe^{3+}$$

O-toluidine
Benzocaine
Nitroglycerin
Nitroprusside

Figure 9.4

- ○ Unexplained cyanosis and hypoxia will occur at high levels of methemoglobin
  - SpO_2 will read approximately 85% regardless of true PaO_2
- ○ Reversed with methylene blue 1–2 mg/kg IV over 5–30 minutes
- Nerve damage/paresthesia
  - More common with higher percent local [6] anesthetic concentration

9.3 Topical Local Anesthetics

- *Fiberoptic intubations covered on page 302*
- Cocaine was the first used
- Many are available over the counter
- Most effective on a dry surface as the medication will be better absorbed
- Can be ester or amide
- Indications
  - Needle-phobic patients
  - Awake fiberoptics
  - Prior to IV placement
  - Prior to local anesthetic injection
  - Assist with intraoral radiographs
  - Minimally invasive intraoral procedure
- Contraindications
  - Allergy
  - While not a contraindication, care should be taken to avoid local anesthetic toxicity, especially in children as unknown amount may be absorbed

Types

- Spray
  - Cetacaine®
    - Made up of ester anesthetics
    - Benzocaine 14.0%
    - Butamben 2.0%
    - Tetracaine 2.0%
    - Unmetered spray so very easy to overdose
- Jelly
  - Lidocaine
    - 2% or 5%
    - Used to lubricate ETT, usually NETT prior to awake fiberoptic intubations
- Viscous
  - Lidocaine
  - Used for patients to gargle and numb posterior pharyngeal structures prior to awake fiberoptic intubations
- Ointment
  - Lidocaine
    - Usually 5%
    - Useful prior to intraoral injection or as lollipop prior to awake FO intubation
- Patch
  - Eutectic mixture of local anesthetics (EMLA)
    - Lidocaine 2.5%
    - Prilocaine 2.5%
  - Uses
    - Numb skin prior to IV start
    - Mild surgical procedures
- Gel/Topical
  - Oraqix®
    - Lidocaine 2.5%
    - Prilocaine 2.5%
    - Injected into tooth sulcus prior to scaling and root planning
    - Also available intraorally as a patch
  - Benzocaine
    - Usually 20%
    - Used prior to local anesthesia injection

9.4 Vasoconstrictors

- Most local anesthetics cause vasodilation via direct smooth muscle relaxation of arterioles. Vasoconstrictors assist in keeping the local anesthetic in the site longer by reducing vascular uptake
  - Cocaine is the only local anesthetic that causes peripheral vasoconstriction
- Types
  - Epinephrine
    - Most commonly
      - 1:50 000
      - 1:100 000 (Figure 9.5)
      - 1:200 000
  - Levonordefrin – alpha-methylnorepinephrine
    - Most commonly 1:20 000

Dosing Equivalencies
1:100 000 = 1 g/100 000 ml = 1000 mg/100 000 ml = 10 mcg/ml

Figure 9.5

	Max dose of epinephrine (mcg)
Healthy adult patient (>45 kg)	200 mcg – unmonitored Observe cardiovascular response in monitored patient
Medically compromised adult Especially CV	40 mcg – monitored Observe cardiovascular response in monitored patient

- Indications
  - ↑ Duration of block
  - ↑ Efficacy of the block
  - Hemostasis
  - ↓ Peak systemic absorption of local anesthetic
- Contraindications/Cautions
  - Cardiovascular patients
    - Unstable/unstable angina pectoris
    - Recent MI
    - Recent CABG/PCI
    - Refractory arrhythmias
    - Untreated or uncontrolled hypertension
    - Untreated or uncontrolled heart failure
    - Uncontrolled diabetes mellitus
  - Uncontrolled or untreated hyperthyroidism
  - Sulfite sensitivity
    - Antioxidant for vasoconstrictor
  - Pheochromocytoma
  - Drug interactions [7]:
    - Nonspecific beta blockers
      - Possible severe hypertension with reflex bradycardia due to unopposed α_1 effects
    - COMT inhibitors
      - Exaggerated epinephrine effects
    - TCAs
      - High dose >50 mg increased epinephrine cardiovascular effects
    - MAOIs
      - Stress/pain of injection may lead to exaggerated BP/HR; no direct effect
    - Acute cocaine ingestion
    - Phenothiazine compounds
      - High-dose epinephrine hypotension possible
- Board Facts
  - Hemodent is aluminum chloride with no vasoconstrictor
  - Epinephrine containing retraction cord may be absorbed systemically

9.5 Local Anesthesia for the Trigeminal Nerve (CN V)

- *Complete list of cranial nerve innervations on pages 31–34*
- Trigeminal nerve sensory distribution (Figure 9.6)

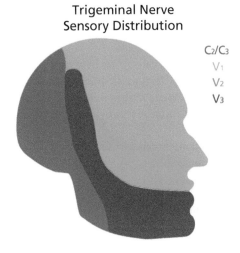

Trigeminal Nerve
Sensory Distribution

C₂/C₃
V₁
V₂
V₃

Figure 9.6

Ophthalmic Nerve (V₁)

- Smallest of the branches
- Innervation
  - Sensory only:
    - o Scalp
    - o Eye
    - o Nose
    - o Forehead
- Supraorbital Nerve Block
  - Palpate the foramen
    - o Intersection of the medial one-third and the lateral two-thirds of the orbit, usually in the sagittal plane with the pupil
  - Create a wheal with 0.5–1 ml of anesthetic solution
  - Apply firm pressure

- Supratrochlear Nerve Block
  - Can be blocked immediately after the supraorbital by advancing the needle 1 cm toward the midline and injecting additional 0.5–1 ml of anesthetic solution
  - Apply firm pressure after each block

Maxillary Nerve (V₂)

- Innervation
  Sensory only (Figure 9.7)
    - o Inferior orbit
    - o Nasal cavity
    - o Maxillary teeth and soft tissues
    - o Maxillary sinus

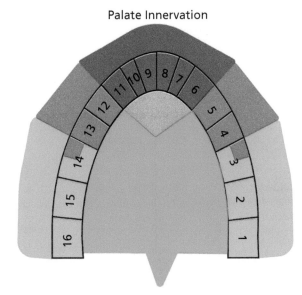

Palate Innervation

Anterior Superior Alveolar n.
Middle Superior Alveolar n.
Nasopalatine n.
Greater & Lesser Palatine nn.
Posterior Superior Alveolar n.

Figure 9.7

- Maxillary Nerve Block
  - Intraoral approach
    - Palpate greater palatine foramen
    - Advance long needle into foramen
    - Aspirate and inject
    - May cause injury to nerve, artery, and/or vein
  - Extraoral approach
    - Suprazygomatic is recommended as having fewer complications
    - Done with ultrasound and/or nerve stimulator
- Infraorbital Nerve Block
  - Inferior palpebral, the lateral nasal, and the superior labial nerves
  - Extraoral approach
    - Palpate foramen, leaving finger there, inject in a caudad and medial direction
  - Intraoral approach
    - Palpate foramen, leaving finger there
    - Needle is inserted into the buccal mucosa at the level of the canine or the first premolar and directed upward and outward into the canine fossa
  - Apply firm pressure after the block
- Greater Palatine Nerve Block
  - Inject at the greater palatine foramen
  - Innervation
    - Hard palate posterior to canine
    - Portion of soft palate
- Lesser Palatine Nerve Block
  - Inject at the greater palatine foramen
  - Innervation
    - Portions of soft palate
- Nasopalatine Nerve Block
  - Inject at the nasopalatine foramen
  - Innervation
    - Lingual of maxillary canines, lateral incisors, and central incisors
- Posterior Superior Alveolar Nerve Block
  - Insert long needle to the buccal of the maxillary second molars
    - Innervation
      - Maxillary molars and buccal tissues

- Middle Superior Alveolar Nerve Block
  - Insert long needle to the buccal of the maxillary second premolar
    - Innervation
      - Maxillary premolar and buccal tissue
      - Mesiobuccal root of maxillary first molar
- Anterior Superior Alveolar Nerve Block
  - Insert long needle to the buccal of the maxillary canine
    - Innervation
      - Maxillary central incisors, lateral incisors, canines, and buccal tissue

Mandibular Nerve (V₃)

- Largest of the branches
- Sensory
  - Lower third of the face
  - Floor of the mouth and mandible
  - Mandibular teeth and soft tissues
  - Entire tongue
- Motor
  - Masseter
  - Temporalis
  - Pterygoids
  - Anterior belly of digastric
  - Mylohyoid
- Mandibular Nerve Blocks [8, 9]
  - Halsted
    - "Standard" inferior alveolar nerve block
  - Gow-Gates
    - Indications:
      - History of inferior alveolar nerve block failure
      - Evidence of anatomical variability
      - Evidence of accessory innervation of mandibular molars
  - Akinosi–Vazirani
    - Indications:
      - Same as above with:
      - Presence of trismus or difficulty in seeing intraoral landmarks

9.6 Natural Guarded Airway (NGA)

- Natural guarded airway (NGA) is the new term for what has been traditionally called "open airway" or "natural airway"

Airway Barriers

- Use of a "throat screen" or "throat pack," to protect the airway from aspiration of dental objects, intraoral irrigation, blood, and debris
- During preoperative airway exam, make note of loose dentition and removable objects
  - Tooth damage is the most common outpatient general anesthesia claim
- Proper airway barriers may help prevent aspiration, laryngospasm, and bronchospasm
- Types of Barriers
  - Physical barriers
    o Throat screen
      - For NGA
      - Placed in region of tonsillar pillars
    o Throat pack
      - For intubated cases
      - Placed in hypopharynx
    o C-sponge
    o Rubber dam
      - Still requires a throat screen or pack
  - Water isolation instruments
    o Isolite/Isovac
      - Provides suction and bite block and possibly illumination
    o Rubber dam
    o Well-trained assistant
    o High volume suction
    o Operator may "cut dry" especially if primary dentition, but pulpal damage possible

Lost Objects

- Ligate small objects with floss to allow retrieval if misplaced in the airway (Figure 9.8)
- Consider a "count" system for disposables such as for gauze and cotton rolls

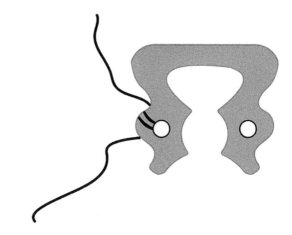

Figure 9.8

- May need to refer patient to radiology to rule out aspiration if unable to locate
- Commonly Lost Objects:
  - 2×2 gauzes
  - Cotton rolls
  - Dental impression materials
  - Implant drivers
  - Brackets
  - Crowns/inlays
  - Teeth
  - Rubber dam clamps

- Common Locations for Lost Objects:
  - Out of the mouth
    - Floor
    - On/behind patient
    - Gauze
  - Suction
  - Posterior pharynx
  - Palatal fold
  - Larynx
  - Lungs
  - Stomach

NGA Positioning

- Utilize a noninvasive oxygen delivery system
- Have patient in a supine or semi-supine position
- Triple Airway Maneuver
  - Jaw thrust
  - Head tilt
  - Chin lift

- Ramp
  - May be helpful in patients prone to obstruction
- Shoulder Roll
  - May assist in patients prone to obstruction as well as give the operator better surgical conditions
- ↑ Difficulty for NGA:
  - History or suspicion of sleep apnea
    - STOPBANG
  - Enlarged tonsils and/or adenoids
  - Craniofacial abnormalities
  - Odontogenic infection
  - ↑ BMI
  - Neuromuscular disorders
- Consider Airway Adjunct
  - Nasopharyngeal airways (NPA)
  - Oral pharyngeal airways (OPA)
- Always have an advanced airway and a Bag Valve Mask (BVM) prepared and immediately available in case further intervention is required

9.7 Noninvasive Oxygen Delivery Systems

Nasal Cannula (Figure 9.9)

- 4% increase in FiO_2 concentration per l increase in O_2 flow above room air
- $FiO_2 - (0.2 + 0.04 \times L/min)$ (max 0.4)

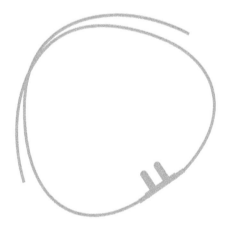

Figure 9.9

- Advantages
  - Practical and inexpensive for most head and neck procedures
  - Respiratory/ventilatory function can be assessed by CO_2 scavenging, but CO_2 levels may not be accurate
- Disadvantages
  - Cannot provide positive pressure ventilation
  - Can cause nasal irritation
  - Cannot utilize N_2O due to lack of scavenging
- Ineffective
  - Chronic sinusitis
  - Mouth breathing
  - Deviated septum
  - Choanal atresia

Nasal Hood

- $FiO_2 \sim 0.5$–0.6 when flow is greater than minute ventilation
- Advantages
  - Inexpensive, practical for most dental procedures
  - Able to titrate N_2O, if used
  - Respiratory/ventilatory function can be assessed by CO_2 scavenging, but CO_2 levels may not be accurate
- Disadvantages
  - Difficult to provide positive pressure ventilation
    - High-flow O_2
    - Close mouth
    - Press nasal mask to face
    - Squeeze bag
- Ineffective
  - Chronic sinusitis
  - Mouth breathing
  - Deviated septum
  - Choanal atresia

Face Mask

- Generally used for extraoral procedures, postoperatively or in emergent situations
- Simple Face Mask
  - 35–50% FiO_2 delivery
  - Minimum of 6 L/min flow to prevent CO_2 rebreathing
- Partial Rebreather Mask
  - Up to 60% FiO_2 delivery
  - Adjust flow to maintain reservoir bag inflation
- Nonrebreather Mask (Figure 9.10)
  - Up to 90% FiO_2 delivery with 10–15 L/min flow
- Advantages
  - Higher concentration of FiO_2 achievable than nasal hood and cannula
  - Respiratory function can be assessed by CO_2 scavenging, but CO_2 levels may not be accurate

Non-Rebreather Mask with
Supplemental Oxygen Reservoir

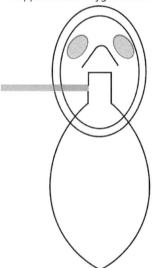

Figure 9.10

- Disadvantages
  - Unable to provide positive pressure ventilation
  - Cannot use N_2O
  - Cannot provide positive pressure ventilation
  - Realistically, unable to do during any lengthy intraoral procedure

High-Flow Nasal Cannula [10]

- Nasal cannula with the capability to humidify oxygen
- Capable of flow rates that exceed the inspiratory pressure of the patient

- Advantages
  - Allows delivery of 100% FiO_2 while maintaining the patient's ability to utilize the mouth to talk or eat
  - May also be used to lengthen times of apnea in preparation for intubation
- Disadvantages
  - Generally not available in office setting or ASC
  - Cannot use N_2O
  - Unable to provide positive pressure ventilation

Bag Valve Mask

- Portable and useful for emergency ventilation when patient obstructs or becomes apneic
- Contains a non-rebreathing valve
- FiO_2 close to 1.0 with O_2 flows >10 L/min and reservoir bag
- Advantages
  - Allows for positive pressure ventilation
  - Can be attached to advanced airways, if needed
- Disadvantages
  - Cannot use N_2O

9.8 Airway Adjuncts

Oral Pharyngeal Airways (OPA)

- Provide airway patency by displacing the tongue from the posterior pharyngeal wall (Figure 9.11)

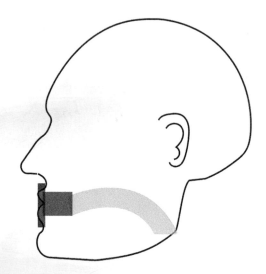

Figure 9.11

- Sizing
  - Many systems are color coded
  - Sizing is typically in millimeters
  - Length is estimated by measuring from the commissure of the mouth to the angle of the mandible
- Uses
  - Only use with deeply sedated or unconscious patients
  - Not tolerated in conscious/semiconscious patients
  - Beneficial for mask ventilation prior to intubation, especially in edentulous patients
  - Requires moderate mouth opening
- Complications
  - Coughing
  - Bronchospasm
  - Gagging
  - Emesis
  - Laryngospasm

- Techniques
  - Ensure that tongue is not pushed posteriorly
  - Check that soft tissues are not pinched between the airway and teeth
  - Technique 1
    o Insert OPA inverted along the hard palate to posterior pharynx
    o Rotate 180° behind tongue
    o Insert until flange is at level of lips
  - Technique 2
    o Use tongue blade to displace tongue from posterior pharynx
    o Use jaw thrust or lift
    o Insert airway along tongue blade

Nasopharyngeal Airways (NPA)

- Provides airway patency and relieves obstruction associated with nasal cavity (Figure 9.12)

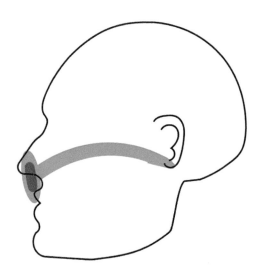

Figure 9.12

- Sizing
  - 2–4 cm longer than the oral airway
  - Sizing is typically in French
    - French size × 0.33 = outer diameter in millimeters
  - Length is estimated by measuring distance from nares to meatus of the ear
- Uses
  - Better tolerated than OPA in semiconscious or awake patients
- Complications/Contraindications:
  - Laryngospasm
  - Prominent adenoids
  - Frequent epistaxis
  - Basilar skull fracture
  - Coagulopathy
- Technique
  - Prior to insertion, should lubricate to reduce nasal trauma
  - Consider using lidocaine jelly for patients who are awake or semiconscious
  - Angle parallel to the plane of the tongue or nasal floor
  - Insert along nasal floor beneath the inferior turbinate

9.9 Supraglottic Airways

- Indications
  - Extraoral procedures
  - Short cases
  - Intraoral procedure if flexible stalk is used
  - Emergency airway
- Contraindications
  - Poor mouth opening
  - Pharyngeal pathology
  - Pharyngeal obstruction
  - ↑ Risk of aspiration
  - ↓ Pulmonary compliance
  - Morbid obesity
    - ○ Hypoventilation due to inability to generate larger inspiratory pressures
- Complications [11, 12]
  - Easily dislodged or displaced especially with head and neck manipulation
    - ○ Distal tip can curl up on itself and reduce ventilation efficacy
  - Nerve damage
    - ○ Recurrent laryngeal n.
    - ○ Trigeminal n.
    - ○ Hypoglossal n.
  - Abrasion and bleeding of pharyngeal tissues
  - Gastric insufflation
    - ○ Especially at ventilation pressures >20 cm H_2O
    - ○ ↑ Risk of vomiting and aspiration

Face Mask Ventilation

- Typically, not an option for longer, more involved oral surgical procedures
- May be a viable option for short, uncomplicated intraoral procedures (extraction of pediatric teeth) if surgery and anesthesia take turns with the airway or for shorter procedures outside of the oral cavity
- Head strap and prongs on face mask will aid in placement and retention

Laryngeal Mask Airway (Figure 9.13)

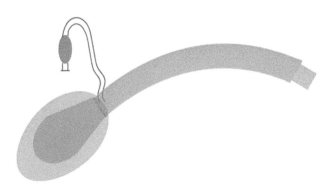

Figure 9.13

- Inflatable device
- Does not provide a completely secure airway
- Peak inspiratory pressure < 20 cm H_2O to avoid insufflation of stomach
- Types
  - Standard rigid tube
  - Flexible tube (anode like)
  - Intubating (Fastrach) – allows conversion from LMA to intubation
- Technique
  - Insert the device completely deflated or partially inflated
  - Insert posterior into the pharynx and should feel a "pop" when it drops into place
  - Inflate with a maximum pressure of 20 cm H_2O

- Sizing
  - Manufacturers have different recommendations, but here are general "cut offs"

Size 1	Neonate (1–5 kg)
Size 1.5	Infant (5–10 kg)
Size 2	Small pediatric (10–20 kg)
Size 2.5	Large pediatric (20–30 kg)
Size 3	Small adult (30–50 kg)
Size 4	Medium adult (50–70 kg)
Size 5	Large adult (70 kg+)

King Airway

- Replacement for the Combitube
- Allows direct ventilation through fenestrations at level of the hypopharynx and then through the larynx to trachea
- Single lumen tube (gastric suction port also available)
- Distal balloon occludes the esophagus preventing gastric inflation and regurgitation
- Proximal balloon occludes the oropharynx
- Technique
  - Inserted blindly
- Sizing
  - Manufacturers have different recommendations, but here are general "cut offs"
  - Size recommendation per Ambu®

Size 0	Neonate (<5 kg)
Size 1.0	Infant (5–12 kg)
Size 2	Small pediatric (12–25 kg)
Size 2.5	Large pediatric (25–35 kg)
Size 3	Small adult (4–5 ft)
Size 4	Medium adult (5–6 ft)
Size 5	Large adult (>6 ft)

I-gel®

- Gel-like thermoplastic elastomeric cuff
  - Inflation not needed
- Anatomical seal of the pharyngeal, laryngeal, and perilaryngeal structures while avoiding compressive trauma
- Has a gastric channel for suctioning
- Technique
  - Inserted blindly
- Sizing
  - Manufacturers have different recommendations, but here are general "cut offs"
  - Size recommendation per Intersurgical®

Size 1	Neonate (2–5 kg)
Size 1.5	Infant (5–12 kg)
Size 2	Small pediatric (10–25 kg)
Size 2.5	Large pediatric (25–35 kg)
Size 3	Small adult (30–60 kg)
Size 4	Medium adult (50–90 kg)
Size 5	Large adult (90 kg+)

9.10 Endotracheal Tubes (Figure 9.14)

- Most secure airway
- Regardless of size, all have 15 mm connectors for circuit or BVM adaptor
- ETT size represents internal diameter in millimeters
- Most are cuffed, may be uncuffed (mostly in peds)
- Cuff [13]
  - Prevents aspiration and leaks during positive pressure ventilation (PPV)
  - Becoming more popular than uncuffed
  - Ideal cuff pressure is 20–30 cm H_2O
    - Allows for adequate delivery of PPV
    - ↓ Risk of aspiration
    - ↓ Risk of ventilator-associated pneumonia
- Murphy's Eye
  - Distal to cuff
  - Prevents complete obstruction of the ETT even if bevel is occluded against tracheal wall

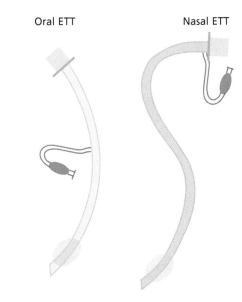

Oral ETT   Nasal ETT

Figure 9.14

Head Movement and ETT Effect

- Literature seems similar for effects regardless if it is NETT or oral ETT
- Head Extension
  - ETT moves cephalad [14]
- Head Flexion
  - ETT moves toward carina [14]
- Head Rotation
  - Unpredictable movement [14]

Oral Endotracheal Tubes

- Less invasive than nasal intubation
- Made of PVC, usually
- Types
  - Straight
  - Preformed (RAE)

- Armored/reinforced/anode
  - Resistant to kinking and biting
  - Used with lasers
- Indications
  - Protected airway for most surgeries not involving the airway
  - Indicated for intraoral procedures when a NETT is contraindicated
- Contraindications
  - Can be cumbersome for some/many intraoral procedures
  - Extremely limited oral opening
  - Interdental fixation
  - Evaluation of occlusion intraoperatively
- Technique
  - Many techniques for placement
  - Many practitioners use stylets for easier guidance

- Sizing (Figure 9.15)

Oral ETT Sizing

	Adults	Pediatrics
Diameter	6–8 mm	$\dfrac{Age}{4} + 4$
Depth	19–23 cm	$(3 \times ETT\ diameter)+1$

Figure 9.15

Nasal Endotracheal Tubes

- Most are preformed
- Most made of PVC
  - Parker Flex is polyurethane
- Straight oral ETTs can be converted to a NETT using a 60° angle connector
- Types
  - "Clear"
    - Straight and preformed
  - Smiths Medical Portex® – blue
    - Straight and preformed, cannot see fogging
    - Slightly larger in length and outer diameter than Clear ETTs
- Indications
  - Intraoral procedures
  - Facial trauma procedures
  - TMJ procedures
  - Implant procedures
  - Orthognathic procedures
- Contraindications
  - Trauma
    - Basilar skull fracture
    - Displace midface fractures
  - Severe nasal obstruction
    - Choanal atresia
    - Chronic/acute sinusitis
  - Some repaired clefts
    - May use Seldinger technique
  - Frequent or severe epistaxis
  - Coagulopathy
  - Anticoagulation therapy
- Technique
  - Consider warming distal 1–1.5 in. of ETT in warm water to lessen potential nasal trauma
    - Careful not to overwarm
    - Probably only needed for clear tubes
  - ETT is inserted parallel to the nasal floor, not in a superior direction
  - Use Magill or Rovenstine forceps, or Aillon tube bender to align tube with glottic opening, being careful not to traumatize adjacent tissues
- Sizing (Figure 9.16)
  - Good rule of thumb is that a NETT will be ½ size smaller than calculated OETT

Nasal ETT Sizing

	Adults	Pediatrics
Diameter	6–7 mm	$\dfrac{Age}{4} + 3.5$
Depth	26–29 cm	$\dfrac{Age}{2} + 15$

Figure 9.16

9.11 Laryngoscopy

Preoxygenation

- Also referred to as "de-nitrogenation" (Figure 9.17)

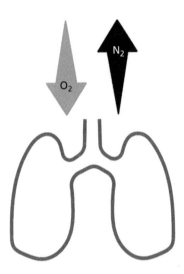

Figure 9.17

- Technique
  - Delivery of 100% oxygen until patient has an ETO_2 concentration of >0.7
  - Done prior to laryngoscopy to allow for a period of apnea without significant desaturation
  - Need to have a good seal around nose and mouth to prevent room air entrainment
  - May need another provider for patient with difficult airway to achieve adequate ventilation
    - May need an airway adjunct device to be successful
  - Consider ETO_2 concentration of >0.8–0.9 in patients who may have difficulty with mask ventilation and/or intubation
    - Beards
    - Edentulous
    - ↑ BMI
    - Facial deformities
    - History of difficult airway
    - OSA

Laryngoscopes

- Blades
  - Reusable and single use types
  - Older ones have light bulbs on blade
  - Newer ones are fiberoptic
  - Common blades
    - Macintosh (Figure 9.18)
      - Curved
    - Miller (Figure 9.18)
      - Straight
    - Wis-Hipple
      - Mostly for peds
    - Phillips
      - Popular for peds

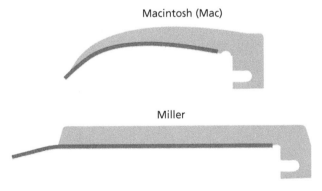

Macintosh (Mac)

Miller

Figure 9.18

- Laryngoscope Handles
  - Reusable and single-use types
  - Older handles have a light bulb on the blade that lights when the blade is engaged with the handle

- Newer handles are fiberoptic with the light source in the handle
- Types
  o Standard
    • Use C batteries, some use D
  o Penlight
    • Uses AA batteries
    • Useful for small hands
  o Stubby
    • Useful in OB or obese patients
- Video Laryngoscopes
  - Fiberoptic display of laryngeal and pharyngeal structures obtained on either remote screen or screen built into device
    o Initially utilized for difficult airways; now used routinely
  - Variety of types from different companies
    o King™
    o GlideScope™, GlideGo™
    o McGrath™
    o UEScope™
    o Storz™

Complications and Preventions During Laryngoscopy and Intubation

Complication	Prevention
Esophageal intubation	Proper technique
	Use of video laryngoscope
	Monitor ETCO$_2$
Endobronchial intubation	Place ETT to adequate depth
	Listen for bilateral breath sounds
Damage to perioral structures	Proper technique
Dislocated mandible	Avoid excessive opening and force
Hypertension Tachycardia Intracranial hypertension Intraocular hypertension	Intubate at an adequate depth of anesthesia
	Consider lidocaine, esmolol, or clevidipine to temporarily prevent hemodynamic response
Laryngospasm	Intubate at an adequate depth of anesthesia
	Consider paralytics
Retropharyngeal dissection	Avoid excessive force during NETT placement
Laryngeal damage	Use appropriately sized NETT
Cuff perforation	Primarily occurs during nasal intubation
	Avoid excessive force during nasal passage navigation
	Fully deflate cuff prior to placement

Complications and Preventions While Patient is Intubated

Complication	Prevention
Unintentional extubation Endobronchial intubation	Record initial depth placement
	Ensure operator interference with ETT is minimal
	Secure ETT appropriately
Mucosal inflammation and ulceration	Avoid excessive cuff pressures
	Use appropriately sized ETT
	Consider testing cuff pressure intermittingly throughout case especially if N$_2$O is used
ETT obstruction	Do not put excessive bends in the ETT
	Pass suction catheter to detect
	If catheter cannot pass, consider ETT exchange
Damage to ETT cuff	From surgery
	Use reinforced tubes/foil if laser is used
Airway fire	Timeout for fire risk assessment
	Use <30% FiO$_2$ when ignition source is present
	Adequate ETT seal
	High volume suction

Complications and Preventions Following Extubation

Complication	Prevention
Sore throat Tracheal stenosis Edema Hoarseness Nerve damage	Proper technique
	Appropriately sized/placed ETT
	Appropriate leak pressure and placement of cuff
Laryngospasm	Extubate awake or at adequate depth of anesthesia
	Suctioning of secretions
Aspiration of gastric contents	Avoid excessive gastric insufflation
	OG/NG suction
	Increased NPO time for at-risk patients
Incomplete reversal of paralytics	Ensure appropriate neuromuscular monitoring
	Titrate long-lasting NMB
Lost airway	Extubate awake
	Have airway adjuncts available

9.12 Fiberoptic Intubation (FOI)

- FOI must be done in a controlled setting with excellent support and availability to surgical airway
- Spontaneous ventilation is maintained while balancing a degree, albeit it "light," sedation for the patient as the priority is not to lose the airway
- Awake fiberoptics primarily discussed here
- Indications
  - Previous difficult airway
  - Predictors of difficult airway
  - Previous major head and neck surgery
  - Previous head and neck radiation therapy
  - Head and neck trauma
  - Odontogenic or other infection compromising airway
  - Pathology involving the neck and airway tissues
  - Head and neck anatomic anomalies
  - Elevated risk of aspiration
  - Unstable cervical spine injury
- Contraindications
  - No real contraindications other than requiring additional time, and likely, increased discomfort to the patient

Patient Preparation

- Emergency airway cart must be at bed side
- Patient is usually in an upright or semi-supine position
- Sedation
  - Minimal or moderate sedation if the airway allows
  - Dexmedetomidine
  - Benzodiazepines
  - Propofol (low dose)
  - Antisialagogue
    - Glycopyrrolate
      - Given early
      - ↓ Secretions
      - Allow more effective topical anesthesia and visualization
  - Antiemetics

Technique

- Consider airway adjunct for oral FOI
  - Ovassapian
    - Most popular
  - Berman
  - Williams
- Lubricated ETT or NETT is placed over scope
- Scope is advanced through the mouth or naris
- Glottic structures are visualized and maintained in center of visual field
- Scope is advanced under epiglottis
- Scope is advanced through vocal cords to tracheal rings are visualized, near the carina
- ETT or NETT is passed over scope
- Scope is withdrawn confirming scope is within ETT and ETT is below the vocal cords
- Bilateral breath sounds and $EtCO_2$ present, radiology if needed
- Emergency airway cart must be at bed side

Local Anesthesia for Awake Fiberoptics [15]

- Care must be taken to avoid local anesthesia toxicity
  - Topical
    - Nasal atomizer
    - Cotton-tipped applicators
    - NPA
    - Rinse and swizzle
    - Spray
    - Lollipop
    - Gargle
  - Glossopharyngeal Nerve Block
    - Intraoral injection at the base of the palatopharyngeal folds
    - Anesthetizes
      - Posterior 1/3 of tongue
      - Oropharynx
      - Laryngopharynx to the vallecula
      - Anterior epiglottis

- Superior Laryngeal Nerve Block
  - ○ Injections done extraorally at the great horn of the thyroid cartilage
  - ○ Anesthetizes
    - Posterior surface of the epiglottis
    - Glottic inlet to the level of the vocal cords
- Recurrent Laryngeal Nerve Block
  - ○ Transtracheal injection – via cricothyroid membrane after aspirating air into syringe
  - ○ Anesthetizes
    - Vocal cord and area below cords
- Sphenopalatine Ganglion Nerve Block (Nasal Intubation)
  - ○ Pledgets/cotton applicators introduced at 45° angle to hard palate
- Anterior Ethmoidal Nerve Block (Nasal Intubation)
  - ○ Pledgets/cotton applicators introduced along nasal floor until posterior nasal cavity is reached
  - ○ Vasoconstrictors may be used to decrease likelihood of bleeding

9.13 Submental Intubation

- Surgical procedure
- Hospital setting only, very experienced providers
- Indications
  - Substantial facial trauma or reconstruction
  - Avoids drawbacks and complications of nasal intubation and tracheotomy
  - Usually done in conjunction with OMS or ENT surgeon
- Technique
  - Midline and lateral approaches
  - Important to collaborate with surgical team

- Patient is intubated orally with spiral ETT
- Incisions are made intraorally (floor of mouth) and extraorally, connected via blunt dissection
- ETT connector is removed, the tube is grasped with forceps
- ETT is pulled through incision and sutured in place, reconnected to circuit

9.14 Deliberate Hypotensive Anesthesia

- Indications
  - Major oral maxillofacial surgery involving maxillary down-fracture or tumor removal
  - Goals:
    - ○ Improves surgical field operating conditions
    - ○ ↓ Need for blood transfusions
    - ○ ↓ Blood loss
  - With increasing use of tranexamic acid, deliberate hypotensive anesthesia may have less indications
- Contraindications
  - Cardiovascular disease
  - Advanced age
  - Renal impairment
- Hemodynamic Goals:
  - Most important to achieve during down-fracture of maxilla
  - MAP between 50 and 65 mmHg
  - SBP between 80 and 90 mmHg
  - Urinary output 1 ml/kg/h to ensure adequate renal perfusion
- Technique
  - Consider need for arterial line and/or urinary catheter
  - There are many methods, but here are some of the more common agents, short-acting agents are preferred:
    - ○ Propofol
    - ○ Beta blockers
      - Esmolol
      - Labetalol
    - ○ Calcium channel blockers
      - Clevidipine
    - ○ Hydralazine
    - ○ Dexmedetomidine
    - ○ Opioids
      - Remifentanil
    - ○ Inhalational agents
      - Sevoflurane
  - Consider limiting:
    - ○ IV fluids
      - As long as adequate urinary output
    - ○ Sympathetic agents
      - Ketamine
      - Adrenergic agonists
      - Desflurane
- Complications
  - Many of the complications are due to prolonged hypotension
    - ○ ↓ Spinal cord perfusion
      - Cerebral thrombosis
      - Hemiplegia
    - ○ Renal insufficiency
      - Acute tubular necrosis
    - ○ Myocardial ischemia or infarction
    - ○ Retinal artery thrombosis
      - Blindness
    - ○ Rebound hypertension [16]

9.15 Legal Considerations

Terms

- Law
  - A body of rules of conduct of binding legal force and effect, prescribed, recognized, and enforced by a controlling authority.
- Statue
  - An act of a legislature that declares, proscribes, or commands something; a specific law, expressed in writing
- Guideline
  - A statement or other indication of policy or procedure by which to determine a course of action
- Advisory
  - Statement issued to give recommendation, advice, or warning.

Statutes

- Anesthesia Provider Specific
  - Depending on the credentials of the anesthesia provider (MD/DO vs. DDS/DMD vs. CRNA vs. AA)
- Location Specific
  - Relating to the venue in which the procedures are being performed (all regulatory bodies are not listed):
    - Dental offices
      - Dental Practice Act
    - ASCs
      - AAAHC
      - AAAASF
    - Hospitals
      - JCAHO
- Insurance Specific
  - Different insurers may have different statutes such as Medicaid or Medicare may differ from Delta Dental
  - Example: You cannot charge a CMS patient a late fee

- The Jurisprudence Exam
  - Usually a requirement for licensure
  - Each state has its own exam that covers their statutes
  - Covers basic practitioner legal knowledge

Informed Consent

- The Nuremberg Code
  - Written to protect humans from unauthorized medical treatment and experimentation without consent [17]
  - Subsequently, the term "informed consent" began to be used after the case Salgo v. Leland [18]
- Each state will generally have different standards, requirements, and obligations to meet valid informed consent and generally falls into two types:
  - The patient-based approach
    - The court would ask if the patient was given all the material information necessary to make an informed decision
  - The physician-based approach
    - The court asks if the physician lived up to the standard disclosure generally followed by the community
- Informed Consent Validity
  - Was the patient given all the relevant information to make an educated decision?
    - Usually evaluated by the predominate approach used in that state, as mentioned above
  - Did the patient have capacity to consent to the proposed treatment both medically and legally?
    - Voluntariness
    - Capacity
    - Agreement
    - Guardianship
- Battery
  - The unlawful touching of one person by another
  - When informed consent does not fit all the above criteria

Negligence

- The failure to exercise a reasonable degree of care which results in harm to another
- Our duty to the patient is usually established once the doctor–patient relationship begins *AND* the DA begins the treatment
- Basic Elements of Negligence
  - Duty
  - Breach of that duty
  - Actual and proximate causation
  - Damage

Lawsuit

- A civil lawsuit will need to prove that with > 50% probability, each of the elements of negligence was satisfied
  - The burden is on the plaintiff (patient) to prove each of these elements
- Usually by showing evidence of substandard care
- The patient must show causation, meaning the breach of duty by the DA was the reason for the alleged injury

- Example: the rash on a patient's arm was from placing an IV and securing it with tape known to cause a rash, yet the DA did not attempt to place an IV in the arm, and instead placed it in the foot, there would be no causation
- There must be an injury that shows physical damage to the body
  - Emotional damage alone does not usually qualify
- Tooth damage is the most common claim filed against anesthesiologists

Liability Insurance

- Occurrence
  - Insures for the time period of when the incident occurred
  - Did the insured have an active policy when the incident actually occurred, even years later
- Claims Made
  - Insures for when the claim was filed
  - Did the insured have an active policy when the claim was made
  - Tail coverage is recommended once the policy expires

References

1 Yasaei, R., Rosani, A., and Saadabadi, A. (2023). *Meperidine*. StatPearls.

2 Chang, H.Y., Togias, A., and Brown, R.H. (2007). The effects of systemic lidocaine on airway tone and pulmonary function in asthmatic subjects. *Anesth. Analg.* 104 (5): 1109–1115, tables of contents https://doi.org/10.1213/01. ane.0000260638.57139.87.

3 Boynes, S., Riley, A., and Milbee, S. (2014). Evaluating complications during intraoral administration of local anesthetics in a rural, portable special needs dental clinic. *Spec. Care Dentist.* 34 (5): 241–245. https://doi.org/10.1111/scd.12059.

4 Giovannitti, J.A., Rosenberg, M.B., and Phero, J.C. (Aug 2013). Pharmacology of local anesthetics used in oral surgery. *Oral Maxillofac. Surg. Clin. North Am.* 25 (3): 453–465, vi. https://doi.org/10.1016/j.coms.2013.03.003.

5 Ramazani, N. (2016). Different aspects of general anesthesia in pediatric dentistry: a review. *Iran. J. Pediatr.* 26 (2): e2613. https://doi.org/10.5812/ijp.2613.

6 Hillerup, S., Jensen, R.H., and Ersbøll, B.K. (2011). Trigeminal nerve injury associated with injection of local anesthetics: needle lesion or neurotoxicity? *J. Am. Dent. Assoc.* 142 (5): 531–539. https://doi.org/10.14219/jada. archive.2011.0223.

7 Balakrishnan, R.E.V. (2013). Contraindications of vasoconstrictors in dentistry. *Biomed. Pharmacol. J.* 6 (2): https://doi.org/10.13005/bpj/435.

8 Huff, T., Weisbrod, L.J., and Daly, D.T. (2023). *StatPearls.* StatPearls.

9 Haas, D.A. (2011). Alternative mandibular nerve block techniques: a review of the Gow-Gates and Akinosi-Vazirani closed-mouth mandibular nerve block techniques. *J. Am. Dent. Assoc.* 142 (Suppl. 3): 8S–12S. https://doi.org/10.14219/jada.archive.2011.0341.

10 Wong, D.T., Dallaire, A., Singh, K.P. et al. (2019). High-flow nasal oxygen improves safe apnea time in morbidly obese patients undergoing general anesthesia: a randomized controlled trial. *Anesth. Analg.* 129 (4): 1130–1136. https://doi.org/10.1213/ANE.0000000000003966.

11 Thiruvenkatarajan, V., Van Wijk, R.M., and Rajbhoj, A. (2015). Cranial nerve injuries with supraglottic airway devices: a systematic review of published case reports and series. *Anaesthesia* 70 (3): 344–359. https://doi.org/10.1111/anae.12917.

12 Gordon, J., Cooper, R.M., and Parotto, M. (2018). Supraglottic airway devices: indications, contraindications and management. *Minerva Anestesiol.*

84 (3): 389–397. https://doi.org/10.23736/S0375-9393.17.12112-7.

13 Viswambharan, B., Kumari, M.J., Krishnan, G., and Ramamoorthy, L. (2021). Under or overpressure: an audit of endotracheal cuff pressure monitoring at the tertiary care center. *Acute Crit. Care* 36 (4): 374–379. https://doi.org/10.4266/acc.2021.00024.

14 Kim, J.T., Kim, H.J., Ahn, W. et al. (2009). Head rotation, flexion, and extension alter endotracheal tube position in adults and children. *Can. J. Anaesth.* 56 (10): 751–756. https://doi.org/10.1007/s12630-009-9158-y.

15 Collins, S.R. and Blank, R.S. (2014). Fiberoptic intubation: an overview and update. *Respir. Care* 59 (6):

865–878; discussion 878-80. https://doi.org/10.4187/respcare.03012.

16 Tegegne, S.S., Gebregzi, A.H., and Arefayne, N.R. (2021). Deliberate hypotension as a mechanism to decrease intraoperative surgical site blood loss in resource limited setting: a systematic review and guideline. *Int. J. Surg. Open* 29: 55–65.

17 Nuremberg Code. The Doctor's Trial: The Medical Case of the Subsequent Nuremberg Proceedings. United States Holocaust Memorial Museum Online Exhibitions. Retrieved 13 February 2019.

18 *Salgo v. Leland Stanford Jr. Univ. Bd. of Trustees*, 317 P. 2d 170, 181 (Cal. App. Ct. 1957).

Section 10
Oral Maxillofacial Surgery

10.1   Odontogenic Infections

OMS Knowledge Updates, Home Study Program, Volume 1, Part I 1994; 1994 American Association of Oral and Maxillofacial Surgeons, all rights reserved, Printed in the United States
"Anatomy and Surgery of Deep Fascial Space Infections of the Head and Neck"—Thomas R. Flynn, DMD, pp. 79–107

- Etiology/Risk Factors
  - Poor oral hygiene
  - Socioeconomic
  - Drug addiction
    - Crystal meth
  - Trauma
  - Radiation therapy
  - Chemotherapy
    - Bisphosphonates
- Evaluation
  - Pain
  - Swelling
    - Localized
    - Extended
    - Fluctuant (abscess)
    - Cellulitis
  - Location (Figure 10.1)
  - Trismus
    - Progression of infection through communicating fascial spaces cause inflammation to masticatory muscles
  - Febrile
  - Stridor
  - Dysphagia/Dyspnea
    - Progression of infection through communicating fascial spaces cause airway inflammation, swelling, and stricture.
    - Leaning forward as you breathe (tripoding)

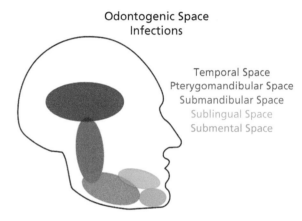

Odontogenic Space Infections

Temporal Space
Pterygomandibular Space
Submandibular Space
Sublingual Space
Submental Space

Figure 10.1

  - Periapical radiograph(s)
  - Panorex
  - CT scan
    - Anatomic fascial spaces involved in the progression of the infection
      - Ludwig's angina
        - Bilateral submandibular and sublingual spaces with submental space involvement
    - Anatomic evaluation of the airway
- Treatment
  - Antibiotics
    - Specifically broad-spectrum penicillins in combination with beta lactamase inhibitors [1]
  - Root canal therapy
  - Extraction
  - Incision and drainage
  - Culture and sensitivity
- Primary Concerns
  - Difficult airway
  - Sepsis

Anesthesia for Dental and Oral Maxillofacial Surgery, First Edition. Spencer D. Wade, Caroline M. Sawicki, Megann K. Smiley, Michael A. Cuddy, Steven Vukas, and Paul J. Schwartz.
© 2024 John Wiley & Sons, Inc. Published 2024 by John Wiley & Sons, Inc.

- Anesthesia Management
  - Consider difficult airway
    - *Difficult airway covered on page 258*
  - Anesthesia is dependent on severity of airway compromise and invasiveness of procedure
  - No specific anesthetic technique intraoperatively
  - Airway concerns should guide the timing of extubation
    - Cuff deflation with ETT tube occlusion to see if patient can breathe around the ETT tube
    - Insertion of hollow tube exchanger into the ETT tube prior to extubation to delivery oxygen and guide reinsertion of ETT tube if the airway is not self-sustainable

10.2 Orthognathic Surgery

OMS Knowledge Updates, Self Study Program, Volume Two, May 1998, 1998 American Association of Oral and Maxillofacial Surgeons, all rights reserved, Printed in the United States
"Stability of Mandibular Osteotomies"—Kirk L. Fridrich, DDS, MS and Brian R. Smith, DDS, MS, pp. 33–44.

OMS Knowledge Update, Home study program, Volume 1, Part II, November 1995; 1995 by the American Association of Oral and Maxillofacial Surgery, all rights reserved; Printed in the United States
"Treatment of Skeletal Asymmetries in the Adult"—Gregory M. Ness, DDS and Peter Larsen, DDS, pp. 3–13.

- Developmental hyper or hypoplasia of the mandible or maxilla may occur without syndromic involvement (Figure 10.2)

- Evaluation
  - Facial Thirds (Figure 10.3)
  - Occlusal analysis
  - Diagnostic models on articulator
  - Angle classification
    o Overbite
    o Overjet
    o Open bite
    o Crossbite
    o Width of maxilla and mandible relative to each other
  - Cephalometric analysis
  - CT scan and Panorex
    o Evaluation of dentition
    o Evaluation of root apices proximity vital structures
    o Evaluation of ramal height
    o Evaluation of mandibular and maxillary bone width
    o Evaluation of pathology

Maxillary Hypoplasia	Maxillary Hyperplasia
Binder Syndrome Crouzon's Syndrome Cleft Lip/Palate Angelman Syndrome Fetal Alcohol Syndrome	Long Face Syndrome Leontiasis Ossea
Mandibular Hypoplasia	Mandibular Hyperplasia
Cri du Chat Syndrome Marfan Syndrome Progeria Pierre Robin Sequence Treacher Collins Syndrome Achondroplasia	Condylar Hyperplasia

Figure 10.2 Adapted from Bakathir et al. [2].

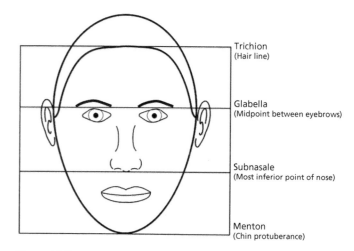

Figure 10.3

Types of Surgery

Maxillary Surgery	Mandibular Surgery
Le Fort I Maxillary Osteotomy	Bilateral Sagittal Split Osteotomy (BSSO)
Surgically Assisted Rapid Palatal Expansion (SARPE)	Vertical Ramus Osteotomy (VRO)
Maxillary Assisted Rapid Palatal Expansion (MARPE)	Subapical Osteotomy
	Genioplasty

Figure 10.4

- Treatment
  - Surgery (Figure 10.4)
- Anesthesia Management
  - Consider difficult airway especially for patients with mandibular hypoplasia [3]
  - Prophylactic antiemetic medications to reduce PONV
  - General anesthesia with NETT
    - Deflation of ETT tube balloon or damage to ETT during surgical treatment
    - ETT pressure necrosis of the nasal tip
  - For cases where electrocautery is to be used:
    - High volume suction
    - $FiO_2 < 0.3$
    - Electrocautery induced fire that travels down the ETT tube
  - Potential for large blood loss
    - Down-fracture of maxilla in Le Fort I maxillary osteotomy
    - Retromandibular vein bleed during intraoral vertical ramus osteotomy of mandible
    - Facial a. injury during BSSO of mandible
    - Consider type and screen
    - Consider foley catheter to measure urine output
    - Consider deliberate hypotensive anesthesia
      - *Deliberate hypotensive anesthesia covered on page 305*
  - For patients in MMF
    - Wire cutters immediately available for airway intervention
    - Awake extubation

10.3   Obstructive Sleep Apnea

Oral and Maxillofacial Surgery Clinics of North America, "Oral and Maxillofacial Treatment of Obstructive Sleep Apnea," Volume 7, Number 2, May 1995; W. B. Saunders Company, The Curtis Center, Independence Square, West Philadelphia, PA, 19106
"Medical Considerations in Surgery for Sleep Apnea"—David G. Davila, MD, pp. 205–219

Oral and Maxillofacial Surgery Clinics of North America, "Oral and Maxillofacial Treatment of Obstructive Sleep Apnea," Volume 7, Number 2, May 1995; W. B. Saunders Company, The Curtis Center, Independence Square, West Philadelphia, PA, 19106
"Continuous and Bilevel Positive Airway Pressure Therapy in Sleep Disorder Breathing"—Patrick Strollo, Jr., MD, Mark H. Sanders, MD, and Ronald A. Stiller, MD, PhD, pp. 221–230

Oral and Maxillofacial Surgery Clinics of North America, "Oral and Maxillofacial Treatment of Obstructive Sleep Apnea," Volume 7, Number 2, May 1995; W. B. Saunders Company, The Curtis Center, Independence Square, West Philadelphia, PA, 19106
"Adjunctive Surgical Procedures in Obstructive Sleep Apnea"—Robert F. Guyette, DMD, MD and Peter D. Waite, MPH, DDS, MD, pp. 301–310

Oral and Maxillofacial Surgery Clinics of North America, "Oral and Maxillofacial Treatment of Obstructive Sleep Apnea," Volume 7, Number 2, May 1995; W. B. Saunders Company, The Curtis Center, Independence Square, West Philadelphia, PA, 19106
"Maxillomandibular Advancement Surgery: A Cure for Obstructive Sleep Apnea Syndrome"—Peter D. Waite, MPH, DDS, MD and Shashindar M. Shettar, MD, pp. 327–336

- Etiology/Risk Factors (Figure 10.5)
  - Signs/Symptoms (Figure 10.6)
    - Waking up with headache, dry mouth, or sore throat
      - Primarily from obstructive sleep apnea

Sleep Apnea Risk Factors

Obstructive Sleep Apnea	Central Sleep Apnea
More Common	Less Common
Relaxation of Upper Airway Musculature	Dysfunction of the Brainstem's Ability to Control Breathing
Risk Factors	**Risk Factors**
Male	Male
>50 years of age	> 60 years of age
High BMI	Cardiovascular Disease
Hypertension	Opioid Use
Narrowed Airway	Cheyne-Strokes Respiratory Pattern
Chronic Nasal Congestion	Arnold-Chiari Malformation
Smoking	CVA
Diabetes	Direct Spinal Cord Injury
Family History	
Asthma	

Figure 10.5

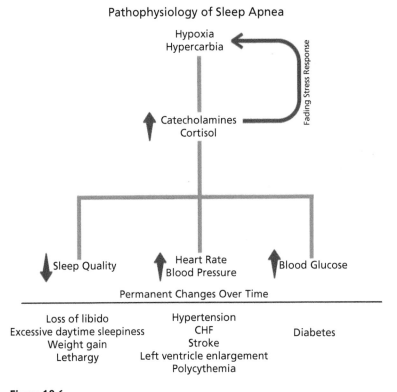

Figure 10.6

- Diagnosis (Obstructive Sleep Apnea)
  - STOPBANG
    o Screening tool
    o *STOPBANG covered on page 77*
  - Polysomnography is the gold standard for diagnosis
    o Complete night study
    o Apnea hypopnea index (AHI)
      - The AHI is the average number of apneic or hypopneic events lasting a minimum of 10 seconds per hour of sleep recorded during polysomnography

Severity	Apnea hypopnea events (per hour)
Normal	<5
Mild OSA	5–15
Moderate OSA	15–30
Severe OSA	>30

    o Also monitored/included:
      - ECG
      - SpO$_2$
      - Snoring microphone
      - EEG

- Electrooculography
- Electromyography
- Treatment
  - Depends on OSA severity and underlying pathophysiology
  - Weight loss
  - Supplemental oxygen
  - Pharyngeal exercises
  - CPAP
  - BiPAP
  - Acetazolamide
  - Surgery
    o Maxillary and mandibular advancement
      - Bimaxillary protrusion
        o Le Fort I maxillary osteotomy with advancement
        o BSSO with advancement/rotation of mandible
      - Hyoid suspension
      - Genioplasty
      - Uvulopalatopharyngoplasty (UPPP)
      - Hypoglossal nerve stimulator
- Primary Concerns
  - Difficult airway [4]
  - Cardiac dysfunction
    o ↑ Risk of systemic HTN
    o ↑ Risk of pulmonary HTN

- – Respiratory acidosis
- – ↑ Risk of GERD [5]
- – ↑ Risk of bronchoconstriction [6]
- ● Evaluation
  - – Previous airway records, if available
  - – STOPBANG score
  - – polysomnogram
    - ○ AHI
  - – Consider cardiologist consult
    - ○ Likely longstanding HTN
    - ○ EKG to rule out underlying cardiac dysfunction
    - ○ Echocardiogram in severe cases
  - – Consider ABG
    - ○ PaCO$_2$
    - ○ Metabolic compensation, if present
    - ○ PaO$_2$
  - – Consider CBC
  - – Consider CMP
  - – Consider preoperative spirometry [7]
  - – Home equipment settings, if applicable
- ● Anesthesia Management [8]
  - – Consider difficult airway [4]
  - – For those with hypoglossal nerve stimulators, consider deactivating prior to general anesthesia [9]
  - – General anesthesia with NETT
  - – ↑ Risk of bronchoconstriction [6]
    - ○ Consider steroids
    - ○ Consider bronchodilators
  - – Avoid long-acting narcotics
  - – Consider:
    - ○ Local anesthetics
    - ○ Dexmedetomidine
    - ○ Fentanyl
    - ○ Remifentanil

- ○ Remimazolam
- ○ Ketamine
- ○ NSAIDs
- ○ Tylenol
- ○ Sevoflurane
- – Extubation
  - ○ Awake
  - ○ Recommended in a non-supine position
    - ● Semi-upright or lateral preferred
  - ○ Ensure full reversal of neuromuscular agents
- – Postoperatively
  - ○ Avoid postoperative respiratory depressants
  - ○ May have increased analgesic requirement postoperatively due to increased opioid receptor expression [10]
  - ○ OSA symptoms should improve, but patients should be on continuous pulse oximeter with nasal cannula as indicated by SpO$_2$
  - ○ Postoperative course may require:
    - ● Additional admission time for observation of surgical sites
    - ● Medical stability
      - ○ SpO$_2$
      - ○ CBC
      - ○ CMB
      - ○ ABG [11]
    - ● Evaluation of surgical effectiveness
      - ○ Oxygen saturation during sleep
      - ○ In-hospital sleep study
- – After discharge
  - ○ CPAP parameters should be reevaluated with a new sleep study
  - ○ Consider avoiding CPAP postoperatively in oral-antral communication

10.4   Oral Reconstruction

Bone Grafting and Implant Restorations

"Soft Tissue and Esthetic Considerations in Implant Therapy"—
Anthony Sclar, DMD; Quintessence Publishing Co., Inc. 2003. 551 Kimberly, Carol Stream Drive, Il 60188; pp. 13–41.

OMS Knowledge Update, Home Study Program, Volume 1, Part I, 1994; 1994 American Association of Oral and Maxillofacial Surgeons, all rights reserved, Printed in the United States
"Diagnostic and Treatment – Planning Considertions for the Partially Edentulous Implant Patient"—
Steven G. Lewis DMD, pp. 3–18

OMS Knowledge Update, Home Study Program, Volume 1, Part I, 1994; 1994 American Association of Oral and Maxillofacial Surgeons, all rights reserved, Printed in the United States
"Diagnosis and Treatment Planning for the Edentulous Overdenture Patient"—Isreal Finger BDS, MSc, Med, DDS and Johnathan Penchas, DMD, pp. 19–26

OMS Knowledge Update, Home Study Program, Volume 1, Part I, 1994; 1994 American Association of Oral and Maxillofacial Surgeons, all rights reserved, Printed in the United States
"Esthetic Considerations and Treatment Planning for the Single Tooth Implant Restoration"—Daniel Y. Sullivan, DDS; pp. 27-33

OMS Knowledge Update, Home Study Program, Volume 1, Part I, 1994; 1994 American Association of Oral and Maxillofacial Surgeons, all rights reserved, Printed in the United States
"Onlay Bone Grafting with Implants"—Thomas A. Collins, DDS, MS, pp. 35–45

OMS Knowledge Update, Home Study Program, Volume 1, Part I, 1994; 1994 American Association of Oral and Maxillofacial Surgeons, all rights reserved, Printed in the United States
"Bone Grafting the Sinus and Nasal Floor"—Kenji W. Higuchi, DDS, MS, pp. 47–53

- Etiology/Risk Factors
  - Caries
  - Periodontal disease
  - Neoplasm
  - Congenital
    - Dentinogenesis imperfecta
    - Amelogenesis imperfecta
    - Ectodermal dysplasia
- Evaluation
  - Areas devoid of tooth structure
  - Deficient bone height
  - Deficient bone width
  - Soft tissue defects of small and large volume
  - Diagnostic casts of the maxilla and mandible
  - Establish vertical dimension of occlusion
  - Periapical radiographs
  - Panorex
  - CT scan
    - Analysis of bone volume
    - Analysis of vital structures
      - Inferior alveolar nerve canal
      - Maxillary sinuses
    - Accurate location and dimensions of pathology

- Treatment
  - Execution of treatment plan determined from collected data
    o Preprosthetic surgery
      - Extractions
      - Soft tissue grafting
        o Bone grafting
    o Implant placement
      - Fully guided surgery
      - Partially guided surgery
      - Soft tissue grafting
      - Bone grafting

- Anesthesia Management
  - Consider difficult airway especially if patient has had previous head and neck radiation and/or extensive surgical resection
  - Anesthetic depth based on patient tolerance and extent of surgery

10.5 Temporomandibular Joint Disorders

OMS Knowledge Updates, Home Study Program, Volume 1, Part I; August 1994; 1994 by American Association of Oral and Maxillofacial Surgery, All rights reserved, Printed in the United States of America
"Diagnostic Imaging"—Per-Lennart Westesson, DDS, PhD, pp. 67–86

OMS Knowledge Update, Self Study Program, Volume Three 2001; 2001 by the American Association of Oral and Maxillofacial Surgery, All right reserved, Printed in the United States of America
"Conservative and Presurgical Management of TMJ Disorders"—David Lustbader, DMD, pp. 29–40

OMS Knowledge Update, Self Study Program, Volume Three 2001; 2001 by the American Association of Oral and Maxillofacial Surgery, All right reserved, Printed in the United States of America
"Arthrocentesis of the TMJ"—Kevin R. Haddle, DDS, MD, pp. 41–51

OMS Knowledge Update, Self Study Program, Volume Three 2001; 2001 by the American Association of Oral and Maxillofacial Surgery, All right reserved, Printed in the United States of America
"Current Concepts in TMJ Arthroscopy"—Daniel Spagnoli, DDS, PhD, Michael Koslin, DMD, Steven Gollehon, MD, DDS, Renato Mazzonetto, DDS, PhD, pp. 53–72

- Etiology/Risk Factors
  - Degenerative joint disease
  - Arthritis
    - Rheumatoid
    - Osteoarthritis
    - Trauma
    - Pathology
  - Female [12]
    - Late teens
  - Psychogenic [13]
    - Anxiety
    - Psychosis
- Evaluation
  - Anatomic evaluation (Figure 10.7)
  - Presence of pain
  - Functional excursions

Temporomandibular Joint Anatomy

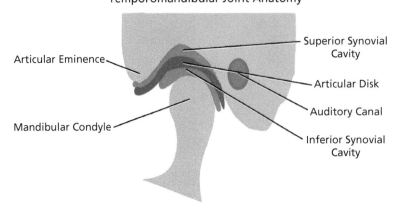

Figure 10.7

- Locking
  o Open vs. closed
- Maximum incisal opening
- Crepitus
- MRI
  o T1 weighted images
    • Highlights fat content of tissues
    • Better anatomic delineation
  o T2 weighted images
    • Highlight water-containing structures
    • Delineation of inflammation and effusion

Wilkes Staging of Internal Derangement

Stage I	Early reducing disk displacement
Stage II	Late reducing disk displacement
Stage III	Nonreducing disk displacement – acute/subacute
Stage IV	Nonreducing disk displacement – chronic
Stage V	Nonreducing disk displacement – chronic with osteoarthrosis

- Combines clinical symptomology and MRI findings
- Treatment
  - Soft diet
  - Rest
  - Heat
  - Physical therapy
    o Increase maximum incisal opening (MIO)
      • 35–40 mm on average
    o Lateral excursions
      • 4–6 mm
    o Protrusive excursions
      • 4–6 mm
  - Appliances/splints
  - NSAIDs
  - Steroids
  - Surgery
    o Brisement procedure
      • Gradual traction to TMJ to increase MIO under local anesthesia, minimal/moderate IV sedation

  o Arthrocentesis
    • Lavage joint space to remove inflammatory mediators
    • Limited lysis of adhesions
  o Arthroscopy
    • Greater visualization of anatomy and disease
    • Lavage of joint space
    • Extensive lysis of adhesions
    • Evaluation for future treatment
    • Biopsy
    • Meniscal repair
  o Arthroplasty
    • Direct vision of anatomy and pathology
    • More extensive surgical access
  o Total joint reconstruction
    • Recurrence of intractable TMJ dysfunction
    • Alloplastic joint reconstruction
    • Autograft reconstruction
      o Costochondral graft
      o Total joint prosthesis
- Anesthesia Management
  - Consider difficult airway especially in those with restrictive openings [14, 15]
  - For awake fiberoptic intubation, consider low-dose midazolam, remifentanil, dexmedetomidine, and/or low-dose propofol to facilitate with intubation in conjunction with profound topicalization [16]
    o Best to avoid long-lasting or nonreversible agents in case of emergency
  - No long-acting paralytics to allow assessment of CN VII
  - Arthrocentesis
    o Anesthetic depth based on patient tolerance and extent of surgery
    o Can likely be performed under local anesthesia with or without minimal or moderate sedation
  - Arthroscopy
    o General anesthesia with NETT
  - Arthroplasty
    o General anesthesia with NETT
  - Total joint reconstruction
    o General anesthesia with NETT

10.6 Trauma

- In Cases of Nonelective Surgery
  - NPO may be violated
    - Rapid sequence intubation
    - *Aspiration management covered on page 263*
  - Preoperative work up may not be ideal
    - If no type and cross available
      - O negative is the universal donor for pRBCs
    - If no PT/PTT/INR/platelets values available
      - Consider transfusion based on clinical picture
  - C-spine precautions may need to be considered
    - In-line traction
    - Sandbags

Frontal Sinus Fracture (Figure 10.8)

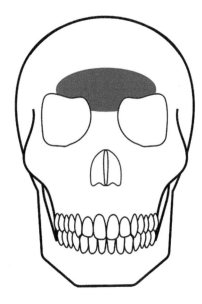

Figure 10.8

- Evaluation
  - Clinical examination
  - CT
  - Evaluate for presence of CSF
    - β_2 transferrin

- Glucose reading less than 30 mg/dl
- Ring/halo sign
  - Annular ring appearance on filter paper
  - Displaced fracture or comminuted fracture of the posterior table of frontal sinus
    - Possible cerebral injury
  - Impaired drainage of the frontal sinus via the nasofrontal duct into the hiatus semilunaris of the middle meatus
- Treatment
  - Observation
  - Surgery
    - Open reduction with rigid fixation of the anterior table
    - Cranialization of the frontal sinus or obliteration of the frontal sinus with obstruction of the nasofrontal duct opening
- Anesthesia Management
  - General anesthesia with oral ETT

Zygomaticomaxillary Complex (ZMC) Fracture (Figure 10.9)

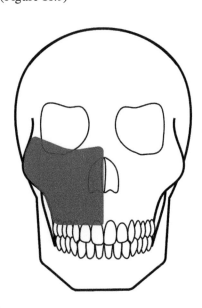

Figure 10.9

- Evaluation
  - Clinically observed cosmetic deformity
    - Depressed zygoma
  - Entrapment of inferior rectus muscle
    - Deficient upward gaze
  - Subconjunctival hematoma
  - CT
    - ZMC fracture and displacement
    - Zygomaticofrontal suture
    - Orbital walls and floor
    - Maxillary sinus
- Treatment
  - Observation
  - Surgery
  - Open reduction with rigid internal fixation
    - Orbital floor reconstruction
- Anesthesia Management
  - General anesthesia with oral ETT
  - Consider difficult airway
    - Depressed zygomatic arch fracture may interfere with coronoid process, thus limiting oral opening for intubation
  - Possible activation of the oculocardiac reflex [17] (Figure 10.10)

Oculocardiac Reflex

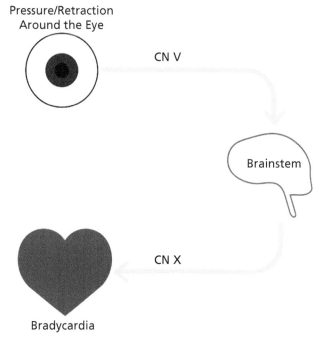

Figure 10.10

- Surgical manipulation
- Pressure from corneal protectors
- Have anticholinergics immediately available
- Can lead to bradycardia and, in rare cases, asystole
- Treat by immediate cessation of the triggering cause

Nasal-Orbital-Ethmoid (NOE) Complex Fracture (Figure 10.11)

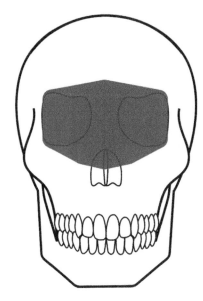

Figure 10.11

- Evaluation
  - Same as ZMC fracture
  - Traumatic telecanthus
    - Increased intercanthal distance from normal
    - Measured medial canthus to medical canthus
    - Medial canthal tendon displacement
- Treatment
  - Observation
  - Surgery
    - Medial canthopexy
- Anesthesia Management
  - General anesthesia with oral ETT
  - Oculocardiac reflex (Figure 10.10)
  - Intranasal cocaine utilized
    - 4–10% topical solution
    - Used for vasoconstrictive and analgesic properties
    - Potentially exacerbate hemodynamic consequences

Nasal Fracture (Figure 10.12)

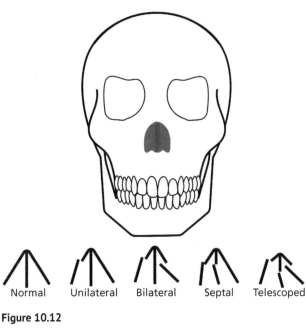

Figure 10.12

- Evaluation
  - Clinically significant displacement
    o Cosmetic deformity
  - Obstruction
    o Nasal septum deviation
  - Presence of epistaxis
  - Nasal bone plain films
  - CT
    o Displacement of bones in three dimensions
- Treatment
  - Observation
  - Surgery
    o Closed reduction
      • Nasal splints utilized
    o Open reduction with rigid internal fixation
      • Nasal splints utilized
- Anesthesia Management
  - Anesthetic depth based on patient tolerance and extent of surgery
  - Local anesthesia with IV sedation
  - General anesthesia with oral ETT
  - Caution when applying full face mask oxygen
    o Preoperatively
      • May cause intense pain to patient
    o Postoperatively
      • May disturb the nasal fracture reduction

Maxillary Fractures (Figure 10.13)

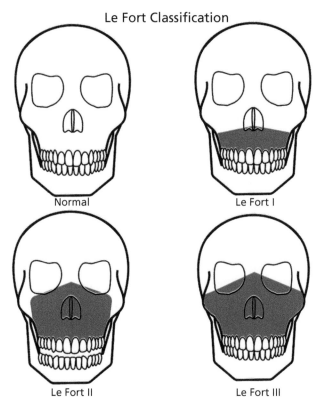

Figure 10.13

- Evaluation
  - Le Fort I
    o Disjunction of the maxilla horizontally from the cranial base
    o Above the apices of the dentition, across the maxillary sinuses, pterygoid plates, and nasal septum
  - Le Fort II
    o Fracture extends across the nasal bones, nasal septum, medial orbital wall, inferior orbital rim and continues to below the zygomatic buttress
  - Le Fort III
    o Complete midface disjunction involving both medial and lateral orbital walls
  - Clinical exam
    o Mobility of the maxilla and adjacent anatomic structures determine the level of the Le Fort fracture
    o Malocclusion
  - CT
    o Analyze involved anatomic structures and degree of fracture displacement

- Treatment
  - Surgery
    - ○ Closed reduction
      - Only for nondisplaced Le Fort I fracture
      - Maxillomandibular fixation (MMF)
    - ○ Open reduction with rigid internal fixation
      - Reconstruction of significant defects with bone graft or reconstruction plates
- Anesthesia Management
  - Le Fort I
    - ○ General anesthesia with NETT
      - NETT required as need to be able to complete MMF at the conclusion of the surgery
  - Le Fort II/III
    - ○ General anesthesia
    - ○ May need oral ETT with submental dissection if there is a lack of adequate space for the ETT to allow for proper establishment of occlusion
      - *Submental intubation covered on page 304*
    - ○ Tracheostomy

Mandibular Fractures (Figure 10.14)

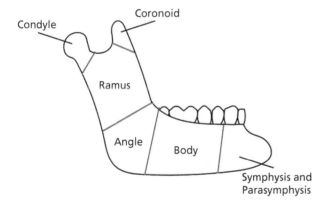

Figure 10.14

- Fractures can occur in multiple locations of the mandible depending on the direction and force of the traumatic injury
  - Ipsilateral
  - Contralateral

- Evaluation
  - Clinical exam
    - ○ Trismus
    - ○ Malocclusion
    - ○ Intraoral lacerations
    - ○ Deviation on opening
    - ○ Segment mobility
  - Panorex
  - CT
    - ○ Analysis degree of fracture displacement
- Treatment
  - Treatment based on:
    - ○ Location of fracture
    - ○ Degree of fracture displacement
    - ○ Concomitant fractures of the mandible
  - Surgery
    - ○ Closed reduction
      - Only for nondisplaced single fractures of mandible or isolated condyle fracture
      - MMF
    - ○ Severely comminuted mandibular fractures
      - MMF
    - ○ Displaced mandibular fractures
      - Open reduction with rigid internal fixation
      - Possible MMF
- Anesthesia Management
  - General anesthesia
  - Consider difficult airway
    - ○ Consider tracheostomy under local anesthesia in some situations
  - Airway management depends on the fracture(s) location
    - ○ Mandible without midface fractures
      - Nasotracheal ETT
    - ○ Midface without occlusion component
      - Oral ETT
    - ○ Midface ± mandible fracture with occlusion component especially if access to the nasal area is required [18]
      - Oral with submental dissection
      - With or without cannula to maintain soft tissue passage
      - Surgical access to the nasal region is required
      - Base of skull fracture with presence of cerebrospinal fluid
      - Elective tracheostomy after oral intubation

10.7 Cricothyrotomy (Figure 10.15)

- Should be a procedure that an anesthesia provider can feel comfortable with in the case of a cannot intubate, cannot ventilate scenario [19]
- This is always an urgent procedure

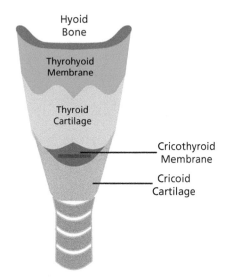

Figure 10.15

- Etiology/Risk Factors
  - Life-threatening upper airway obstruction
    - Tumor
    - Odontogenic infection
    - Trauma
    - Difficult airway

- Evaluation
  - Anatomic landmarks
    - Thyroid cartilage prominence
- Procedure (Percutaneous)
  - Place shoulder roll to extend the neck
  - Insertion of 14-gauge angiocath into airway through cricothyroid membrane with assistance of 10 ml syringe with 2–3 ml of saline
    - A "bubbling" effect will be eliciting when aspirating within the airway
  - Connect angiocath to a 3 ml syringe which can then be connected to a 7.0 ETT adaptor
  - Attach to device
    - Anesthesia machine
    - Ambu bag – valve – mask
  - Should only be used as a temporary bridge until final surgical airway can be established
- Procedure (Surgical)
  - Horizontal incision and sharp dissection
    - Can use an angiocath as a guide to cricothyroid membrane if placed
  - Dissection through layers of cervical fascia
  - Dissection through pre-tracheal fascia
  - Horizontal incision at cricothyroid membrane
  - Spread of airway at cricothyroid membrane with large hemostat
  - Placement of ETT
  - Inflation of cuff once CO_2 return is noted
  - Secure to skin with sutures
  - Commercially available cricothyrotomy kit

10.8 Tracheostomy

- Can be an elective or emergent procedure
- Etiology/Risk Factors
  - Tumor
  - Odontogenic infection
  - Trauma
  - Difficult airway
  - Surgery involves upper airway/larynx
- Evaluation
  - Obstruction
  - Clinical exam
  - CT scan
- Procedure
  - Extension of neck using shoulder roll
  - Horizontal (elective procedure)/vertical incision (emergent procedure)
  - Dissection through layers of cervical fascia
  - Dissection through pre-tracheal fascia
  - Utilize proper instrumentation and anatomic planes to prevent a false passage or pneumothorax
  - Retraction or bisection of thyroid isthmus to expose trachea
  - Incision at tracheal ring #2 or #3 1/3 the liminal dimension of the trachea
  - Once into the trachea, withdraw the ETT so the tip is superior to the incision
  - Placement of tracheostomy tube
  - Inflate cuff once CO_2 is noted
  - Secure with sutures
  - Only after the inserted trach is deemed functional should the ETT be removed
- Anesthesia Management
  - Depending on surgical procedure and patient tolerance, may choose to perform tracheostomy under local initially
  - For procedures where tracheostomy is performed after induction
    - o Maintain airway patency using an ETT
    - o Cuff may be punctured if trachea is incised
    - o ETT is "withdrawn" just slightly until the tip of the tube is above the tracheal opening but left in place until the procedure is finished and the surgeon and anesthesiologist agree that the surgical airway is functional.

10.9   Facial Plastic Surgery

Rhytidectomy (Face Lift)

- Etiology/Risk Factors
  - Older age
  - Wrinkles
  - Loss of skin elasticity
- Evaluation
  - Psychologically
    - o Well-adjusted
    - o Realistic expectations
    - o Previous experience with plastic surgery
  - Clinical exam
  - Presurgical photographs
  - Postsurgical photographs
  - Relative contraindications
    - o Uncontrolled hypertension
    - o Diabetes
    - o Bleeding disorders
    - o Keloid formations
- Anesthesia Management
  - Anesthetic depth based on patient tolerance and extent or procedure
    - o General anesthesia with oral ETT
    - o Moderate-deep sedation with local anesthesia
  - No paralytic to monitor CN VII function
  - Tumescent solution may be utilized
    - o *Local anesthesia toxicity covered on page 270*
  - Strict control of perioperative hemodynamics and postoperative pain, nausea, and vomiting to reduce hematoma formation [20]
  - Smooth emergence with minimal laryngeal stimulation

Blepharoplasty (Figure 10.16)

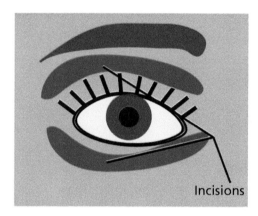

Figure 10.16

- Etiology/Risk Factors
  - Functional
    - o Reduced visual fields
    - o Blepharoptosis Accumulation of excess skin
  - Adenexal conditions
    - o Brow-forehead ptosis
    - o Thyroid dysfunction
    - o Lacrimal gland ptosis
  - Protrusion of periorbital fat
    - o Orbital septum weakness
    - o Musculus orbicularis oculi hypertrophy
    - o Horizontal lid laxity
  - Dermatochalasis
    - o Redundance or relaxation of skin

- Evaluation
  - Abnormal visual acuity test
  - Extraocular movements and balance
  - Corneal exam
  - Intraocular exam
  - Lacrimal function (Schirmer's test)
  - Visual field tests at rest and with excess skin retraction
- Treatment
  - Surgery
- Anesthesia Management
  - Anesthetic depth based on patient tolerance and extent of procedure
    - Most commonly performed under minimal, moderate sedation, or deep sedation with local anesthetic
    - General anesthesia in extreme circumstances unless combined with simultaneous additional facial plastic procedures
  - Oculocardiac reflex can be activated (Figure 10.10)

Rhinoplasty

- Etiology/Risk Factors
  - Developmental deformity
  - Obstruction
    - Nasal polyps
    - Deviated septum
    - Turbinate hypertrophy
    - Nasal valve obstruction/incompetence
  - Trauma

- Evaluation
  - Timing of surgery based on age-appropriate growth completion on average
    - Females
      - >15 years of age
    - Males
      - >17 years of age
  - Psychologically
    - Well-adjusted
    - Realistic expectations
  - Manual exam (Cottle test)
  - Nasal endoscopy
  - Nasal speculum
  - CT scan
    - Facial bones
  - Rhinomanometry
- Treatment
  - Surgery
- Anesthesia Management
  - Anesthetic depth based on patient tolerance and extent or procedure [21, 22]
    - General anesthesia with oral ETT
    - Moderate sedation with local anesthesia
      - Greater palatine (V_2) block
      - External branch of anterior ethmoid n.
      - Infraorbital n.
      - Supratrochlear n.
      - Infratrochlear n.
  - Topical cocaine in 4–10% solution or local anesthetics containing a vasoconstrictor
    - Possible hemodynamic consequences

Further Reading

1 OMS Knowledge Update
   a. Volume One – Part One and Part Two
   b. Volume Two
   c. Volume Three
2 OMS Reference Guide second edition
3 Fonseca, R. et al. (2013). *Book: Oral and Maxillofacial Trauma*, 4e. St. Louis, MO: Elsevier/Sanders.

4 Miloro, M. et al. (2012). *Peterson's Principles of Oral and Maxillofacial Surgery*, 3e.
5 Waite, P. D. Oral and Maxillofacial Treatment of Obstructive Sleep Apnea.
6 Sclar, A.G. Soft Tissue and Esthetic Considerations in Implant Therapy
7 Oral and Maxillofacial Surgery Clinics of North America, W. B. Saunders Company, 7, Number 2 May 1995

References

1 Baum, S.H., Ha-Phuoc, A.K., and Mohr, C. (2020). Treatment of odontogenic abscesses: comparison of primary and secondary removal of the odontogenic focus and antibiotic therapy. *Oral Maxillofac. Surg.* 24 (2): 163–172. https://doi.org/10.1007/s10006-020-00835-w.

2 Bakathir, A.A., Margasahayam, M.V., and Al-Ismaily, M.I. (2008). Maxillary hyperplasia and hyperostosis cranialis: a rare manifestation of renal osteodystrophy in a patient with hyperparathyroidism secondary to chronic renal failure. *Saudi Med. J.* 29 (12): 1815–1818.

3 Raj, D. and Luginbuehl, I. (2014). Managing the difficult airway in the syndromic child. *Contin. Educ. Anaesth. Crit. Care Pain* 15 (1): 7–13:https://doi.org/10.1093/bjaceaccp/mku004.

4 Seet, E., Chung, F., Wang, C.Y. et al. (2021). Association of obstructive sleep apnea with difficult intubation: prospective multicenter observational cohort study. *Anesth. Analg.* 133 (1): 196–204. https://doi.org/10.1213/ANE.0000000000005479.

5 Wu, Z.H., Yang, X.P., Niu, X. et al. (2019). The relationship between obstructive sleep apnea hypopnea syndrome and gastroesophageal reflux disease: a meta-analysis. *Sleep Breath.* 23 (2): 389–397. https://doi.org/10.1007/s11325-018-1691-x.

6 Alkhalil, M., Schulman, E., and Getsy, J. (2009). Obstructive sleep apnea syndrome and asthma: what are the links? *J. Clin. Sleep Med.* 5 (1): 71–78.

7 Clavellina-Gaytán, D., Velázquez-Fernández, D., Del-Villar, E. et al. (2015). Evaluation of spirometric testing as a routine preoperative assessment in patients undergoing bariatric surgery. *Obes. Surg.* 25 (3): 530–536. https://doi.org/10.1007/s11695-014-1420-x.

8 Cozowicz, C. and Memtsoudis, S.G. (2021). Perioperative management of the patient with obstructive sleep apnea: a narrative review. *Anesth. Analg.* 132 (5): 1231–1243. https://doi.org/10.1213/ANE.0000000000005444.

9 Soberon, J.R., Murray Casanova, I., and Wright, J. (2022). Anesthetic implications for patients with implanted hypoglossal nerve stimulators: a case report. *Cureus* 14 (1): e21424. https://doi.org/10.7759/cureus.21424.

10 Kaczmarski, P., Karuga, F.F., Szmyd, B. et al. (2022). The role of inflammation, hypoxia, and opioid receptor expression in pain modulation in patients suffering from obstructive sleep apnea. *Int. J. Mol. Sci.* 23 (16): https://doi.org/10.3390/ijms23169080.

11 Lermuzeaux, M., Meric, H., Sauneuf, B. et al. (2016). Superiority of transcutaneous CO_2 over end-tidal CO_2 measurement for monitoring respiratory failure in nonintubated patients: a pilot study. *J. Crit. Care* 31 (1): 150–156. https://doi.org/10.1016/j.jcrc.2015.09.014.

12 Sharma, S., Gupta, D.S., Pal, U.S., and Jurel, S.K. (2011). Etiological factors of temporomandibular joint disorders. *Natl. J. Maxillofac. Surg.* 2 (2): 116–119. https://doi.org/10.4103/0975-5950.94463.

13 Dıraçoğlu, D., Yıldırım, N.K., Saral, İ. et al. (2016). Temporomandibular dysfunction and risk factors for anxiety and depression. *J. Back Musculoskelet. Rehabil.* 29 (3): 487–491. https://doi.org/10.3233/BMR-150644.

14 Arslan, Z., Ozdal, P., Ozdamar, D. et al. (2016). Nasotracheal intubation of a patient with restricted mouth opening using a McGrath MAC X-blade and Magill forceps. *J. Anesth.* 30 (5): 904–906. https://doi.org/10.1007/s00540-016-2205-2.

15 Gaszynska, E., Wieczorek, A., and Gaszynski, T. (2014). Awake endotracheal intubation in patients with severely restricted mouth opening- alternative devices to fiberscope: series of cases and literature review. *Open Medicine* 9 (6): 768–772.

16 Eftekharian, H.R., Zarei, K., Arabion, H.R., and Heydari, S.T. (2015). Remifentanil, ketamine, and propofol in awake nasotracheal fiberoptic intubation in temporomandibular joint ankylosis surgery. *J. Craniofac. Surg.* 26 (1): 206–209. https://doi.org/10.1097/SCS.0000000000001243.

17 Uda, H., Sugawara, Y., Sarukawa, S., and Sunaga, A. (2014). The oculocardiac reflex in aponeurotic blepharoptosis surgery. *J. Plast. Surg. Hand Surg.* 48 (3): 170–174. https://doi.org/10.3109/2000656X.2013.836529.

18 de Souza, A.A.B., Araújo, S.C.S., Martins, G.H. et al. (2022). New device for submental endotracheal intubation: a prospective cohort study. *J. Oral Maxillofac. Surg.* 80 (12): 1927–1942. https://doi.org/10.1016/j.joms.2022.08.013.

19 Fradet, L., Iorio-Morin, C., Tissot-Therrien, M. et al. (2020). Training anaesthetists in cricothyrotomy techniques using video demonstrations and a hands-on practice session: a shift towards preferred surgical approaches. *Br. J. Anaesth.* 125 (1): e160–e162. https://doi.org/10.1016/j.bja.2019.11.021.

20 Cason, R.W., Avashia, Y.J., Shammas, R.L. et al. (2021). Perioperative approach to reducing hematoma during Rhytidectomy: what does the evidence show? *Plast. Reconstr. Surg.* 147 (6): 1297–1309. https://doi.org/10.1097/PRS.0000000000007943.

21 Steinbacher, D.M. (2019). *Aesthetic Orthognathic Surgery and Rhinoplasty*. Wiley-Blackwell:xxiii, 622 pages.

22 Jumaily, J.S., Jumaily, M., Donnelly, T., and Asaria, J. (2022). Quality of recovery and safety of deep intravenous sedation compared to general anesthesia in facial plastic surgery: a prospective cohort study. *Am. J. Otolaryngol.* 43 (2): 103352. https://doi.org/10.1016/j.amjoto.2021.103352.

Index

Anesthesia for Dental and Oral Maxillofacial Surgery, First Edition. Spencer D. Wade, Caroline M. Sawicki, Megann K. Smiley, Michael A. Cuddy, Steven Vukas, and Paul J. Schwartz.
© 2024 John Wiley & Sons, Inc. Published 2024 by John Wiley & Sons, Inc.